Color Atlas of Female Genital Tract Pathology

Pranab Dey

Color Atlas of Female Genital Tract Pathology

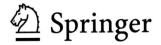 Springer

Pranab Dey
Department of Cytology and Gynecologic Pathology
Post Graduate Institute of Medical Education and Research
Chandigarh
India

ISBN 978-981-13-1028-7   ISBN 978-981-13-1029-4   (eBook)
https://doi.org/10.1007/978-981-13-1029-4

Library of Congress Control Number: 2018953338

This Springer imprint is published by the registered company Springer Nature Singapore Pte Ltd.
The registered company address is: 152 Beach Road, #21-01/04 Gateway East, Singapore 189721, Singapore

To Shree Shree Satyananda Giri, Rini and Madhumanti

Preface

Pathology of the female genital tract is one of the important areas in histopathology. In this book, I have highlighted various neoplastic and non-neoplastic lesions of the female genital tract with the help of numerous gross and microscopic figures. I have followed the World Health Organization classification of tumours of the female genital tract and have arranged the lesions accordingly. The book contains the salient diagnostic features of cytology, histopathology, immunohistochemistry, molecular pathology and differential diagnosis of each lesion with selected references. This is a practical and illustrated approach of the pathology of female genital tract lesions. I strongly believe that this Atlas will help the post-graduate students and also the practicing pathologists.

Chandigarh, India   Pranab Dey
2018 April

Acknowledgements

Firstly, I am thankful to Dr. Naren Aggarwal, who gave me the proposal and inspired me to write this book. I also wish to express my thanks to Ms. Jagjeet Kaur Saini, Ms. Beauty Christobel and the team at Springer particularly Ms Shanjini Rajasekaran, Project Manager of Springer who helped me in every stage of this book.

I also wish to express my thanks to my teacher Professor Arvind Rajwanshi and the late Professor Subhas Kumari Gupta.

It is my great pleasure to mention the name of my friend Dr. Suvradeep Mitra, Assistant Professor of Pathology and Laboratory Medicine, AIIMS, Bhubaneswar, India. Dr. Suvradeep helped me to execute my plan in reality. I want to sincerely thank Dr. Uma Nahar Saikia, Professor of Histopathology, PGIMER, Chandigarh, India, who provided me many valuable microphotographs.

My heartiest thanks to my wife Rini and daughter Madhumanti who are always my continuous sources of inspiration.

I am grateful to the Almighty God who always provides me the courage and wisdom in every sphere of my life.

Contents

Abbreviations

AFP	Alpha fetoprotein
AGCT	Adult granulosa cell tumour
BP	Bullous pemphigoid
CA	Condyloma acuminatum
CD	Cluster differentiation
CEA	Carcinoembryonic antigen
CIN	Cervical intraepithelial neoplasia
CHM	Complete hydatidiform mole
CK	Cytokeratin
CMV	Cytomegalovirus
DES	Diethylstilbestrol
DPAM	Disseminated peritoneal adenomucinosis
d-VIN	Differentiated type of vulvar squamous intraepithelial neoplasia
EBV	Epstein-Barr virus
EIN	Endometrial intraepithelial neoplasia
EMA	Epithelial membrane antigen
ER	Oestrogen receptor
ESS	Endometrial stromal sarcoma
EST	Endodermal sinus tumour
FATWO	Female adnexal tumour of probable Wolffian duct origin
FIGO	International Federation of Gynecology and Obstetrics
FTA-ABS	Fluorescent treponemal antibody absorption test
GCDFP	Gross cystic disease fluid protein
HCC	Hepatocellular carcinoma
hCG	Human chorionic gonadotropin
HDAC	Histone deacetylases
HGSC	High-grade serous carcinoma
HPF	High power field
HPV	Human papilloma virus
HSIL	High-grade squamous intraepithelial lesion
HSV	Herpes simplex virus
IUCD	Intrauterine contraceptive device
JGCT	Juvenile granulosa cell tumour
LCNET	Large cell neuroendocrine tumours
LEEP	Laser vaporization and loop electrosurgical excision
LGSC	Low-grade serous carcinoma
LP	Lichen planus
LS	Lichen sclerosis
LSC	Lichen simplex chronicus
LSIL	Low-grade squamous intraepithelial lesion
MBT	Mucinous borderline tumour
MC	Molluscum contagiosum

MDA	Minimal deviation adenocarcinoma
MFI	Maternal floor infract
MPF	Massive perivillous fibrin
NSE	Neuron-specific enolase
PAS	Periodic acid Schiff
PAX 8	Paired box gene 8
PCR	Polymerase chain reaction
PLAP	Placental alkaline phosphatase
PMCA	Peritoneal mucinous carcinomatosis
PR	Progesterone receptor
PSTT	Placental site trophoblastic tumour
PTD	Persistent trophoblastic disease
PTEN	Phosphatase and tensin homologue
RPR	Rapid plasma regain test
SBT	Serous borderline tumour
SBT-MP	Serous borderline tumour of micropapillary variant
SF 1	Serodiagnostic factor 1
SIL	Squamous intraepithelial lesion
SLCT	Sertoli-Leydig cell tumour
STIC	Serous tubal intraepithelial carcinoma
STUMP	Smooth muscle tumours of uncertain malignant potential
TTF 1	Thyroid transcription factor 1
UCS	Uterine carcinosarcoma
u-VIN	Usual type of vulvar squamous intraepithelial neoplasia
VAIN	Vaginal intraepithelial neoplasia
VDRL	Venereal disease research laboratory test
VIN	Vulvar squamous intraepithelial
YST	Yolk sac tumour

About the Author

Pranab Dey is a professor in the Department of Cytology and Gynecologic Pathology at the Postgraduate Institute of Medical Education and Research, Chandigarh. Professor Dey completed his M.D. (pathology) at the Postgraduate Institute of Medical Education and Research, Chandigarh, and FRCPath (cytopathology) at the Royal College of Pathologists, London. He has conducted several research projects and has pioneered works on DNA flow cytometry, image morphometry, mono-layered cytology and cytomorphologic findings of various lesions on cytology smears. He is a well-published author, has published several books, and numerous articles in international journals in the field of gynaecologic pathology and cytology and is a member of various societies.

Classification of tumours of vulva according to World Health Organization (WHO) is highlighted in Fig. 1.1a [1].

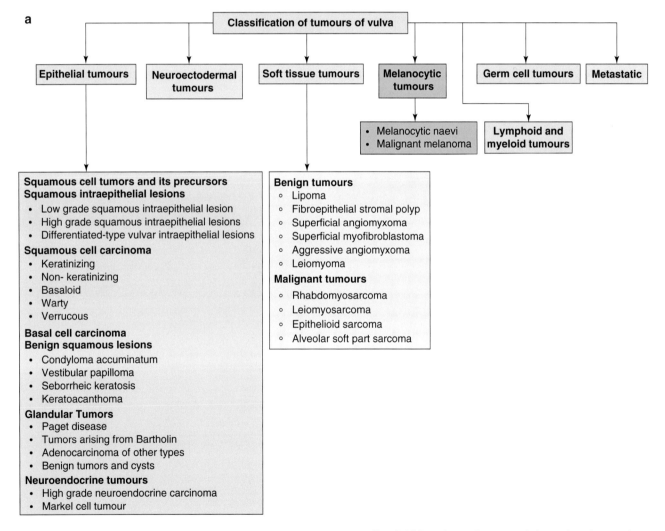

Fig. 1.1 (**a**) Classification of tumours of vulva. (**b**) Lichen planus: Band like lymphocytic infiltration in the dermo-epidermal junction. (**c**) Lichen planus: Higher magnification showing predominant chronic inflammatory cells. (**d**) Lichen planus: Compact orthokeratosis and no parakeratotic cells. (**e**) Lichen planus: Civatte bodies stained by IgG antibody (see *red arrow*). (Courtesy Professor Uma Nahar, PGIMER, Chandigarh)

© Springer Nature Singapore Pte Ltd. 2019

P. Dey, *Color Atlas of Female Genital Tract Pathology*, https://doi.org/10.1007/978-981-13-1029-4_1

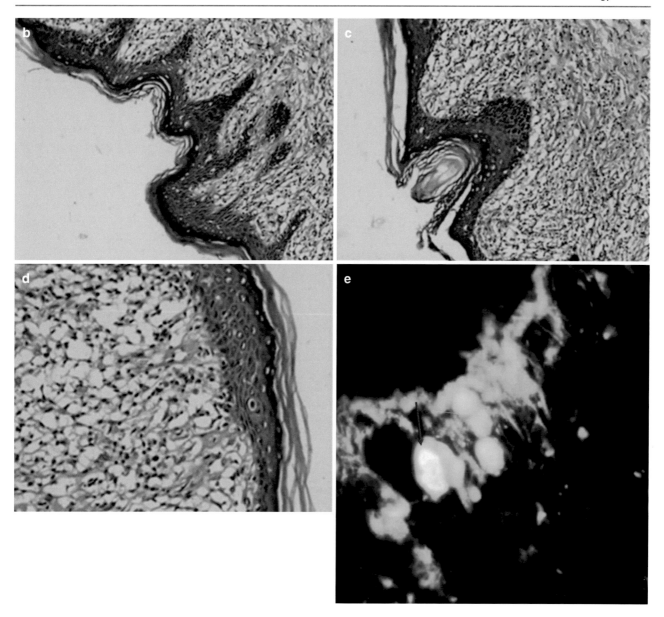

Fig. 1.1 (continued)

Inflammatory Diseases of Vulva

Non-Infectious Inflammation of Vulva

Lichen Planus

Image gallery: Fig. 1.1b–e.

Abbreviation: Lichen Planus (LP)

Definition: This is a chronic inflammatory dermatological lesion characterized by "band like lymphocytic infiltrate" in the dermo-epidermal junction along with basal cell degeneration and wedge-shaped hypergranulosis of the epidermis.

Etiopathogenesis

- Exact etiology not known
- Probably a T cell related autoimmune disease

Clinical features

- Itching
- Burning pain
- Dyspareunia
- Whitish plaques
- Koebner's phenomenon: Lesion appears at the site of previous trauma

Gross appearances

- Small papules in vulva with white lines which is known as "Wickham's striae"
- Hyperpigmented after a few months

Histopathology

- "Band like infiltration" of chronic inflammatory cells in the upper dermis
- Inflammation does not extend to the epidermis
- Degenerated basal cells of the epidermis
- Eosinophilic colloid bodies within the papillary dermis
- Compact orthokeratosis: No parakeratotic cells are present in the cornified layer
- Wedge shaped hyperplasia of granular layer

Ancillary tests

- Immunofluorescence:
  - Deposition of fibrinogen in the dermo-epidermal junction
  - Occasionally IgM, IgG and C3 deposition in the dermo-epidermal junction
  - Necrotic keratinocytes are stained by IgM, IgG and C3. The round homogenous bodies are known as Civatte bodies

Key diagnostic features of Lichen planus: See Box 1.1.

Box 1.1 Key Features of Lichen Planus
- Band like infiltration of lymphohistiocytic cells in dermo-epidermal junction
- Degenerated basal keratinocytes
- Compact orthokeratosis
- Irregular acanthosis
  - Hyperkeratosis and wedge shaped hyperplasia of granular layer
  - Eosinophilic colloid bodies within the papillary dermis

Immunofluorescence: Deposition of fibrinogen in the dermo-epidermal junction.

Differential diagnosis

- Lichen sclerosis: No band like infiltration of inflammatory cells and absence of sclerosis
- Lichenoid drug eruption: Predominant eosinophils in the inflammatory component
- Bullous lesion: Formation of bullae and absence of inflammation

Treatment:

- It is a self-limited disease and is cured within a year
- Tropical corticosteroid (clobetasol propionate ointment)
- Systemic corticosteroid if the lesion is severe

Prognosis: Spontaneous remission.

Lichen Sclerosus

Image gallery: Fig. 1.2a–d.

Abbreviations: Lichen Sclerosis: LS

Definition: LS is a chronic fibrosing inflammatory dermatological lesion which shows homogenization and loss of collagen in the upper dermis.

Etiopathogenesis

- Idiopathic
- Possibly autoimmune disease

Clinical features and Gross appearances

- Pruritus
- Pain
- Dyspareunia
- Porcelain white skin
- Thinned skin easy to bleed
- At times "figure of eight" appearance

Histopathology

- Papillary dermis shows homogenization and loss of collagen
- Epidermal thinning and loss of the rete ridges
- Linear band like inflammation in dermis below the sclerosis

Key diagnostic features of Lichen sclerosis: See Box 1.2.

Differential diagnosis

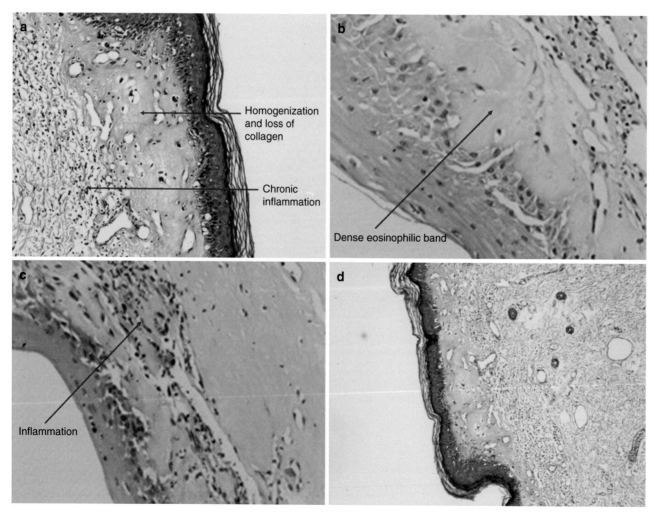

Fig. 1.2 (**a**) Lichen sclerosis: Homogenization and loss of collagen in upper dermis. (**b**) Lichen sclerosis: Higher magnification shows dense eosinophilic band. (**c**) Lichen sclerosus: Inflammatory cell infiltration under the epidermis. (**d**) Lichen sclerosus: Thinner epidermis and loss of rete ridges. In addition loss of collagen in the upper dermis. (**e**) Comparison of lichen planus and lichen sclerosus

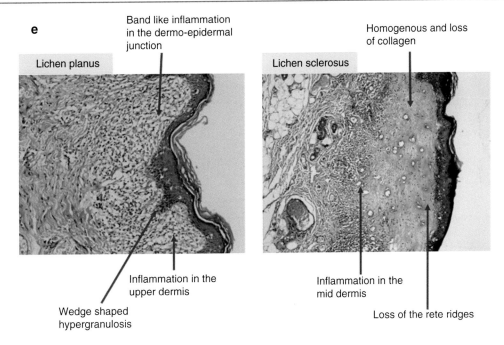

Fig. 1.2 (continued)

Box 1.2 Key Features of Lichen Sclerosis
- Homogenization and loss of collagen in papillary dermis
- Marked hyperkeratosis
- Epidermal atrophy and loss of rete pegs in mature state
- Linear band like inflammation of lymphohistiocytes in the dermis below the sclerosis

- Lichen planus: See Table 1.1 and Fig. 1.2e.
- Morphea: Absence of basal cell degeneration and hyperkeratosis in morphea

- Radiation induced fibrosis: History of radiation, bizarre looking atypical fibroblasts and thick walled blood vessels are noted in radiation induced fibrosis.

Cancer risk

- Risk of malignancy in 5% cases

Treatment and prognosis

- Chronic course with improvement and worsening
- Periodical follow up necessary to note any dysplastic changes
- Long term tropical corticosteroid
- Sedation in night time to relieve from itching
- Rarely surgery in grossly disfigured external genitalia

Table 1.1 Distinguishing features of Lichen sclerosis versus lichen planus

Features	Lichen sclerosis	Lichen planus
Inflammation	Lymphocytic infiltration is seen in dermis below the sclerosis	Band like infiltration of lymphohistiocytic cells in dermo-epidermal junction
Wedge shaped hyperplasia of granular layer	Absent	Present
Loss of collagen giving amorphous eosinophilic material	Present	Absent
Colloid bodies	Absent	Present

Lichen Simplex Chronicus

Image gallery: Fig. 1.3.

Abbreviation: Lichen Simplex Chronicus (LSC)

Synonyms: Squamous Cell Hyperplasia, Hyperplastic dystrophy

Definition: LSC is a nonspecific chronic inflammatory disease of skin characterised by epidermal hyperplasia, dermal fibrosis, and chronic inflammation.

Etiopathogenesis

- Repeated physical injury on a chronic pruritic lesions

Clinical features and Gross appearances

- Pruritus
- Thickened skin
- Reddish scaly skin
- Long standing itching may cause hyperpigmentation

Histopathology

- Non-specific changes
- No atypia of squamous cells in epidermis
- Hyperkeratosis
- Parakeratosis
- Chronic inflammation in dermis
- Collagenous vertical band in dermis

Differential diagnosis

- Psoriasis: Psoriasis shows parakeratosis, hypergranulosis and polymorphs collection in the epidermis.
- Infection: Various fungal infections such as tinea cruris, candidal infection etc.

Key diagnostic points of LSC: See Box 1.3.

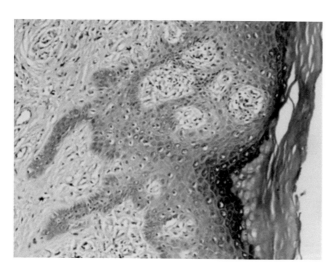

Fig. 1.3 Lichen simplex chronicus: Hyperkeratosis of the epidermis along with mild inflammation in the dermis

---

Box 1.3 Key Diagnostic Features of Lichen Simplex Chronicus
Histopathology

- Hyperkeratosis
- Parakeratosis
- Chronic inflammatory cells in dermis
- Collagenous vertical band in dermis

Note: These histopathological features are non-specific.

Treatment

- Protection of skin
- Antipruritic agents
- Local corticosteroids
- Treatment of underlying infections if any

Psoriasis

Image gallery: Fig. 1.4a, b.

Definition: Psoriasis is a chronic, relapsing hyper proliferative dermatitis with regular epidermal hyperplasia.

Clinical features and Gross appearances

- Symmetrical well circumscribed plaque
- Erythematous area with a silvery scale on top
- Auspitz sign: Pin point bleeding if the silvery scale is removed
- Affects 1–4% of Caucasian population
- Common sites in vulva: Lateral area of the labia majora

Genetic predisposition and etiology

- Autosomal dominant trait
- The gene is PSORS1, and present in 6p21.3
- Possibly immunological dysfunction is related with psoriasis

Histopathology

- Epidermal spongiosis: Oedema in the epidermal layer
- Papillary dermal oedema and vascular congestion
- Perivascular lymphocyte rich dermatitis
- Rete ridges become widened and elongated
- Parakeratosis with neutrophilic infiltration and loss of cells in the granular layer
  - Munro's microabscess: Polymorphs are collected in the epidermis forming small abscesses

Differential diagnosis

- Chronic fungal infection: Candidiasis of the vulva often mimic psoriasis. Special stain such as Periodic Acid Schiff's stain (PAS) may demonstrate the fungi.
- Psoriasiform drug reaction: Inflammatory infiltrate is usually rich in eosinophils in drug reaction.
- Seborrheic dermatitis: Epidermal spongiosis, and thinning of the suprapapillary plate favours psoriasis.
- Lichen simplex chronicus: Acanthosis and hyperkeratosis and thicker suprapapillary plates favour LSC (Fig. 1.4c).

Key diagnostic points of Psoriasis: See Box 1.4.

Treatment

- Mild: Topical application of steroids, emollients and vitamin D analogs
- Severe: Methotrexate, retinoid or phototherapy

Box 1.4 Key Diagnostic Features of Psoriasis

Histopathology

- Epidermal spongiosis
- Munro's microabscess
- Widened and elongated rete ridges
- Parakeratosis
- Absence of granular layer
- Papillary dermal oedema and vascular congestion
- Perivascular lymphocyte rich dermatitis

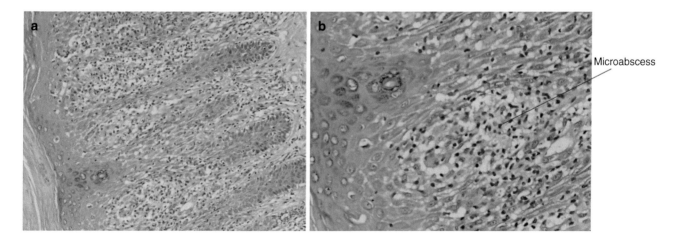

Microabscess

Fig. 1.4 (**a**) Psoriasis: Elongation of rete ridges and perivascular lymphocytic infiltrate. (**b**) Psoriasis: Polymorphs infiltrate in the epidermis forming Munro's microabscess. (**c**) Comparison of psoriasis and Lichen simplex chronicus

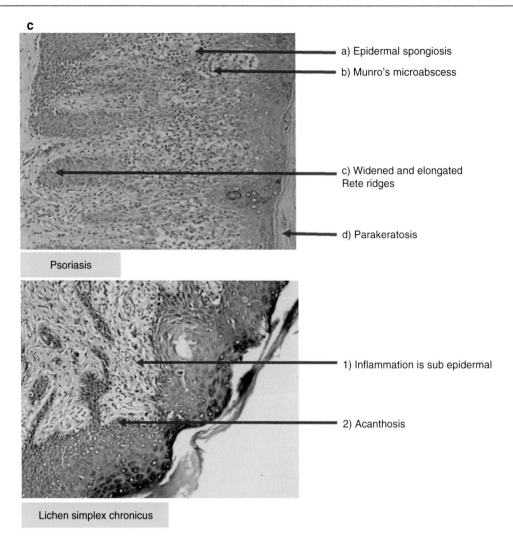

a) Epidermal spongiosis

b) Munro's microabscess

c) Widened and elongated Rete ridges

d) Parakeratosis

Psoriasis

1) Inflammation is sub epidermal

2) Acanthosis

Lichen simplex chronicus

Fig. 1.4 (continued)

Inflammation of Vulva Due to Infection

Herpes Simplex

Image gallery: Fig. 1.5a, b.

Abbreviation: Herpes Simplex Virus: HSV

Definition: Vulvar Herpes is a sexually transmitted ulcerative disease that is caused by herpes simplex virus infection.

Causative agents

- HSV-2 infection is more common
- HSV-1 infection occurs in young patient

Clinical features

- Systemic symptoms such as malaise and fever
- Large number of vesicles to pustules
- Pustules ulcerates
- Painful ulcer

Cytology features

- Multinucleated giant cells
- Homogenization of chromatin

- Characteristic ground glass appearance
- Intranuclear inclusion

Mode of diagnosis

- Cytological scrapping
- HSV serology
- Immunohistochemistry
- Polymerase chain reaction (PCR)

Differential diagnosis

- Different causes of genital ulcers such as chancroid, lymphogranuloma venerum, syphilitic chancre, tuberculosis etc.

Management

- Antiviral agent: acyclovir
- Acyclovir is not effective for latent infection

Key features: Summarizing the key features of herpes simplex in Box 1.5.

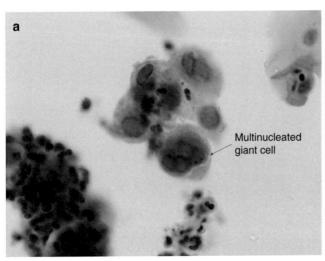
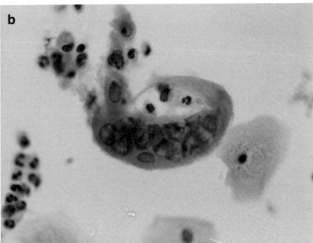

Multinucleated giant cell

Fig. 1.5 (**a**) Herpes simplex: Large mononuclear and multinuclear giant cells in scraping of ulcer in vulva. (**b**) Herpes simplex: The nuclei of the giant cells are compressed with each other and they show ground glass appearance

Box 1.5 Key Features of Herpes Simplex

Causative organism

- HSV 2 and HSV 1

Clinical features

- Large number of vesicles to pustules
- Pustules ulcerates
- Painful ulcer

Cytology

- Multinucleated giant cells
- Homogenization of chromatin
- Characteristic ground glass appearance
- Intranuclear inclusion

Differential diagnosis

- Different causes of genital ulcers

Diagnostic mode

- Cytological scrapping
- HSV serology
- Immunohistochemistry
- Polymerase chain reaction

Treatment

- Antiviral agent: acyclovir

Cytomegalovirus Infection

Image gallery: Fig. 1.6.

Abbreviations: Cytomegalovirus (CMV)

Clinical feature: Ulcerated lesion in the vulvovaginal area

Histopathology and cytology

- Epithelium and vascular endothelial cells show typical large intranuclear viral inclusions.

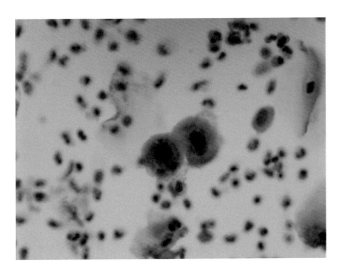

Fig. 1.6 Cytomegalovirus: Cytology smear showing cells with large intranuclear inclusion

Molluscum Contagiosum

Image gallery: Fig. 1.7a, b.

Abbreviations: Molluscum Contagiosum (MC)

Infection: It is a sexually transmitted disease caused by molluscum contagiosum virus.

Clinical features

- Multiple papules
- Flesh coloured
- Central dome shaped notch

Histopathology

- Marked acanthosis
- Molluscum bodies (Henderson-Patterson bodies): Eosinophilic oval shaped viral inclusions

Diagnostic features: See Box 1.6.

> **Box 1.6 Key Diagnostic Features of Molluscum Contagiosum**
> - Characteristic clinical appearance of multiple papules with dome shaped notch
> - Scrapping cytology or histopathology showing Eosinophilic oval shaped viral inclusions i.e., Molluscum bodies (Henderson-Patterson bodies)

Prognosis and treatment

- Spontaneous regression
- Removal of the lesion by
  - Cryosurgery
  - Laser surgery
  - Curetting
  - Topical application of Trichloroacetic acid

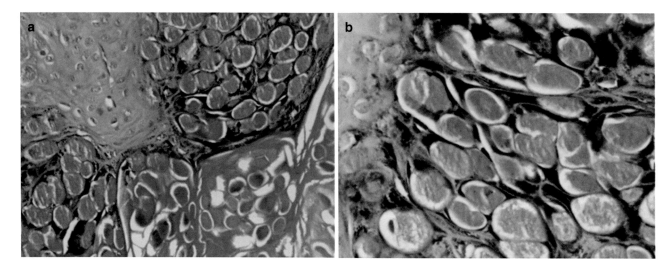

Fig. 1.7 (**a**) Molluscum contagiosum: Eosinophilic oval shaped viral inclusions. (**b**) Molluscum contagiosum: Higher magnification showing the eosinophilic inclusion

Candidal Infection

Image: Fig. 1.8.

Organisms

- Candida albecans is the most common organism
- Others: *Candida glabrata, Candida tropicalis, Candida parapsilosis*

Clinical feature

- Whitish patches
- Intense itching
- Erythema

Cytology

- Slender fungal pseudohyphae
- Fungal spores

Diagnosis

- Cytology scrapping
- Fungal culture

Treatment

- Topical antifungal agent

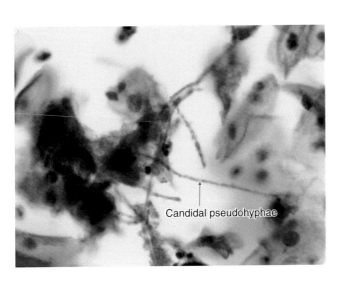

Fig. 1.8 Candidal infection: Long slender candidal pseudohyphae

Syphilis

Image gallery: Fig. 1.9a, b.
   Causative agent: Treponema pallidum.
   Mode of infection spread: Sexually transmitted disease.
   Phases of disease: Primary, secondary and tertiary stage.
   Primary syphilis:

- Characteristic feature is chancre
    - Chancre:
        It appears 10 days to 3 months after the infection
        Painless, clean ulcer.
- Multiple mobile, rubbery lymph nodes develop in the inguinal region
- This is a highly infective stage
- Histopathology: Subepidermal lymphocytes, and plasma cells infiltration along with perivascular inflammation.

Secondary syphilis:

- It develops after weeks to months of the primary infection if not treated
- Patient shows fever, pain in joints and maculopapular lesions.
- Condyloma lata: Plaque like elevated lesions appear in the vulva which is labelled as condyloma lata.
- Histopathology:
    - Dermal infiltration of lymphocytes and plasma cells along with perivascular plasma cell infiltration.
    - Small arterial obliteration

Tertiary syphilis:

- Rarely vulva is affected as nodular soft lesions which is called as gumma

- Histopathology: Central necrosis along with epithelioid cell granulomas

Ancillary tests

- Serological tests: Venereal disease research laboratory test (VDRL), fluorescent treponemal antibody absorption test (FTA-ABS) and rapid plasma regain test (RPR),
- Stain for Treponema pallidum: Warthin –Starry stain

Key diagnostic features of syphilis: See Box 1.7.
Treatment: Penicillin.

Box 1.7 Key Features of Syphilis
- Caused by Treponema pallidum
- Sexually transmitted disease
- Primary, secondary and tertiary stage
- Chancre: Painless, clean ulcer. Characteristic of primary syphilis
- Condyloma lata: About 2 to 3 cm elevated plaque like lesions in the vulva that is seen in secondary syphilis
- Histopathology:
    - Dermal infiltration of lymphocytes and plasma cells along with perivascular plasma cell infiltration.
    - Small arterial obliteration
- Serological tests: VDRL, RPR,FTA-ABS
- Stain for Treponema pallidum: Warthin –Starry stain

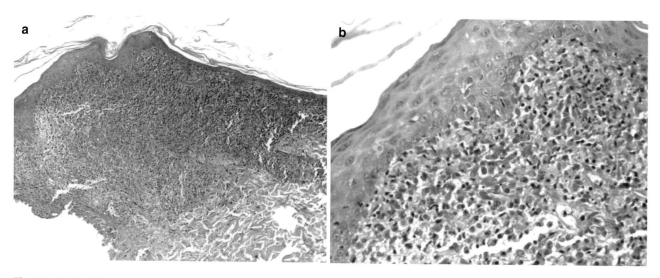

Fig. 1.9 (**a**) Syphilis: Dense lymphoplasmacytic infiltration in the dermis. (**b**) Syphilis: Higher magnifications shows lymphocytes and plasma cells infiltration

Vulvar Inflammation: Miscellaneous

Crohn's Disease

Image gallery: Fig. 1.10.

Definition: It is non caseating granulomatous disease of unknown etiology.

Clinical feature

- Reddish, indurated or ulcerated area
- The ulcer is usually slit like and deep in the vulva
- Patient may also have perianal fistula
- Associated colon and small bowel involvement may be present

Histopathology

- Non caseating epithelioid cell granulomas
- No demonstrable acid fast bacilli on Ziehl Neelsen stain

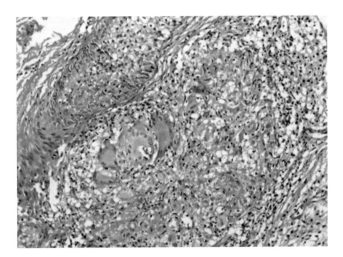

Fig. 1.10 Crohn's disease: Epithelioid cell granulomas and giant cells in the dermis. (Courtesy Professor Uma Nahar, PGIMER, Chandigarh)

Behcet's Syndrome

Image gallery: Fig. 1.11a, b.

Definition: It is a syndrome that consists of aphthous ulcer in the oral cavity, ulcer in the genital tract, and inflammation in eye.

Gross: Deep ulcer in the vulva that repeatedly heals and reappears.

Histopathology:

- Chronic inflammation
- Predominant perivascular location of the inflammatory cells
- Necrosis

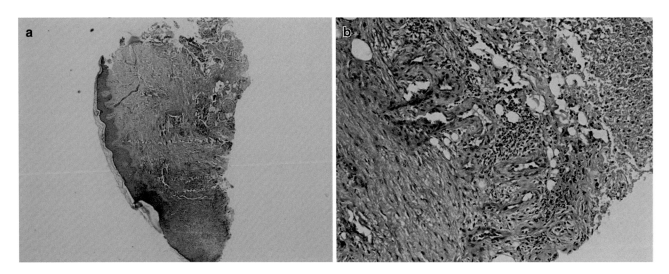

Fig. 1.11 (**a**) Behcet's syndrome: Inflammation in the deeper dermis (Courtesy Professor Uma Nahar, PGIMER, Chandigarh). (**b**) Behcet's syndrome: Predominant perivascular inflammation. (Courtesy Professor Uma Nahar, PGIMER, Chandigarh)

Erythema Multiforme

Image gallery: Fig. 1.12a, b.

Synonym: Stevens–Johnson Syndrome.

Causes: Drug reaction, herpes infection, malignancy etc.

Clinical features:

- Usually young patients
- High fever
- Skin and mucus membranes are affected
- Multiple papules or papulovesicular lesions appear typically after drug ingestion
- More than 10% of the body surface area is involved in erythema multiforme major

Histopathology

- In the dermoepidermal junction perivascular lymphocytic collection is seen

- Vacuolar dermatitis characterised by the presence of vacuoles both above and below the basement membrane
- Epidermis shows necrotic keratinocytes
- In the later stage, subepidermal vesicles appear due to separation of epidermis at the dermoepidermal junction.

Differential diagnosis:

- Fixed drug eruption: Presence of eosinophils and neutrophils

Prognosis and treatment

- Self-limited and spontaneous healing occur within 1 month
- Withdrawal of the triggering factors
- Adequate care of the skin and mucus membrane

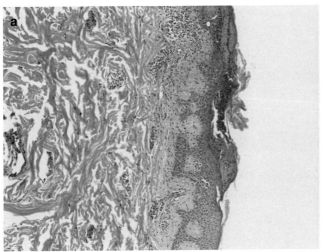
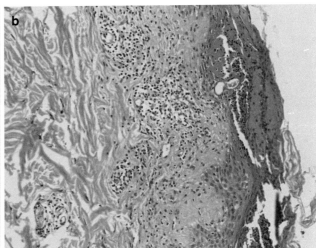

Fig. 1.12 (a) Erythema multiforme: Perivascular lymphocytic infiltration in the dermoepidermal junction. (Courtesy Professor Uma Nahar, PGIMER, Chandigarh). (b) Erythema multiforme: Higher magnification of the lymphocytic infiltration. (Courtesy Professor Uma Nahar, PGIMER, Chandigarh)

Bullous Lesions of Vulva

Pemphigus Vulgaris

Image gallery: Fig. 1.13a, c.

Definition: Pemphigus vulgaris is an uncommon bullous disease of skin characterized by mucosal erosion and suprabasal bullae formation.

Etiopathogenesis: Autoantibody formation against desmoglein, a component of desmosome of the epidermal cells.

Clinical features and Gross appearances

- Multiple recurrent and painful bullae
- Nikolsky's sign: The peripheral border of the bullae are extend if pressure is applied to the margin of the vesicle.

Histopathology

- Suprabasal separation of cells and the intact rows of cells are attached with dermis giving "row of tombstones" appearance.
- Acantholysis
- Bullae contain acantholytic keratinocytes and sparse eosinophils

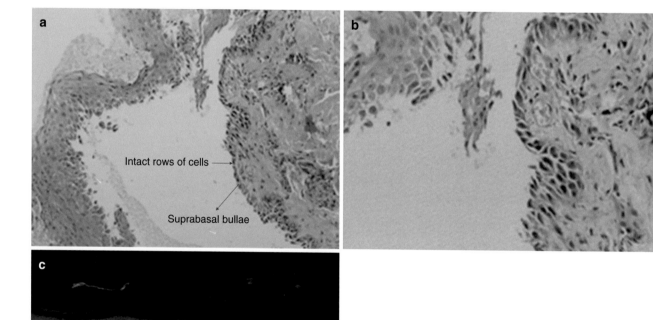

Fig. 1.13 (**a**) Pemphigus vulgaris: Suprabasal bulla formation. (**b**) Pemphigus vulgaris: Intact rows of basal cells are attached with dermis giving "row of tombstones" appearance. (**c**) Pemphigus vulgaris: Basket weave IgG deposit in immunofluorescence (Courtesy Professor Uma Nahar, PGIMER, Chandigarh). (**d**) Comparison of Pemphigus vulgaris and bullous pemphigoid

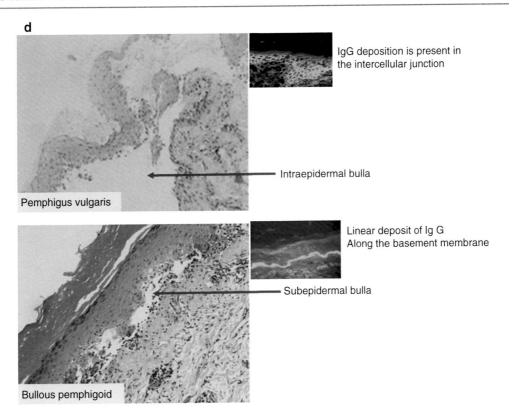

d

IgG deposition is present in
the intercellular junction

Intraepidermal bulla

Pemphigus vulgaris

Linear deposit of Ig G
Along the basement membrane

Subepidermal bulla

Bullous pemphigoid

Fig. 1.13 (continued)

Ancillary Tests

Immunofluorescence: The lace-like deposition of IgG in the intercellular epidermal junction.

Key points of Pemphigus vulgaris: See Box 1.8.

Box 1.8 Diagnostic Key Points of Pemphigus Vulgaris
- Multiple recurrent and painful bullae
- Nikolsky's sign
- Suprabasal separation of cells forming bullae
- Acantholysis
- Bullae contain acantholytic keratinocytes and sparse eosinophils
- *Immunofluorescence*: The lace-like deposition of IgG in the intercellular epidermal junction.

Differential diagnosis

- Bullous pemphigoid: The subepidermal location of bullae and absence of acantholytic cells with linear IgG and C3 demonstration in the basement membrane favour bullous pemphigoid (Fig. 1.13d).
- Other causes of acantholytic disorders of vulva: Hailey-Hailey disease, Darier disease, acantholytic dermatosis.

Treatment

- Topical corticosteroid
- Intraoral corticosteroid
- Occasionally cyclophosphamide, azathioprine or methotrexate.
- Anti CD 20 antibody is also been used against the B cells

Bullous Pemphigoid

Image gallery: Fig. 1.14a.

Abbreviation: Bullous Pemphigoid: BP

Definition: BP is a chronic autoimmune bullous lesion of skin characterized by subepidermal bullae formation.

Etiopathogenesis: BP is caused by formation of autoantibody against plakin which is a constituent of hemidesmosomes.

Clinical features

- Sites: Labia majora and minora, perianal region, arms and legs
- Bullae: Multiple intact blisters
- Nikolsky's sign: Negative

Histopathology

- Subepidermal bullae formation
- There is distinct separation between epidermis and underlying dermis
- The bullae usually contain serum and fibrin

Ancillary tests

- *Immunofluorescence*: IgG and C3 is deposited linearly along the basement membrane

Key diagnostic features of Bullous pemphigoid: See Box 1.9.

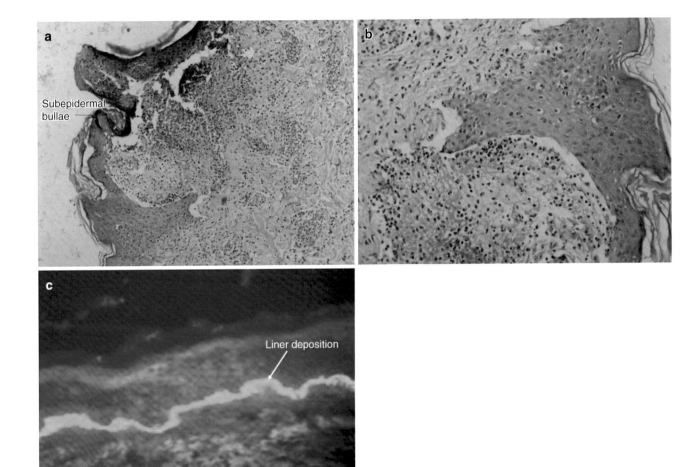

Fig. 1.14 (**a**) Bullous pemphigoid: Sub epidermal bullae formation. (**b**) Bullous pemphigoid: There is distinct separation between epidermis and underlying dermis. (**c**) Bullous pemphigoid: linear Ig G deposition demonstrated by immunofluorescence. (Courtesy Professor Uma Nahar, PGIMER, Chandigarh)

Box 1.9 Key diagnostic features of Bullous pemphigoid
- Subepidermal bullae
- Distinct separation between epidermis and underlying dermis
- *Immunofluorescence*: IgG and C3 is deposited linearly along the basement membrane

Differential diagnosis

- Pemphigus vulgaris: See Table 1.2

Treatment

- Systemic corticosteroid
- Tropical corticosteroid

Table 1.2 Differentiating features between bullous pemphigoid and pemphigus vulgaris

Features	Bullous pemphigoid	Pemphigus vulgaris
Position of bullae	Sub epidermal	Intraepidermal
Suprabasal cells	No acantholysis	Acantholysis present
Immunofluorescence pattern	Lace-like deposition of IgG in the intercellular epidermal junction	IgG and C3 is linearly deposited along the basement membrane

Cysts of Vulva

The lining epithelium of the different vulvar cysts have been highlighted in the Fig. 1.15.

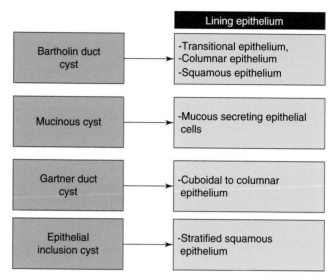

Fig. 1.15 Lining epithelium of different cysts of vulva

Bartholin Duct Cyst

Image gallery: Fig. 1.16a, b.

Source of origin: Bartholin duct.

Location of the cyst: Posterior introitus near the opening of the Bartholin duct.

Cause: Obstruction of the Bartholin duct.

Histopathology:

- Cyst lining: Squamous epithelium, transitional epithelium or columnar epithelium
- Occasionally the epithelium is completely flat
- Wall is formed by dense fibrous tissue

Differential diagnosis:
Other cysts in vulva.

Key diagnostic features of Bartholin duct cyst: see Box 1.10.

Box 1.10 Key Diagnostic Features of Bartholin Duct Cyst
- Cyst lining is formed by squamous epithelium, transitional epithelium or columnar epithelium
- Occasionally the epithelium is completely flat
- Wall is formed by dense fibrous tissue

Treatment: Word catheter placement or Marsupialization.

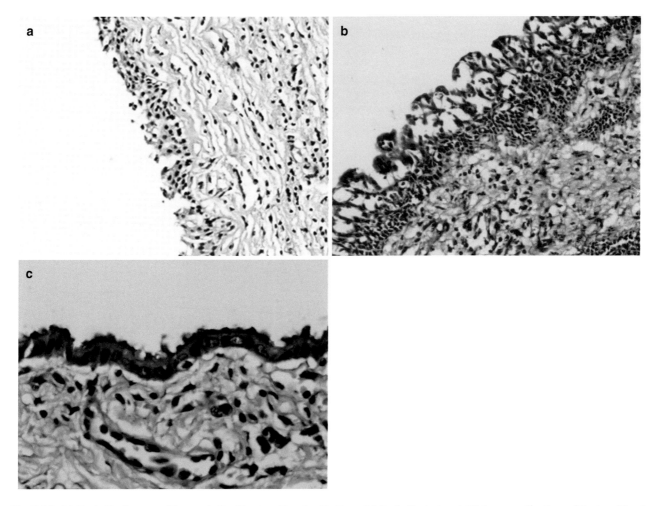

Fig. 1.16 (**a**) Bartholin duct cyst: The cyst is lined by transitional epithelium. (**b**) Bartholin duct cyst: Higher magnifications of the transitional epithelium. (**c**) Bartholin duct cyst: columnar lining of the cyst

Mucinous Cyst

Image gallery: Fig. 1.17a, b.

    Source of origin: Most likely from the minor vestibular gland.
    Location of the cyst: Vestibular region.
    Histopathology:
    The cyst lining

- Mucous secreting cuboidal to columnar epithelium
- Squamous metaplasia may be present in the lining epithelium.

Differential diagnosis: Other cysts in vulva.

Key features: See Box 1.11.

> **Box 1.11 Key Diagnostic Features of Mucinous Cyst**
> - The cyst is present in the vestibular region
> - Mucous secreting cuboidal to columnar epithelial lining
> - Squamous metaplasia may be seen in the lining epithelium.

Treatment: Marsupialization.

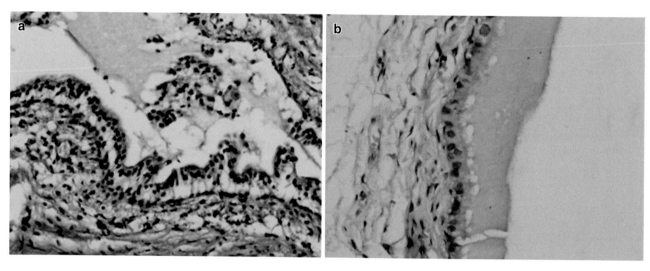

Fig. 1.17 (**a**) Mucinous cyst: Mucous secreting cuboidal to columnar epithelium. (**b**) Mucinous cyst: Higher magnification shows the cuboidal epithelial cells

Gartner Duct Cyst

Image gallery: Fig. 1.18.

Synonym: Gartner duct cyst: Wolffian duct cyst.

Location: Lateral part of vulva.

Histopathology

- The cyst lining: Non-ciliated cuboidal epithelium
- Wall: smooth muscle

Differential diagnosis: Other cysts in vulva.

Key diagnostic features: See Box 1.12.

Treatment: Marsupialization.

Box 1.12 Key Features of Gartner Duct Cyst
- Cyst in the lateral part of vulva
- The cyst lined by non-ciliated cuboidal epithelium
- Wall is formed by smooth muscle

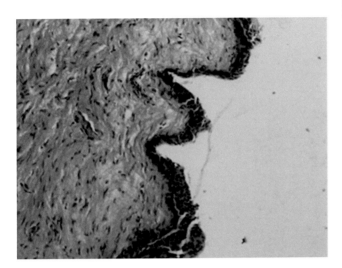

Fig. 1.18 Gartner duct cyst: Cyst wall is lined by Non-ciliodal epithelium

Epithelial Inclusion Cyst

Image gallery: Fig. 1.19a, b.

> *Synonym*: Keratinous cyst.
> *Source of origin*: Skin adnexal gland.
> *Location*: Labia majora and clitoris.
> *Histopathology*:

- Cyst lining: Flat stratified squamous epithelium
- Content: Keratinous material

Key diagnostic points: See Box 1.13.
Treatment: Surgical excision.

Box 1.13 Key Diagnostic Features of Epithelial Inclusion Cyst
- Cyst location: Labia majora and clitoris
- Lining: Flat stratified squamous epithelium
- Contents: Keratinous material

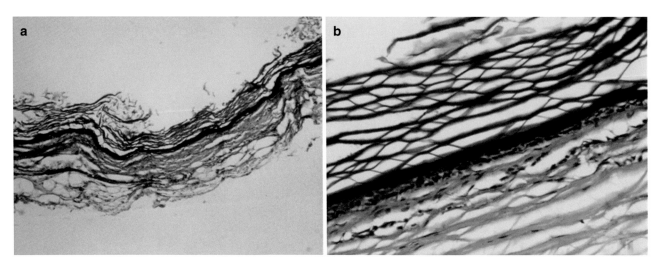

Fig. 1.19 (**a**) Epithelial inclusion cyst: Cyst wall is formed by squamous epithelium. (**b**) Epithelial inclusion cyst: Higher magnifications shows flat stratified squamous epithelial lining of the cyst

Epithelial Tumours

Squamous Cell Tumours

Vulvar Intraepithelial Lesion

Classification of squamous intraepithelial lesion (SIL) of vulva is highlighted in Fig. 1.20.

Usual type of vulvar squamous intraepithelial (u-VIN) lesion is divided into:

(a) Low grade squamous intraepithelial lesion
(b) High grade squamous intraepithelial lesion

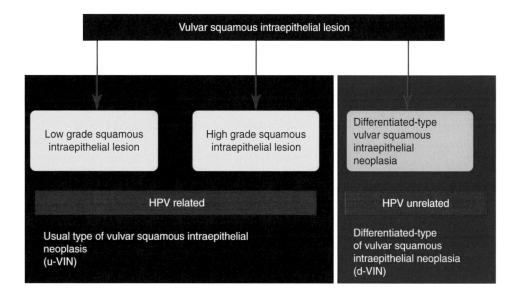

Fig. 1.20 Classification of vulvar squamous intraepithelial lesion

Low Grade Squamous Intraepithelial Lesion (LSIL)

Image gallery: Fig. 1.21a–c.

Definition: Low grade squamous intraepithelial lesion (LSIL) characterized by abnormal nuclei predominantly present in the lower third of the valval epithelium. The lesion is caused by the HPV infection.

Synonym: Vulvar intraepithelial neoplasia grade 1, mild squamous dysplasia.

Clinical features

- Asymptomatic
- Pruritus

Gross appearance

- Single or multiple pale areas
- Papular lesion

Histopathology

- Only lower third of the vulvar epithelium is involved
- Nuclei of the epithelial cells are enlarged, pleomorphic with irregular margin

- Frequent mitosis
- Continuous linear p16 immunostaining positivity (weak or patchy p16 staining indicates negative stain)

Key diagnostic features: See Box 1.14.

Box 1.14 Key Diagnostic Features of Low Grade Squamous Intraepithelial Lesion
- Hyperplastic lining epithelium
- Predominantly lower 1/3rd involved
- Parakeratosis
- Anisonucleosis
- Koilocytosis
- P16 immunostaining: Strong continuous linear positivity of the basal cells

---

Prognosis and treatment

- LSIL usually does not progress to higher grade.
- Simple excision

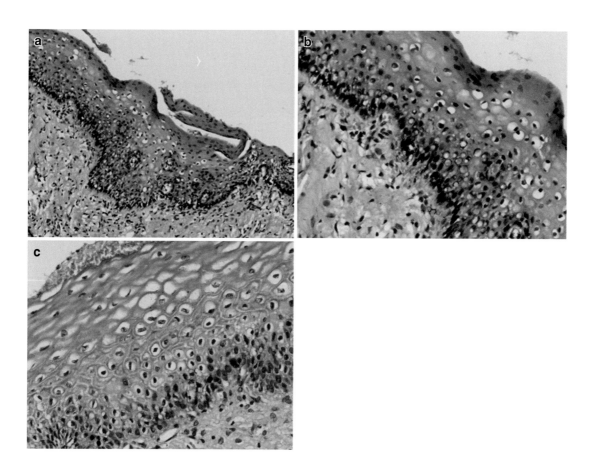

Fig. 1.21 (**a**) Low grade squamous intraepithelial neoplasia: lower third of the epithelium is involved. (**b**) Low grade squamous intraepithelial neoplasia: Mild nuclear enlargement and pleomorphism in the cells of the lower third of the epithelium. (**c**) Low grade squamous intraepithelial neoplasia: Dysplastic cells with Koilocytotic change

High Grade Squamous Intraepithelial Lesion

Image gallery: Fig. 1.22a–c.

Definition: High grade squamous intraepithelial lesion (HSIL) is characterized by nuclear abnormalities in more than the lower third of the valval epithelium. The lesion is related with significant risk of cancer development if it remains untreated.

Synonym: Moderate dysplasia, severe dysplasia, vulvar intraepithelial neoplasia grade 2, vulvar intraepithelial neoplasia grade 3.

Clinical features

- Asymptomatic
- Pruritus

- Mean age is 40 years

Gross appearance

- Usually multifocal
- Erythematous papules
- Elevated hyperpigmented area
- Aceto white area if 3% acetic acid is applied on the lesion

Risk factors

- Smoking
- Immunosuppression

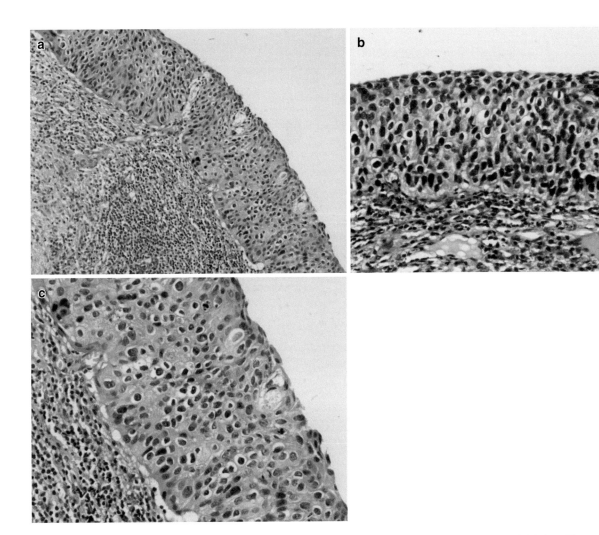

Fig. 1.22 (**a**) High grade squamous intraepithelial lesion: The epithelial cells show loss of polarity and abnormality in more than basal third of the cell layer. (**b**) High grade squamous intraepithelial lesion: The epithelial cells show moderate nuclear enlargement and pleomorphism. (**c**) High grade squamous intraepithelial lesion: The entire thickness of the epithelium shows atypical cells with high nucleocytoplasmic ratio and hyperchromatic nuclei

Association

- Strong association with HPV
- Predominantly HPV 16 (70%)
- Others: HPV 31, 33
- HPV 18 rare

Histopathology

- Thickened epithelial layer
- Hyperkeratosis and acanthosis
- Nuclear abnormality beyond the lower third of the epithelium
- Nuclei: Enlarged, pleomorphic, hyperchromatic
- Absence of cellular maturation
- Crowded nuclei
- Abnormal mitosis
- The lesion may also affects the skin adnexa and may mimic invasion

Ancillary investigations

- HPV: HPV 16 demonstration
- P16 immunostaining: positive in VIN
- Ki 67: High Ki 67 index

Differential diagnosis

- Multinucleated atypia of vulva: Absence of nuclear atypia.
- Reactive non-specific atypia: Negative p16 immunostaining.
- Paget's disease of vulva: Classical Paget's cells that are positive for CK 7, CEA, and CAM 5.2
- Superficial spreading malignant melanoma: Melanoma cells show HMB 45 and Melan A positivity.

- Condyloma: Epithelial cells of lower part are bland looking
- Seborrheic keratosis: No atypia.

Key diagnostic features: See Box 1.15.

Box 1.15 Key Diagnostic Features of High Grade Squamous Intraepithelial Lesion
- Hyperplastic epithelium
- Hyperkeratosis, parakeratosis and acanthosis
- Nuclear atypia is present beyond the lower third of the epithelium
- Enlarged, pleomorphic, hyperchromatic nuclei:
- Absence of cellular maturation
- Abnormal mitosis
- p16: Diffuse block positivity of both nucleus and cytoplasm

Prognosis

- Progression to invasive carcinoma
- Small number of cases may regress

Treatment

- Surgical excision
  - Laser excision
  - Laser vaporization and loop electrosurgical excision procedure (LEEP)
- Medical
  - Topical 5 fluorouracil application

Differentiated Type of Vulvar Squamous Intraepithelial Neoplasia

Image gallery: Fig. 1.23a, b.

Synonym: d-VIN.

Definition: Differentiated type of vulvar squamous intraepithelial neoplasia are HPV-negative lesion characterized by atypical basal cells and abnormal differentiation of the epithelial cells.

Etiology: Chronic vulvar disease causing p53 mutation.

Clinical features

- Rarely identified prospectively
- Usually noted in the margins of the squamous cell carcinoma
- Pruritus, pain

Gross features

- Unifocal
- White or reddish lesion

Histopathology

- Thickened epithelium
- Elongation of rete ridges
- Hyperkeratosis
- Basal cell atypia: Nuclear enlargement, pleomorphism, vesicular chromatin, prominent nucleoli
- Upper layer shows terminal differentiation, however the dyskeratotic cells may be seen there

Ancillary investigations

- P53: Variable positive
- P16: Negative or weak/patchy positive
- Ki 67: Positive cells only in basal and parabasal layer

Key diagnostic features: See Box 1.16.

Box 1.16 Key Diagnostic Features of Differentiated Type of Vulvar Squamous Intraepithelial Neoplasia
- Thickened epithelium with elongation of rete ridges
- Hyperkeratosis
- Terminal differentiation of the squamous cells seen in the upper part of the epithelium
- Basal layer showing the most important features:
  - Abnormal shaped mitosis
  - Nuclear enlargement and pleomorphism
  - Nucleolar prominence
  - Dyskeratotic cells
- Strongly positive for p 53 and negative for p16
- High Ki 67 positivity in the basal cell nuclei

Note: This lesion is likely to be missed. Careful observation of the basal epithelium along with immunostaining may be needed. However p53 is not reliable as it is often negative.

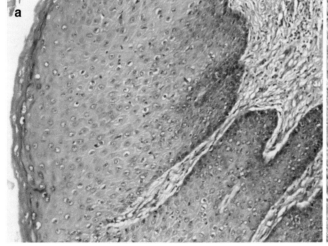
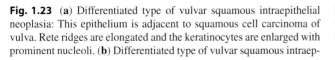
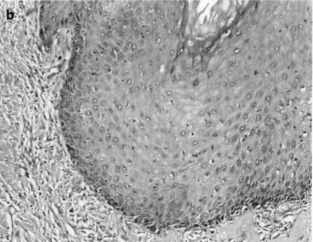

Fig. 1.23 (**a**) Differentiated type of vulvar squamous intraepithelial neoplasia: This epithelium is adjacent to squamous cell carcinoma of vulva. Rete ridges are elongated and the keratinocytes are enlarged with prominent nucleoli. (**b**) Differentiated type of vulvar squamous intraepithelial neoplasia: Basal cell show nuclear atypia, however upper layer of cells show terminal differentiation with few atypical cells. (**c**) Etiopathogenesis of vulvar squamous cell carcinoma

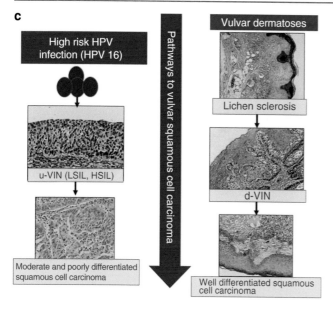

Fig. 1.23 (continued)

Table 1.3 Distinguishing d-VIN from the u-VIN

Features	u-VIN	d-VIN
Terminal differentiation of the epithelium	Grossly deranged	Not affected
Basal layer	It is affected along with other layers	Mainly the cells of this layer is affected and show atypical mitosis, atypia and prominent nucleoli
Mitotic activity	Throughout all the layers of epithelium	Restricted in the basal layer
P16 positivity	Diffuse block positivity	Negative or weakly positive
P 53	Negative	Often positive (>80%)

Differential diagnosis: Usual type of vulvar squamous intraepithelial neoplasm (see Table 1.3).

Prognosis and treatment

- Common association with squamous cell carcinoma
- Risk of progression is unknown
- Complete resection of the lesion

Squamous Cell Carcinoma

Image gallery: Figs. 1.23c and 1.24.

Definition: This is an invasive carcinoma with squamoid differentiation.

Etiology (Fig. 1.23c)

- One pathway: HPV infection, HSIL
- Other pathway: Chronic vulvar diseases (lichen sclerosis, lichen planus etc), differentiated VIN

Clinical features

- Nodular mass
- Ulcer
- Macule
- Bleeding
- Pain

Gross features

- Nodular
- Ulcerated with firm margin

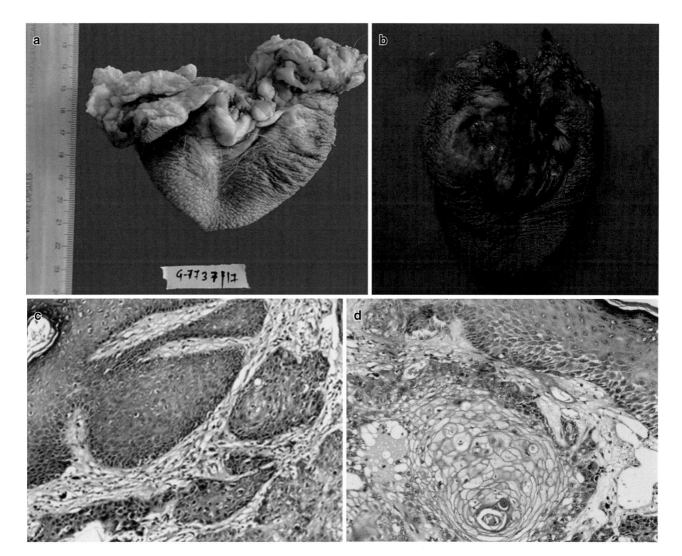

Fig. 1.24 (**a**) Gross photo of vulvar carcinoma: Soft and fleshy growth. (**b**) Gross photo of vulvar carcinoma: Ulcerated fleshy growth. (**c**) Keratinizing Squamous cell carcinoma: Keratin pearl formation. (**d**) Keratinizing Squamous cell carcinoma: Malignant cells forming keratin pearl. (**e**) Keratinizing Squamous cell carcinoma: The cells are polyhedral with central large hyperchromatic nuclei. (**f**) Non-keratinizing Squamous cell carcinoma: Diffuse sheets of malignant squamoid cells. (**g**) Non-keratinizing Squamous cell carcinoma: Sheets of malignant cells with hyperchromatic nuclei. (**h**) Non-keratinizing Squamous cell carcinoma: Malignant cells showing intracellular keratinization. (**i**) Reporting of vulvar carcinoma

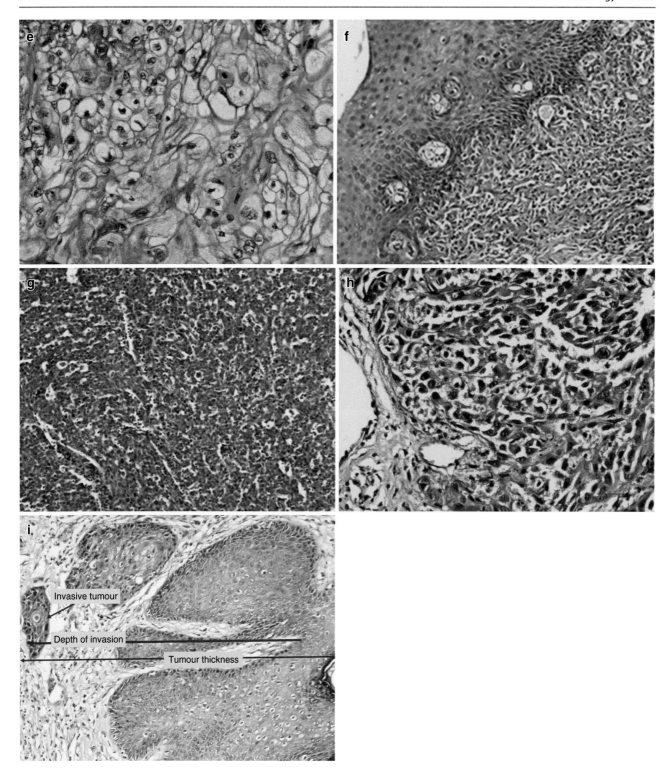

Fig. 1.24 (continued)

Histopathology

Keratinizing Squamous Cell Carcinoma

- Infiltrating nests of cells in the deeper tissue
- Desmoplastic tissue reaction
- Large polyhedral tumour cells
- Hyperchromatic and moderately pleomorphic nuclei
- Keratin pearl's formation

Non-Keratinizing Squamous Cell Carcinoma

- No keratin pearl formation
- Only diffuse sheets of malignant squamous cells present

Reporting of Carcinoma of Vulva (Fig. 1.24i)

- Tumour thickness
- Depth of invasion
- Perivascular and perineural invasion
- Status of tumor margin and deep resection plane
- Presence of VIN
- Status of lymph node

Various Types of Squamous Cell Carcinoma

Basaloid Carcinoma
Image gallery: Fig. 1.25.
Histopathology

- Nests of cells
- Cord like arrangement
- Monomorphic basaloid cells with scanty cytoplasm
- Granular nuclear chromatin
- HPV positive

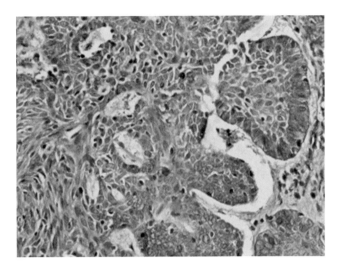

Fig. 1.25 Basaloid carcinoma: Nests of basaloid cells having peripheral palisading arrangement

Verrucous Carcinoma

Image gallery: Fig. 1.26a–c.

Histopathology:

- Well differentiated type of squamous cell carcinoma
- Broad based papillae with bulldozer like pushing margin
- No nuclear atypia in the basal cells
- Blunt looking epithelial stromal junction
- No evidence of any co-existing squamous cell carcinoma

Differential diagnosis (Fig. 1.26d)

- Keratinizing squamous cell carcinoma
  - Moderate nuclear atypia
  - Isolated cell clusters
  - Absent Koilocytosis
  - High mitotic activity
- Condyloma accuminatum
  - Papillary growth

- Minimal nuclear atypia
- Koilocytosis present

Key diagnostic points: See Box 1.17.

Box 1.17 Key Diagnostic Points of Verrucous Carcinoma
- Verruco-papillary lesion
- Absence of nuclear atypia in basal layer
- Nuclei show coarse chromatin and prominent nucleoli
- Blunt epithelial stromal junction
- Broad based large bulbous papillae with pushing pattern of invasion
- No associated squamous cell carcinoma

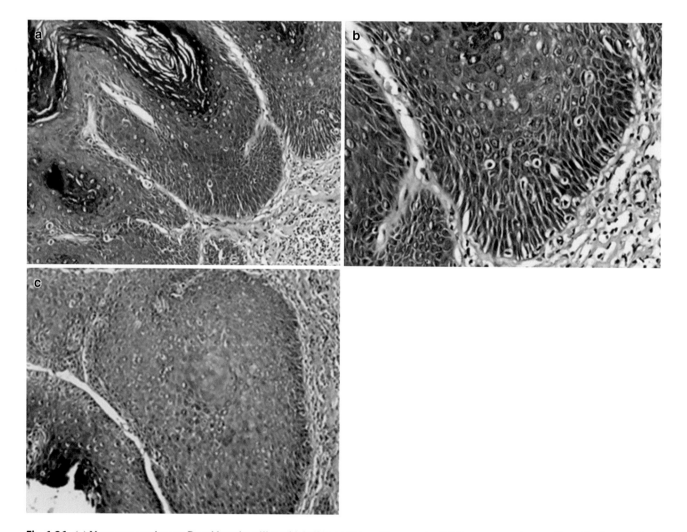

Fig. 1.26 (**a**) Verrucous carcinoma: Broad based papillae with bulldozer like pushing margin. (**b**) Verrucous carcinoma: The cells show minimal nuclear pleomorphism. (**c**) Verrucous carcinoma: Blunt looking epithelial- stromal junction. (**d**) Differential diagnosis of verrucous carcinoma

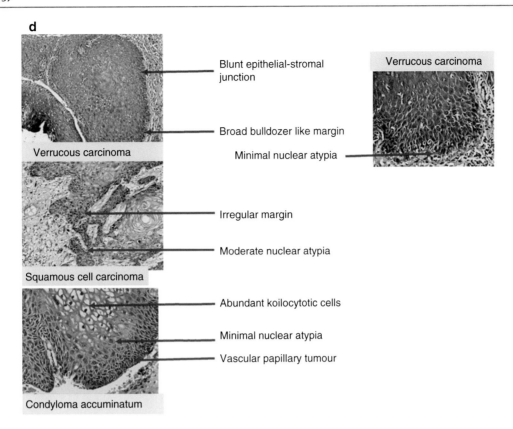

Fig. 1.26 (continued)

Lymphoepithelioma

Image gallery: Fig. 1.27.

Histopathology

- Nests of tumour cells: Islands of undifferentiated cells with ill-defined outer margin
- Dense lymphocytic infiltration around the tumour cells

Differential diagnosis

- Amelanotic melanoma: Adjacent area of squamous cell carcinoma may show VIN and focal squamous differentiation may also be seen. HMB 45 and melan A are positive in melanoma.
- Basaloid squamous cell carcinoma versus small cell carcinoma: Nuclear moulding and crushing artifact are often present in small cell carcinoma. The small cell carcinoma cases are positive for NSE and chromogranin.

Prognosis of vulvar squamous cell carcinoma

- Prognosis depends on the FIGO stage of the carcinoma
- Survival rate:
  - Stage I: 98%
  - Stage IV: 28%
- Other prognostic factors: lymphovascular emboli, depth of invasion, lymph node metastasis

Treatment: Surgical resection: Either partial or total vulvectomy.

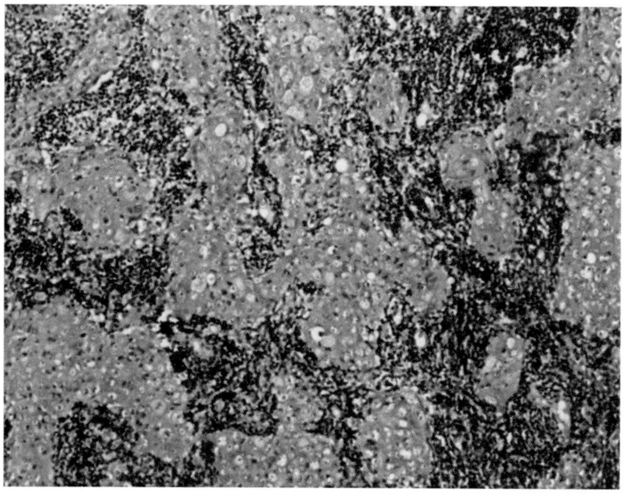

Fig. 1.27 Lymphoepithelioma: Dense lymphocytic infiltration around the tumour cells

Basal Cell Carcinoma

Image gallery: Fig. 1.28a, b.

Definition: This is an invasive tumour that resembles basal cell carcinoma of skin.

Origin: Basal cells of the hair follicles of the vulva.

Clinical features

- Elderly patient
- Pruritus
- Located in the labia majora

Gross features

- Ulcerated
- Nodular mass
- Hypo pigmented area

Histopathology

- Palisading basal cells infiltrating into the deeper tissue
- Oval to mild elongated nuclei
- Minimal nuclear pleomorphism
- Dark basophilic nuclei

Prognosis and treatment

- Relatively good prognosis than squamous cell carcinoma
- Surgical excision with wide resection margin

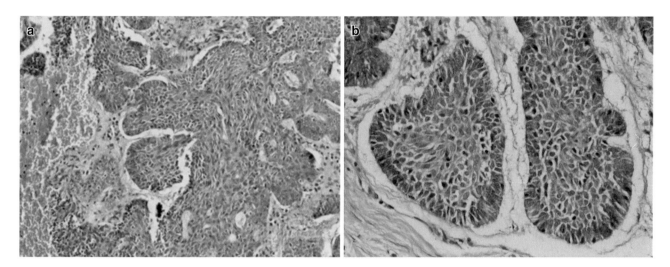

Fig. 1.28 (**a**) Basal cell carcinoma: Multiple nests of tumour cells with peripheral palisading arrangement. (**b**) Basal cell carcinoma: The tumour cells showing monomorphic hyperchromatic nuclei

Benign Tumours of Epithelial Origin

Condyloma Acuminatum

Image gallery: Fig. 1.29a–d.

Synonym: Vulvar wart, papilloma of vulva.

Abbreviation: Condyloma Acuminatum: CA

Definition: Condyloma acuminatum is a benign verrucous papillary lesion of vulva caused by Human papilloma virus infection and is often a precursor lesion of vulvar carcinoma.

Causative factors

- HPV 6 is the commonest infection followed by HPV 11
- Other associated factors are: Diabetes mellitus, immuno-suppression, sexual promiscuity

Clinical features

- Multiple small popular lesions
- Site: Vulva, perianal region, vagina, cervix

- Commonly asymptomatic
- Uncommonly presents with pruritus and bleeding

Gross features

- Exophytic warty
- The warts may merge to form cauliflower like lesion

Histopathology

- Papillae lined by squamous epithelial cells
- Squamous lining shows hyperkeratosis, acanthosis and parakeratosis
- Koilocytotic cells: These cells are seen in the superficial layer. The cells have central enlarged nuclei surrounded by clear halo.
- Basal layer may show increased mitosis. However no atypical mitosis is seen.

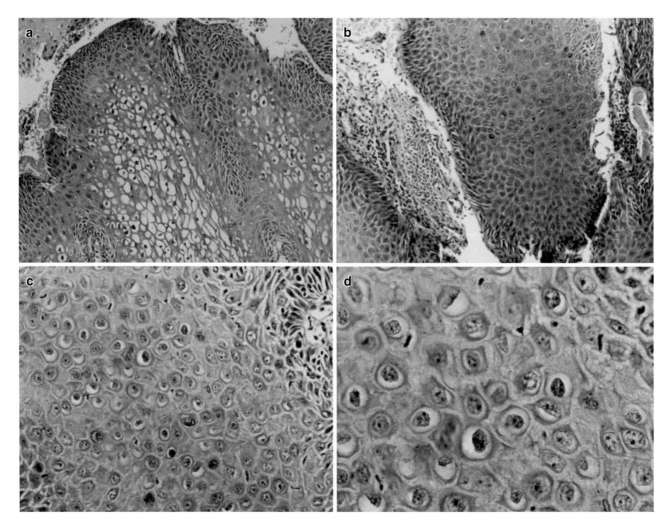

Fig. 1.29 (**a**) Condyloma accuminatum: Multiple verrucous like hyperplasia. (**b**) Condyloma accuminatum: Parabasal hyperplasia of the epithelial cells. (**c**) Condyloma accuminatum: Prominent Koilocytotic changes in the epithelial cell. (**d**) Condyloma accuminatum: Higher magnification showing the detailed features of Koilocytotic cells. The nuclei are enlarged with a perinuclear halo. (**e**) Differential diagnosis of condyloma acuminatum

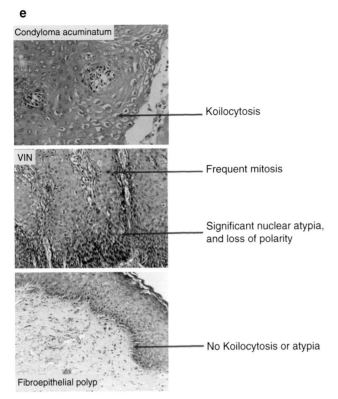

e

Condyloma acuminatum

Koilocytosis

VIN

Frequent mitosis

Significant nuclear atypia, and loss of polarity

No Koilocytosis or atypia

Fibroepithelial polyp

Fig. 1.29 (continued)

Immunohistochemistry

- Increased Ki 67 index in the upper layer
- HPV DNA is positive by in situ hybridization technique

Differential diagnosis (Fig. 1.29e)

- Vulvar intraepithelial lesion (VIN): High mitotic activity and nuclear atypia are the characteristic features of VIN.

- Fibroepithelial polyp: Absence of Koilocytosis and HPV changes in the fibroepithelial polyp.

Box 1.18 Key Diagnostic Points of Condyloma Acuminatum
- Papillary structure covered with squamous cells
- Hyperkeratosis, acanthosis and parakeratosis
- Koilocytotic cells in the superficial layer
- Increased mitosis in basal layer
- High Ki 67 index
- HPV DNA: HPV 6 and 11

Key diagnostic features: See Box 1.18.
Natural history

- CA is a benign lesion and it slowly regresses.
- Only a few cases of CA progress to VIN and subsequently to carcinoma.
- Recurrence of CA is more often seen in immunosuppressive patients.

Management

- Small lesion: Local application of podophyllin or Trichloroacetic acid
- Larger lesion: Electrocautery, cryotherapy, laser ablation, surgical resection

Seborrheic Keratosis

Image gallery: Fig. 1.30a, b.

Location: It is seen in the hairy part of vulva.

Association: Commonly associated with acanthosis nigricans.

Gross appearance: Brownish raised irregular area on skin.

Histopathology:

- Many horny keratinous cyst
- Hyperkeratosis
- Acanthosis
- Papillomatosis

Treatment: Surgical excision.

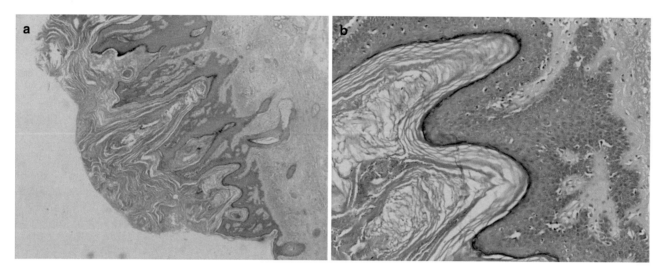

Fig. 1.30 (**a**) Seborrheic keratosis: Acanthosis, hyperkeratosis and papillomatosis of the lining epithelium with many horn cysts. The entire lesion is above the normal epidermis. (**b**) Seborrheic keratosis: Higher magnification showing acanthosis and horny keratin cyst

Glandular Tumours

Paget Disease of Vulva

Definition: It is an intraepithelial adenocarcinoma having apocrine or eccrine glandular differentiation. The tumour shows typical Paget's cell with moderate amount of clear cytoplasm and centrally placed enlarged nuclei.

Origin: Tumour arises from the pluripotent stem cells of the epidermis.

Clinical features:

- Pruritus
- Reddish eczematous lesion
- Located in the labia majora and minora

Classification of Paget disease of vulva: See Fig. 1.31a.
Image gallery: Fig. 1.31b–g.
Histopathology

- Intraepidermal Paget's cells: These cells are present discretely and in small isolated clusters. They are present adjacent to parabasal and basal areas.
- Paget cell:
  - Large cell with abundant clear vacuolated cytoplasm
  - Centrally placed enlarged nuclei with prominent nucleoli
  - PAS positive and diastase resistant cytoplasmic material

Immunostaining

- *Positive for*
  - CK 7
  - CEA
  - Gross cystic disease fluid protein (GCDFP-15)
- *Negative for*
  - HMB 45
  - Melan A
  - S-100 protein
  - Uroplakin
  - CK 20

Differential diagnosis (see Fig. 1.31h)

- Superficially spreading malignant melanoma: Positive for HMB 45, Melan A and S-100 protein
- In situ squamous cell carcinoma: No Paget cells
- Mycosis fungoides: Classical large convoluted cerebriform cells of mycosis fungoides

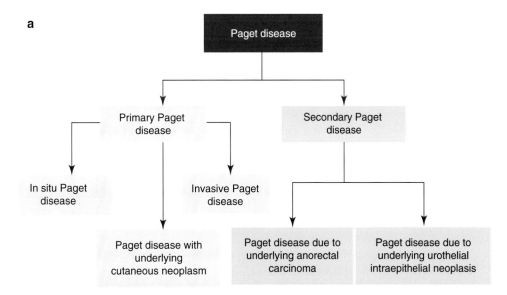

Fig. 1.31 (**a**) Classification of Paget disease. (**b**) Paget's disease: Hyperkeratosis and papillary proliferation of the epidermal layer with multiple nests of Paget cell. (**c**) Paget's disease: Abundant discrete intraepidermal Paget cells. (**d**) Paget's disease: The Paget cells show abundant clear cytoplasm and enlarged round nuclei. (**e**) Paget's disease: Higher magnification showing better cell morphology of Paget cells. The cells have vacuolated cytoplasm. Large nuclei show prominent nucleoli. (**f**) CK 7 immunostaining in Paget vulva. Clusters and discrete Paget cells show strong CK 7 positivity. (**g**) HMB 45 immunostaining in Paget vulva. Note that only basal melanocytes are positive and tumour cells are negative for the stain. (**h**) Differential diagnosis of Paget's disease of vulva

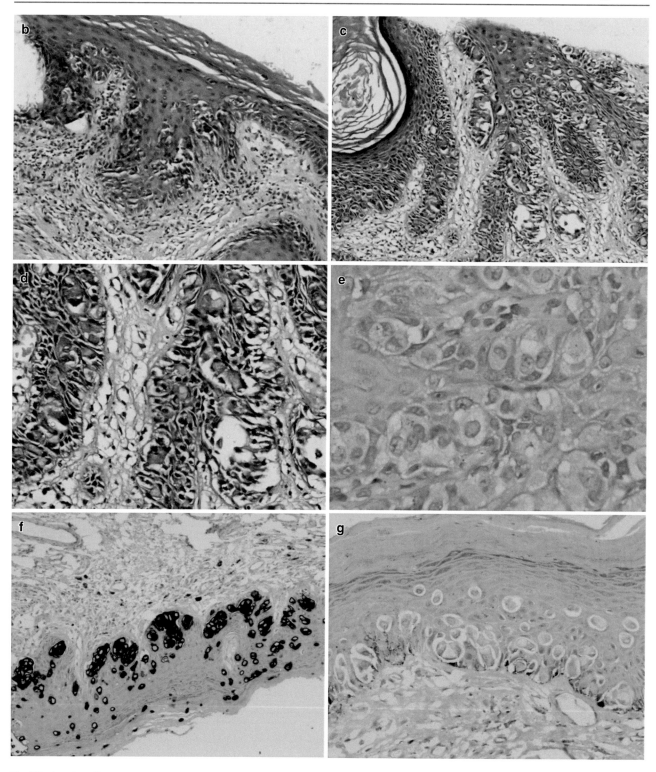

Fig. 31 (continued)

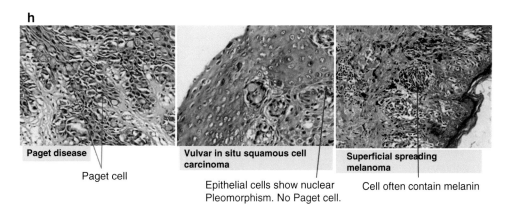

h

Paget disease

Paget cell

Vulvar in situ squamous cell carcinoma

Epithelial cells show nuclear Pleomorphism. No Paget cell.

Superficial spreading melanoma

Cell often contain melanin

Fig. 31 (continued)

Key diagnostic points: See Box 1.19.

Box 1.19 Key Diagnostic Points of Paget Disease of Vulva
- Nests, or isolated Paget's cell in the epidermis
- Paget's cells: Large cells with vacuolated cytoplasm having centrally placed enlarged nuclei
- Occasionally acini like arrangement
- Frequent mitosis
- Positive: CEA, EMA, CAM 5.2 and CK 7
- Negative: CK 20, GCDFP

Prognosis
Non-invasive Paget disease have good prognosis

- Slow and indolent course
- Frequent recurrence (33% cases) after resection
- Disease free survival depends on age, extent of dermal invasion

Treatment

- Surgical resection with 1 cm free margin
- Invasive Paget disease: Inguino femoral lymphadenectomy

Bartholin Gland and Other Specialized Anogenital Glands Tumours

Types of carcinomas originated in Bartholin gland

- Squamous cell carcinoma
- Adenocarcinoma
- Adenosquamous cell carcinoma
- Transitional cell carcinoma
- Adenoid cystic carcinoma

Squamous Cell Carcinomas of Bartholin Gland

Image gallery: Fig. 1.32a, b.
  Histopathology

- Morphology of the squamous cell carcinoma of the Bartholin gland resembles squamous cell carcinoma of any other region

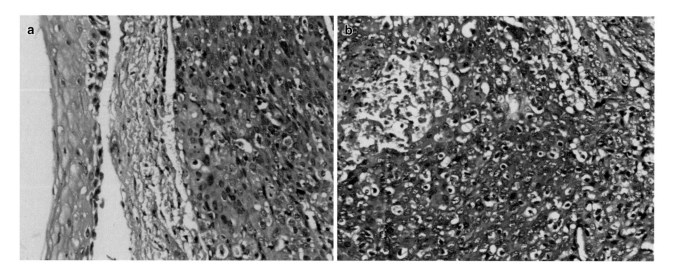

Fig. 1.32 (**a**) Squamous cell carcinoma of Bartholin gland: Diffuse sheets of malignant cells. (**b**) Squamous cell carcinoma of Bartholin gland: Polyhedral cells with central moderately pleomorphic nuclei

Adenoid Cystic Carcinomas

Image gallery: Fig. 1.33a–c.

   Cell of origin: Myoepithelial cells of Bartholin gland.

   Clinical features: Painful nodular mass.

   Histopathology:

- Pattern
  - Cribriform
  - Tubular
  - Solid

- Round monomorphic ducal cells with scanty cytoplasm
- Ductal cells surround the pinkish hyaline stroma
- No atypia or mitosis

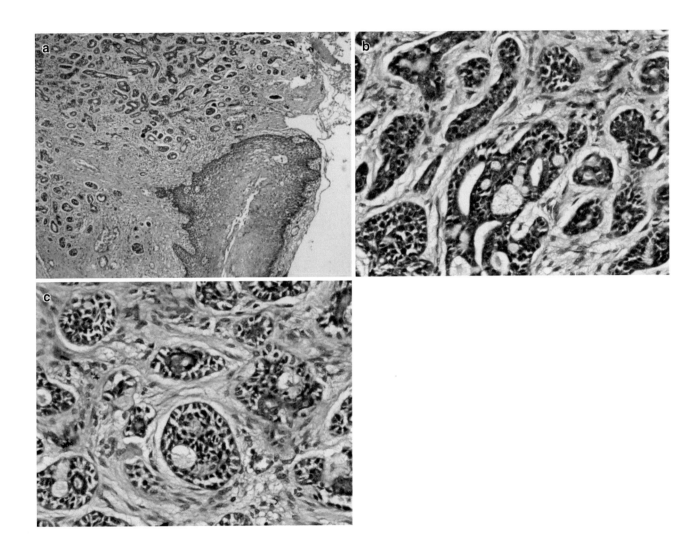

Fig. 1.33 (**a**) Adenoid cystic carcinoma: The tumour underneath the epithelium shoes multiple tubules with cribriform pattern. (**b**) Adenoid cystic carcinoma: Cribriform pattern. (**c**) Adenoid cystic carcinoma: The tubules are lined by small cells with monomorphic hyperchromatic nuclei

Phyllodes Tumours

Image gallery: Fig. 1.34a, b.
   Source of origin: Anogenital glands.
   Clinical features: Mass lesion, 2–3 cm dimeter.
   Histopathology

- Similar to Phyllodes tumour of the breast
- Exuberant stromal material
- Glandular proliferation

- Stroma often encroaches in the gland
- Nuclear pleomorphism, mitosis depend on the type of Phyllodes tumour (benign/borderline/malignant)

Prognosis and treatment

- Prognosis depends on the grade of tumour
- Excision of the swelling is the treatment of choice

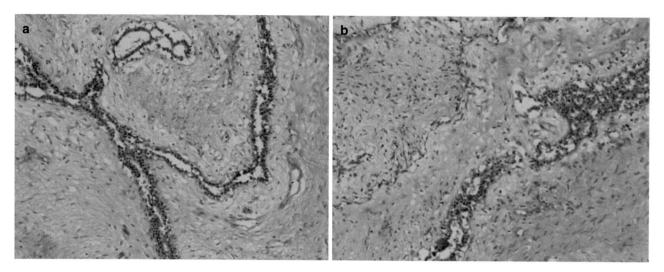

Fig. 1.34 (**a**) Phyllodes tumours: Glands admixed with abundant stromal tissue. (**b**) Phyllodes tumours: Stromal cells showing exuberant proliferation

Papillary Hidradenoma

Image gallery: Fig. 1.35a–c.

Synonym

- Hidradenoma Papilliferum
- Mammary like glandular adenoma

Location

- Labia minora
- Intra-labial sulci

Source of origin

- Apocrine sweat gland

Clinical features

- Small mass less than 2/3 cm in size
- May be cystic
- Often ulcerated

Histopathology

- Well encapsulated
- Multiple tubules and acini
- Complex papillae with central fibrovascular core
- Glands lined by cuboidal or tall columnar cells
- Outer layer of Myoepithelial cell is present
- Mitotic activities are often seen

Differential diagnosis

- Adenocarcinoma: The distinguishing features:
  – Moderate nuclear pleomorphism and mitosis.
  – Hidradenoma is always well circumscribed

Prognosis and treatment

- Benign tumour
- Surgical excision of the swelling

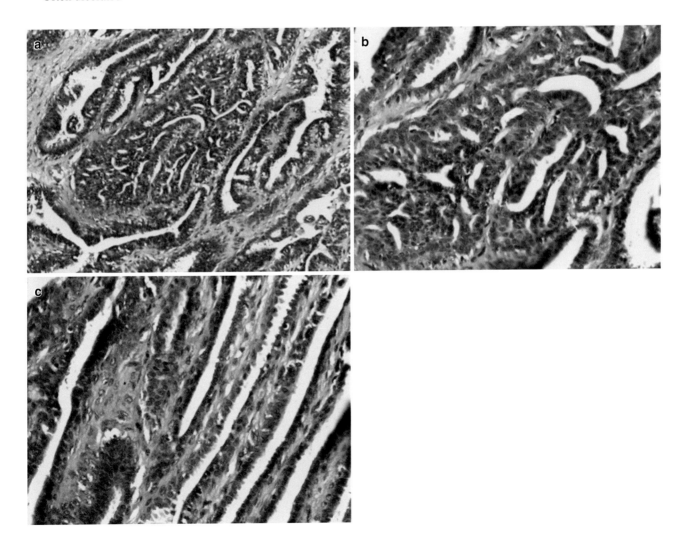

Fig. 1.35 (**a**) Papillary Hidradenoma: Multiple tubular and gland like structures. (**b**) Papillary Hidradenoma: The complex papillary structures may be misinterpreted as adenocarcinoma. (**c**) Papillary Hidradenoma: The tubular lining cells lining are monomorphic and rest on myoepithelial cells

Mixed Tumour of the Vulva

Image gallery: Fig. 1.36a, b.

Clinical features

- Subcutaneous swelling
- Solid mass

Location

- Labia majora
- Near Bartholin's gland

Histogenesis

- Myoepithelial cells in the vulva

Histopathology

- Epithelial cells: In nest, cord, trabeculae
- Stromal cells: Myxoid, cartilaginous and bony area simulates pleomorphic adenoma

Prognosis and treatment

- Benign lesion
- Recurrence may occur
- Development of malignancy is very rare. In case of metastasis only epithelial component metastasize.
- Surgical resection is the treatment of choice

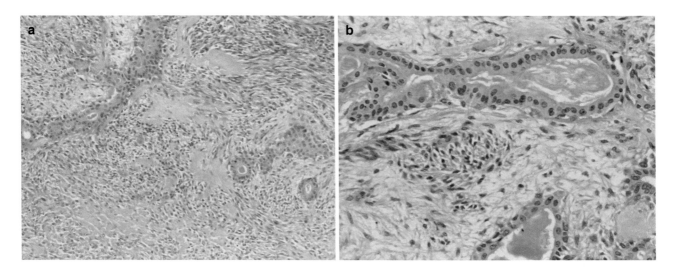

Fig. 1.36 (**a**) Mixed tumour: Glands and chondromyxoid connective tissue stroma with many spindle shaped cells. The tumour resembles pleomorphic adenoma of salivary gland. (**b**) Mixed tumour: Tubular structures embedded in the chondromyxoid stroma

Fibroadenoma

Image gallery: Fig. 1.37.

Clinical features

- Single
- Soft to firm swelling
- Subcutaneous
- Swelling increases during pregnancy

Histogenesis

- Specialized glands in the anogenital region

Histopathology

- Stroma consisting of spindle cells
- Multiple slit like glands

Prognosis and treatment

- Benign tumour
- Incomplete excision may cause recurrence
- Surgical excision is the choice of treatment

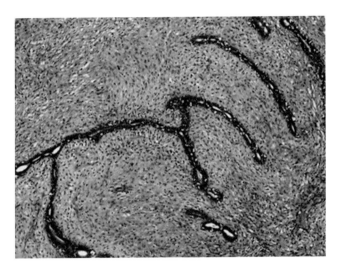

Fig. 1.37 Fibroadenoma of vulva: Multiple slit like glands embedded in the connective tissue

Soft Tissue Tumours of Vulva

Fibroepithelial Polyp

Image gallery: Fig. 1.38a–c.

Definition: It is a slowly growing benign neoplasm covered by stratified squamous epithelium containing stromal tissue.

Clinical features

- Usually seen in the middle aged patient in the reproductive age period
- Common during pregnancy
- Feeling of a mass lesion, bleeding

Gross features

- Usually solitary but may be multiple
- Small pedunculated or sessile flesh coloured mass

Histogenesis

- Subepithelial stromal cells undergo proliferation due to hormonal stimulation

Histopathology

- Surface of polyp: Squamous epithelium that may have hyperkeratosis, papillomatosis and acanthosis.
- Stroma:
- Loose oedematous fibrocollagenous tissue rich in blood vessels.
- Stellate shaped stromal cells and multinucleated cells.
- At the time of pregnancy the stromal cells may show increased cellularity, nuclear pleomorphism and atypical mitosis

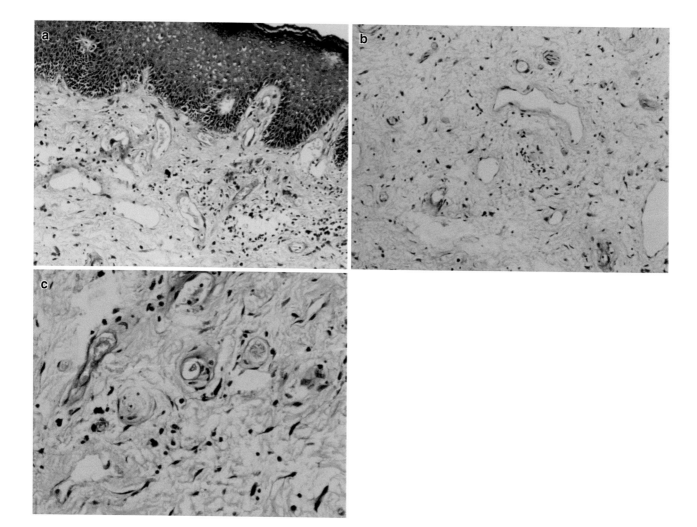

Fig. 1.38 (**a**) Fibroepithelial Polyp: Polyp is lined by epithelial cells with hyperkeratosis and acanthosis. (**b**) Fibroepithelial Polyp: The stromal tissue shows loose fibrocollagenous tissue. (**c**) Fibroepithelial Polyp: Multiple vascular channels in the stroma. The stromal cells are stellate shaped with minimal atypia

Immunocytochemistry

- *Positive*: vimentin, desmin, oestrogen and progesterone receptors

Key diagnostic points: See Box 1.20.

Box 1.20 Key Diagnostic Points of Fibroepithelial Polyp
- Polyp with squamous lining
- Hyperkeratosis, papillomatosis and acanthosis
- Loose oedematous stroma formed by fibrocollagenous tissue
- Stellate shaped stromal cells
- Multinucleated cells.
- *Positive*: Vimentin, desmin, oestrogen and progesterone receptors

---

Differential diagnosis

- *Aggressive angiomyxoma*: Rarely due to torsion the fibroepithelial polyp may undergo torsion and mimic angiomyxoma. No deeper tissue invasion is seen in polyp.
- *Embryonal rhabdomyosarcoma*: Lower age group of the patient, clinical presentation, the presence of cambium layer help in the diagnosis of embryonal rhabdomyosarcoma.

Prognosis

- Benign tumour and usually do not recur but incomplete resection or prolonged hormonal stimulation may cause recurrence of the polyp

Treatment

- Surgical resection of the polyp.

Superficial Angiomyxoma

Image gallery: Fig. 1.39.

    Definition: It is a benign soft tissue tumour of vulva.

    Epidemiology: Uncommon tumour.

    Clinical features

- Commonly in 4th decade
- Slow growing painless tumour
- Polypoid lesion
- Superficially located

Gross features

- Polypoid mass
- Usually less than 5 cm in diameter
- Cut surface: Soft gelatinous

Histopathology

- Lobulated lesions
- Stellate shaped spindle cells with blunt nuclei
- Myxoid stroma
- Blood vessels are thin walled
- Focal polymorphs and lymphocytes present

Immunohistochemistry

- Positive for: CD 34 and vimentin

Differential diagnosis

- Aggressive (deep) angiomyxoma: Deep in location, infiltrative tumour, thick walled blood vessels

    Prognosis: One third of the tumour recurs after resection.

    Treatment: Surgical resection of the tumour.

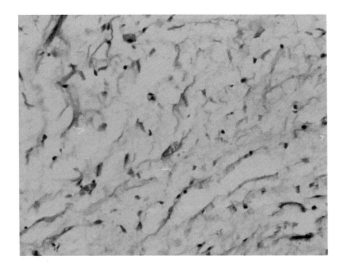

Fig. 1.39 Superficial angiomyxoma: Blunt stellate shaped cells in a myxoid stroma. Note the thin walled vessels

Aggressive (Deep) Angiomyxoma

Image gallery: Fig. 1.40a–f

Definition

It is locally invasive infiltrative low grade soft tissue neoplasm of the vulva that often recurs after resection.

Synonym: Deep angiomyxoma, aggressive angiomyxoma.

Clinical features

- Usually seen in the reproductive age period
- Slowly enlarging mass in the vulva
- Often presents as cystic mass

Gross features

- Usually large
- Poorly circumscribed

- Soft
- Lobulated
- Cystic degeneration

Histopathology

- Infiltrating margins
- Usually sparsely cellular tumour
- Spindle to stellate shaped cells with bland nuclei
- The spindle cells do not show any atypia or mitosis
- The stroma is myxoid
- Many large thick walled blood vessels that are often hyalinised
- Smooth muscle cells within the stroma

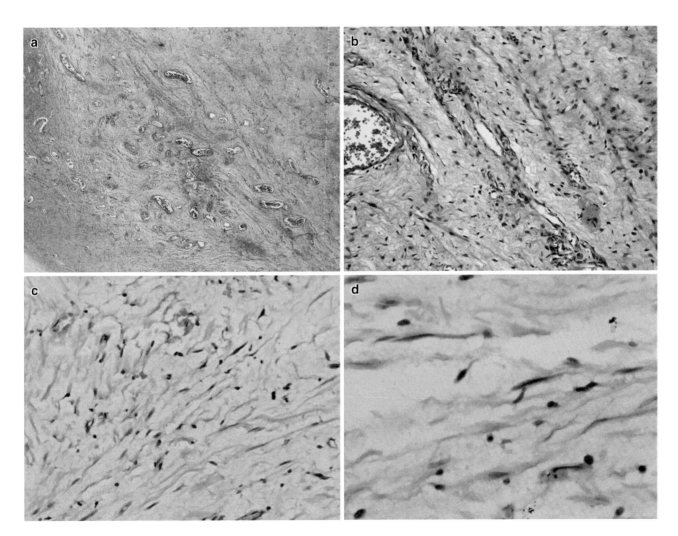

Fig. 1.40 (**a**) Aggressive angiomyxoma: Numerous blood vessels embedded in the myxoid stroma. Note that medium to large sized vessels are present here. (**b**) Aggressive angiomyxoma: Sparsely cellular stroma. (**c**) Aggressive angiomyxoma: Loose myxoid stroma with spindle shaped stromal cells. (**d**) Aggressive angiomyxoma: Stellate shaped stromal cells. (**e**) Aggressive angiomyxoma: Desmin positive cells. (**f**) Aggressive angiomyxoma: Tumour cells show strongly positive vimentin. (**g**) Differential diagnosis of deep angiomyxoma

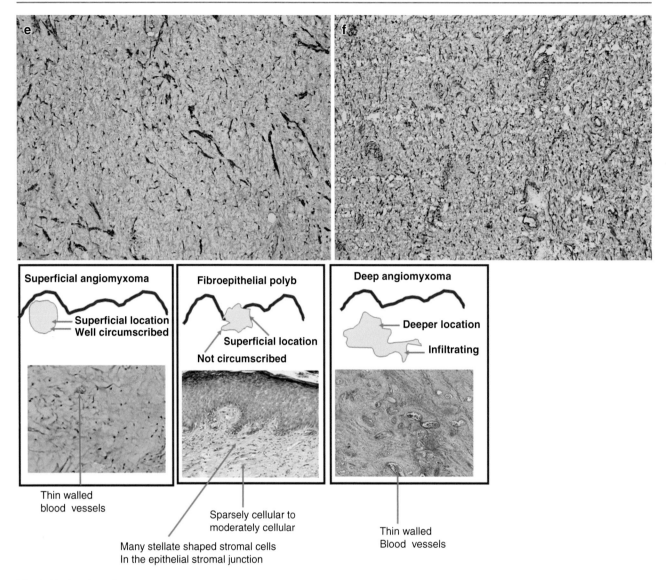

Superficial angiomyxoma

Superficial location

Well circumscribed

Thin walled
blood vessels

Fibroepithelial polyb

Superficial location

Not circumscribed

Sparsely cellular to
moderately cellular

Many stellate shaped stromal cells
In the epithelial stromal junction

Deep angiomyxoma

Deeper location

Infiltrating

Thin walled
Blood vessels

Fig. 1.40 (continued)

Immunohistochemistry

Positive for: CD 34, desmin, vimentin, oestrogen and progesterone receptors. Also positive for HMGA2.

Key diagnostic features: See Box 1.21.

Box 1.21 Key Diagnostic Features of Deep Angiomyxoma

- Poorly circumscribed
- Deep Infiltrating margins
- Usually hypo cellular tumour
- Bland spindle cells with pale delicate cytoplasmic extensions
- No atypia or mitosis
- Myxoid stroma
- Many large thick walled hyalinised blood vessels
- Aggregations of smooth muscle cells around the blood vessels or loosely scattered in the stroma
- Stromal cells are positive for desmin, actin and CD 34

Differential diagnosis

- Superficial angiomyxoma: Well circumscribed and superficial in position (Fig. 1.40g) and negative for desmin.
- Fibroepithelial polyp: Superficial and well circumscribed, no myxoid stroma
- Cellular angiofibroma: Superficial and well circumscribed, cellular with small to medium sized vessels
- Other tumours with myxoid changes: Myxoid fibroma and fibrosarcoma.

Prognosis

- Frequently recurs (40% cases) due to incomplete excision

Treatment:

- Local excision with 1 cm tumour free margins along with free deep resection plane

Leiomyoma

Image gallery: Fig. 1.41a, b.

  Definition: This is a benign smooth muscle tumour.

  Clinical features:

- Commonly seen in 4th or 5th decade of life
- Presents as mass lesion
- Synchronous leiomyoma may be noted

Gross features

- Well circumscribed
- Grey white in cut surface

Histopathology

- Intersecting fascicles of spindle cells
- Spindle cells with monomorphic nuclei
- Blunt ended nuclei
- Moderate amount of eosinophilic cytoplasm

Treatment

- Surgical excision of the swelling
- Incomplete excision may cause recurrence

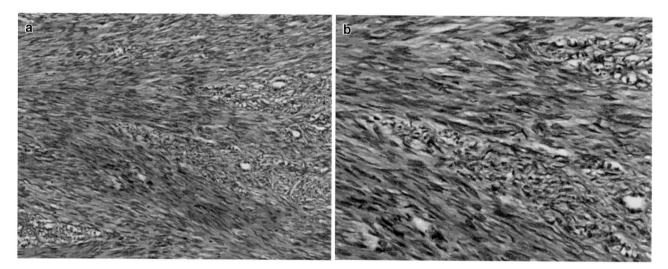

Fig. 1.41 (**a**) Leiomyoma: Small and large fascicles of spindle cells. (**b**) Leiomyoma: Oval to elongated spindle cells with blunt ends

Leiomyosarcoma

Image gallery: Fig. 1.42b.

Definition: This is a malignant tumour with smooth muscle differentiation.

Clinical features

- Patient is elderly in 4th or 5th decade
- Rapidly growing painless mass

Gross features

- Small to large mass
- Cut surface yellow
- Areas of haemorrhage and necrosis

Histopathology

- Spindle cells
- The criteria of malignancy include
  - More than 5 mitosis per 10 high power field
  - Moderate nuclear atypia
  - Growth infiltrating in the deeper tissue
  - More than 5 cm diameter in size

Treatment

- Surgical resection

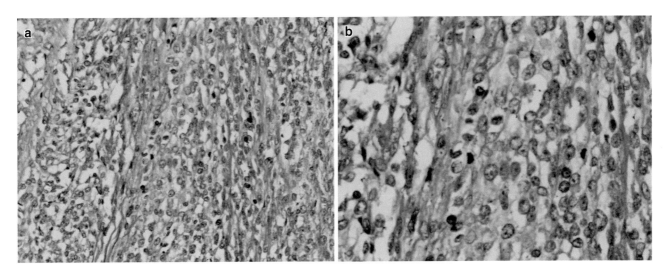

Fig. 1.42 (**a**) Leiomyosarcoma: Bundles of spindle shaped smooth muscle cells with moderate nuclear pleomorphism. (**b**) Leiomyosarcoma Frequent mitotic activity of the tumour cells

Melanocytic Tumours

Melanocytic Naevi

Image gallery: Fig. 1.43a–c.

Definition: This is a benign lesion of melanocytic origin.

Clinical features:

- Patient presents with pigmented lesion in the vulva
- Often asymptomatic and detected incidentally

Histopathology

- Naevus cells are present in epidermis and upper dermis
- Round to oval cells with abundant cytoplasm
- Melanin granules in the cytoplasm

Treatment

- Local surgical excision

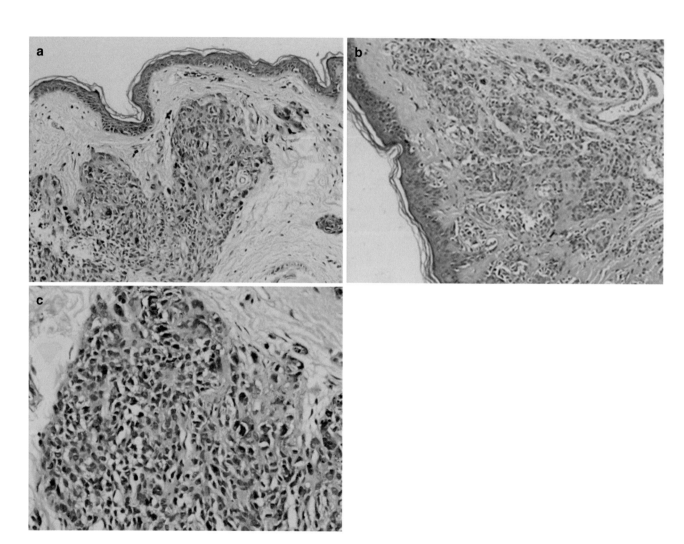

Fig. 1.43 (**a**) Melanocytic naevi: Clusters of melanocytes in the upper dermis. The cells show mild nuclear pleomorphism. (**b**) Melanocytic naevi: Nests of melanocytes in the dermis extending to papillary der-mis. (**c**) Melanocytic naevi: The cells have moderate cytoplasm containing melanin pigment. The nuclei show mild nuclear pleomorphism

Melanoma

Image gallery: Fig. 1.44a–c.

Definition: This is the malignant tumour arising from the melanocytes.

Clinical features

- Pigmented lesion
- Bleeding
- Pruritus
- Dysuria

Gross features

- Pigmented nodular lesion
- Asymmetric margin
- Irregular outline
- Often ulcerated

Histopathology

- Nest or single cells invading in the deeper dermis
- Large epithelioid cells or spindly looking cells
- Moderate to abundant cytoplasm containing melanin pigment
- Large nuclei with prominent nucleoli

Growth pattern

- Mucosal lentiginous: Both radial and vertical extension of the tumour
- Nodular melanoma: Predominantly vertical extension of the growth
- Superficial spreading melanoma: Tumour mainly extends radially

Key diagnostic features: See Box 1.22.

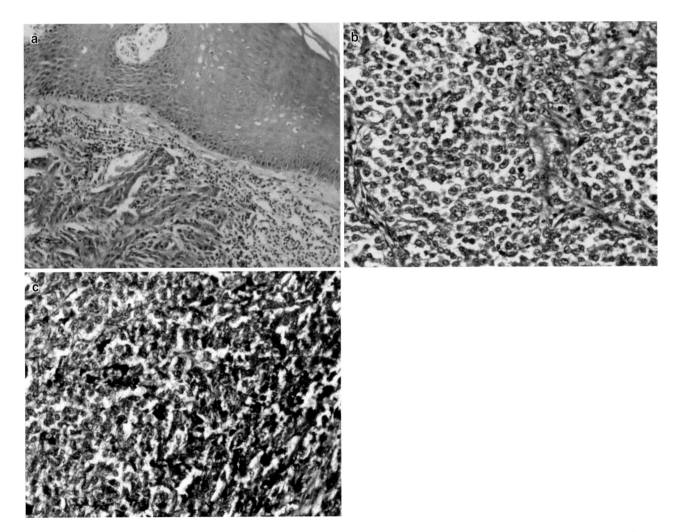

Fig. 1.44 (**a**) Melanoma: The melanin containing tumour cells underneath the epithelium. (**b**) Melanoma: Diffuse sheets of malignant cells. (**c**) Melanoma: The tumour cells have large round nuclei with prominent nucleoli. The cell contains dark brown melanin pigment

Box 1.22 Key Diagnostic Features of Malignant Melanoma

- Nest or single cells within the epidermis
- Maturation of the cells is absent
- The cells have large nuclei with prominent nucleoli having moderate amount of cytoplasm with melanin pigment
- Tumour cells invading in the deeper dermis
- Tumour in the dermis often extends along the nerve and adnexal structure
- Vascular invasion is common
- Tumour cells are positive for Melan A and HMB 45

Differential diagnosis

- Paget disease: Paget cell present, CK 7, CEA positive.
- VIN: Negative for HMB 45 immunostaining.

Prognosis

- Thickness of tumour: Breslow's classification of melanoma invasion
- Depth of invasion: Clark's classification on tumour infiltration
- Adverse prognosis:

   – Breslow's classification T2 and above (more than 1 mm)
   – Vertical growth pattern
   – Ulceration
   – High mitotic activity

Reporting vulvar melanoma: See Box 1.23.

Box 1.23 Reporting Vulvar Melanoma

- Histological subtypes
- Tumour margin involvement
- Invasion: Vascular, perineural
- Mitotic rate per 10 HPF
- The presence of microsatellite lesion
- Depth of invasion: Clark's classification on tumour infiltration
- Tumour thickness by Breslow's classification
- Tumour growth: Radial or vertical
- Any associated precursor lesion

Treatment: Surgical resection with 1 cm tumour free margin.

Lymphoma

Image gallery: Fig. 1.45a, b.

Definition: Lymphoma is the malignant tumour of lymphoid cells.

Clinical features

- Primary lymphoma is very uncommon
- Nodular swelling
- Itching

Gross features

- Nodules
- Ulcerated overlying skin

Histopathology

- The morphology depends on the type of lymphoma
- Diffuse large B cell lymphoma is the most common type
- Others: Follicular lymphoma, marginal zone lymphoma

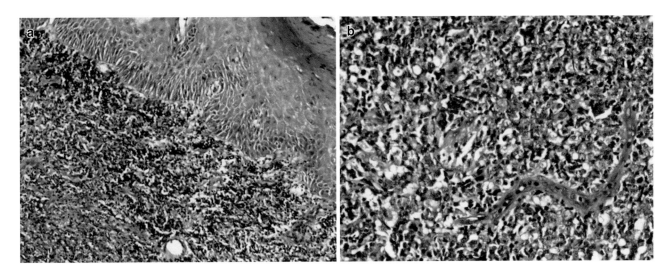

Fig. 1.45 (**a**) Non Hodgkin Lymphoma: Diffuse infiltration of immature lymphoid cells underneath the squamous epithelium in a diffuse large cell lymphoma. (**b**) Non Hodgkin Lymphoma: Discrete lymphoid cells with scanty cytoplasm and round moderately pleomorphic nuclei

Metastatic Tumours

Metastatic Adeno Carcinoma

Image gallery: Fig. 1.46 and 1.47a–f.

Definition: Metastatic adenocarcinoma are developed outside the vulva and secondarily deposited in vulva.

Primary sites

- Cervix
- Breast
- Gastrointestinal tract

Histopathology

- Morphology resembles the primary tumour

Miscellaneous lesions

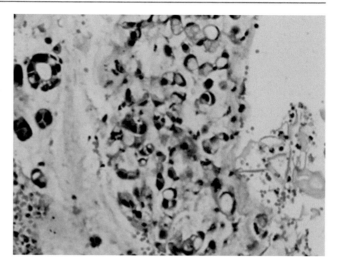

Fig. 1.46 Metastatic adeno carcinoma: Metastatic signet ring cell carcinoma in the vulva from carcinoma of the stomach

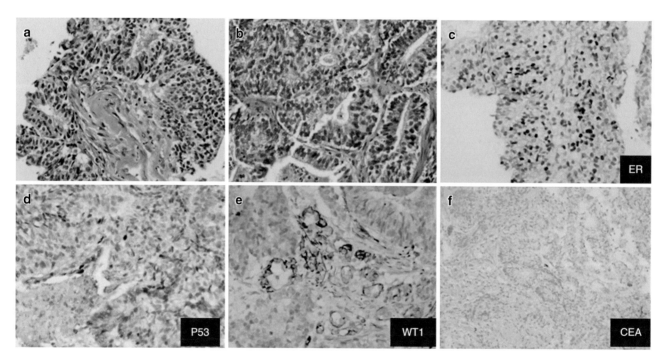

Fig. 1.47 (**a–f**) Metastatic uterine adenocarcinoma in vulva showing strong nuclear positivity of ER and negative for p53, WT 1 and CEA

Endometriosis

Image gallery: Fig. 1.48a, b.

Clinical features

- Near episiotomy wound
- Reddish nodule
- Enlarged and decrease in relation to menstruation

Histopathology

- Endometrial glands
- Stroma
- Evidence of old haemorrhage like pigment laden macrophages

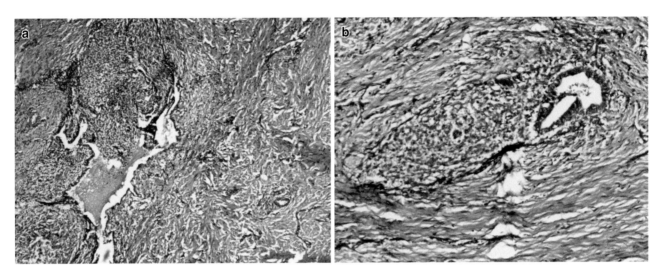

Fig. 1.48 (**a**) Endometriosis of vulva: Endometrial glands and stroma in the deeper dermis of vulva. (**b**) Endometriosis of vulva: Higher magnification shows the endometrial glands embedded in the endometrial stroma

Ectopic Breast

Image gallery: Fig. 1.49.

Clinical features

- Diffuse enlargement
- Prominent at the time of pregnancy

Histopathology

- Benign ductal elements and stromal tissue

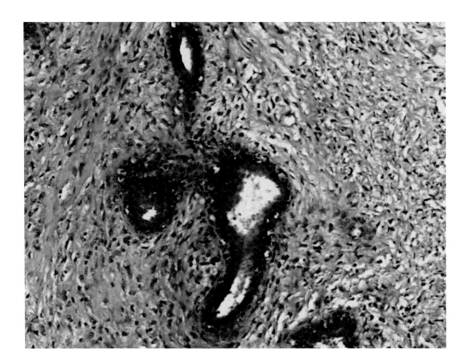

Fig. 1.49 Ectopic breast: Normal looking breast tissue in the vulva

Reference

1. Kurman RJ, Carcangiu ML, Herrington S, Young RH. Tumours of vulva. In: WHO classification of tumours of female genital reproductive organs. 4th ed. Lyon: International Agency for Research on Cancer; 2014.

Suggested Reading

Akhyani M, Chams-Davatchi C, Naraghi Z, Daneshpazhooh M, Toosi S, Asgari M, Malekhami F. Cervicovaginal involvement in pemphigus vulgaris: a clinical study of 77 cases. Br J Dermatol. 2008;158(3):478–82.

Alkatout I, Schubert M, Garbrecht N, Weigel MT, Jonat W, Mundhenke C, Günther V. Vulvar cancer: epidemiology, clinical presentation, and management options. Int J Womens Health. 2015;7:305–13.

Allbritton JI. Vulvar neoplasms, benign and malignant. Obstet Gynecol Clin N Am. 2017;44(3):339–52.

Barret M, de Parades V, Battistella M, Sokol H, Lemarchand N, Marteau P. Crohn's disease of the vulva. J Crohns Colitis. 2014;8(7):563–70.

Breslow A. Thickness, cross-sectional areas and depth of invasion in the prognosis of cutaneous melanoma. Ann Surg. 1970;172:902–6.

Carter J, Elliott P, Russell P. Bilateral fibroepithelial polypi of labium minus with atypical stromal cells. Pathology. 1992;24:37–9.

de Deus JM, Focchi J, Stávale JN, de Lima GR. Histologic and biomolecular aspects of papillomatosis of the vulvar vestibule in relation to human papillomavirus. Obstet Gynecol. 1995;86(5):758–63.

Del Pino M, Rodriguez-Carunchio L, Ordi J. Pathways of vulvar intraepithelial neoplasia and squamous cell carcinoma. Histopathology. 2013;62(1):161–75.

Epstein WL. Molluscum contagiosum. Semin Dermatol. 1992;11:184–9.

Feakins RM, Lowe DG. Basal cell carcinoma of the vulva: a clinicopathologic study of 45 cases. Int J Gynecol Pathol. 1997;16:319–24.

Fetsch JF, Laskin WB, Lefkowitz M, et al. Aggressive angiomyxoma: a clinicopathologic study of 29 female patients. Cancer. 1996;78:79–90.

Friedrich EG Jr, Wilkinson EJ. Mucous cysts of the vulvar vestibule. Obstet Gynecol. 1973;42:407–14.

Galloway DA, McDougall JK. Alterations in the cellular phenotype induced by herpes simplex viruses. J Med Virol. 1990;31(1):36–42.

Guerrero A, Venkatesan A. Inflammatory vulvar dermatoses. Clin Obstet Gynecol. 2015;58(3):464–75.

Haefner HK, Tate JE, McLachlin CM, Crum CP. Vulvar intraepithelial neoplasia: age, morphological phenotype, papillomavirus DNA, and coexisting invasive carcinoma. Hum Pathol. 1995;26(2):147–54.

Heller DS. Benign Tumours and tumour-like lesions of the vulva. Clin Obstet Gynecol. 2015;58(3):526–35.

Hoogendam JP, Smink M. Gartner's duct cyst. N Engl J Med. 2017;376(14):e27.

Hsu ST, Wang RC, Lu CH, Ke YM, Chen YT, Chou MM, Ho ES. Report of two cases of adenoid cystic carcinoma of Bartholin's gland and review of literature. Taiwan J Obstet Gynecol. 2013;52(1):113–6.

Huff SC, Weston WL, Tonnesen MG. Erythema multiforme: a critical review of characteristics, diagnostic criteria, and causes. J Am Acad Dermatol. 1983;8:763–75.

Irvin PW, Legallo RL, Stoler MH, Rice LW, Taylor PT Jr, Andersen WA. Vulvar melanoma: a retrospective analysis and literature review. Gynecol Oncol. 2001;83:457–65.

Kapila S, Bradford J, Fischer G. Vulvar psoriasis in adults and children: a clinical audit of 194 cases and review of the literature. J Low Genit Tract Dis. 2012;16(4):364–71.

Katz Z, Goldchmit R, Blickstein I. Post-traumatic vulvar endometriosis. Eur J Pediatr Surg. 1996;6(4):241–2.

Khandpur S, Verma P. Bullous pemphigoid. Indian J Dermatol Venereol Leprol. 2011;77(4):450–5.

Kondi-Pafiti A, Grapsa D, Papakonstantinou K, Kairi-Vassilatou E, Xasiakos D. Vaginal cysts: a common pathologic entity revisited. Clin Exp Obstet Gynecol. 2008;35(1):41–4.

Kurman RJ, Carcangiu ML, Herrington S, Young RH: Tumours of vulva. WHO classification of tumours of female genital reproductive organs. 4th ed. International agency for research on Cancer, Lyon; 2014.

Lam C, Funaro D. Extramammary Paget's disease: summary of current knowledge. Dermatol Clin. 2010;28(4):807–26.

Lee S, Nodit L. Phyllodes tumour of vulva: a brief diagnostic review. Arch Pathol Lab Med. 2014;138(11):1546–50.

Lehtinen M, Hakama M, Aaran RK, Aromaa A, Knekt P, Leinikki P, Maatela J, Peto R, Teppo L. Herpes simplex virus type 2 infection and cervical cancer: a prospective study of 12 years of follow-up in Finland. Cancer Causes Control. 1992;3:333–8.

Lewis FM. Vulval lichen planus. Br J Dermatol. 1998;138(4):569–75.

Liu G, Li Q, Shang X, Qi Z, Han C, Wang Y, Xue F. Verrucous carcinoma of the vulva: a 20 year retrospective study and literature review. J Low Genit Tract Dis. 2016;20(1):114–8.

Malik M, Ahmed AR. Involvement of the female genital tract in pemphigus vulgaris. Obstet Gynecol. 2005;106(5 Pt 1):1005–1.

Marzano DA, Haefner HK. The bartholin gland cyst: past, present, and future. J Low Genit Tract Dis. 2004;8(3):195–204.

Mucitelli DR, Charles EZ, Kraus FT. Vulvovaginal polyps. Histologic appearance, ultrastructure, immunocytochemical characteristics, and clinicopathologiccorrelations. Int J Gynecol Pathol. 1990;9:20–40.

Nielsen GP, Rosenberg AE, Koerner FC, et al. Smooth-muscle tumours of the vulva. A clinicopathological study of 25 cases and review of the literature. Am J Surg Pathol. 1996;20:779–93.

Nielsen GP, Young RH. Mesenchymal tumours and tumour-like lesions of the female genital tract: a selective review with emphasis on recently described entities. Int J Gynecol Pathol. 2001;20(2):105–27.

Nucci MR, Fletcher CD. Vulvovaginal soft tissue tumours: update and review. Histopathology. 2000;36:97–108.

O'Mahony C. Genital warts: current and future management options. Am J Clin Dermatol. 2005;6:239–43.

Oi RH, Munn R. Mucous cysts of the vulvar vestibule. Hum Pathol. 1982;13(6):584–6.

Özbudak IH, Akkaya H, Akkaya B, Erdoğan G, Peşterelı HE, Karavelı FŞ. Phyllodes tumour of the vulva: report of two cases. Turk Patoloji Derg. 2013;29(1):73–6.

Pincus SH. Vulvar dermatoses and pruritus vulvae. Dermatol Clin. 1992;10(2):297–308.

Pirog EC. Pathology of vulvar neoplasms. Surg Pathol Clin. 2011;4(1):87–111.

Ragnarsson-Olding BK, Nilsson BR, Kanter-Lewensohn LR, et al. Malignant melanoma of the vulva in a nationwide, 25–year study of 219 Swedish females: predictors of survival. Cancer (Phila). 1999;86:1285–93.

Raspagliesi F, Ditto A, Paladini D, et al. Prognostic indicators in melanoma of the vulva. Ann Surg Oncol. 2000;7(10):738–42.

Rorat E, Wallach RC. Mixed tumours of the vulva: clinical outcome and pathology. Int J Gynecol Pathol. 1984;3:323–8.

Rufforny I, Wilkinson EJ, Liu C, Zhu H, Buteral M, Massoll NA. Human papillomavirus infection and p16(INK4a) protein expression in vulvar intraepithelial neoplasia and invasive squamous cell carcinoma. J Low Genit Tract Dis. 2005;9(2):108–13.

Salehin D, Haugk C, William M, Hemmerlein B, Thill M, Diedrich K, Friedrich M. Eur J Gynaecol Oncol. 2012;33(3):306–8. Leiomyosarcoma of the vulva.

Samim F, Auluck A, Zed C, Williams PM. Erythema multiforme: a review of epidemiology, pathogenesis, clinical features, and treatment. Dent Clin N Am. 2013;57(4):583–96.

Scurry J, van der Putte SC, Pyman J, Chetty N, Szabo R. Mammary-like gland adenoma of the vulva: review of 46 cases. Pathology. 2009;41(4):372–8.

Simonetta C, Burns EK, Guo MA. Vulvar dermatoses: a review and update. Mo Med. 2015;112(4):301–7.

Steeper TA, Rosai J. Aggressive angiomyxoma of the female pelvis and perineum: report of nine cases of a distinctive type of gynecologic soft-tissue neoplasm. Am J Surg Pathol. 1983;7:463–75.

van der Linden M, Meeuwis KA, Bulten J, Bosse T, van Poelgeest MI, de Hullu JA. Paget disease of the vulva. Crit Rev. Oncol Hematol. 2016;101:60–74.

van der Putte SCJ. Mammary-like glands of the vulva and their disorders. Int J Gynecol. 1994;13:150–60.

Venkatesan A. Pigmented lesions of the vulva. Dermatol Clin. 2010;28(4):795–805.

Veraldi S, Schianchi-Veraldi R, Marini D. Hidradenoma papilliferum of the vulva: report of a case characterized by unusual clinical behavior. J Dermatol Surg Oncol. 1990;16(7):674–6.

Vettraino IM, Merritt DF. Crohn's disease of the vulva. Am J Dermatopathol. 1995;17:410–3.

Wang Q, Cracchiolo B, Heller DS. Lymphoma presenting as a mass of the vulva: report of a case of a rare vulvar neoplasm not treated by surgery. J Low Genit Tract Dis. 2017;21(2):e26–7.

Woida FM, Ribeiro-Silva A. Adenoid cystic carcinoma of the Bartholin gland: an overview. Arch Pathol Lab Med. 2007;131(5):796–8.

Yang EJ, Kong CS, Longacre TA. Vulvar and anal intraepithelial Neoplasia: terminology, diagnosis, and ancillary studies. Adv Anat Pathol. 2017;24(3):136–50.

Pathology of Vagina

2

Classification of tumours of vagina by World Health Organization is highlighted in Fig. 2.1a, b [1].

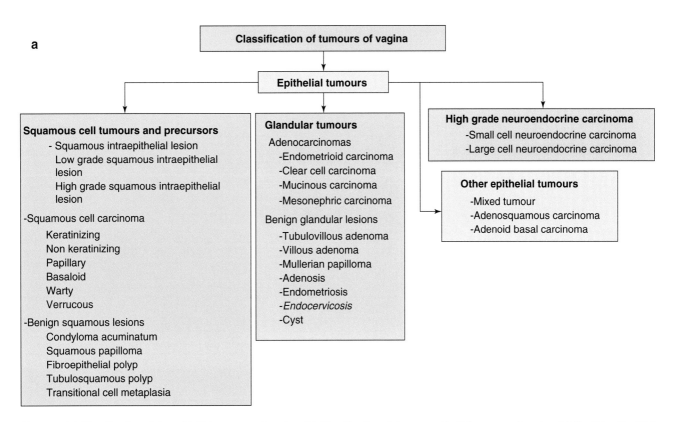

Fig. 2.1 (**a**) Classification of the epithelial tumours of vagina. (**b**) Classification of the non-epithelial tumours of vagina. (**c**) Candida: Candidal pseudohyphae and spore. (**d**) Candida: Slender and long pseudohyphae

© Springer Nature Singapore Pte Ltd. 2019
P. Dey, *Color Atlas of Female Genital Tract Pathology*, https://doi.org/10.1007/978-981-13-1029-4_2

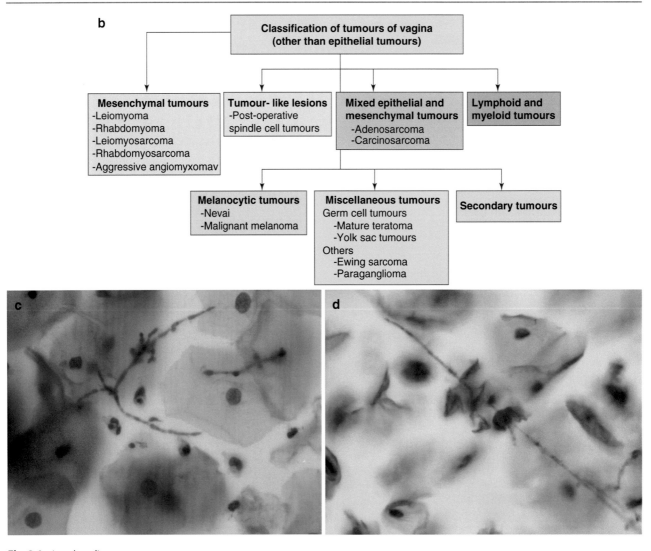

Fig. 2.1 (continued)

Infectious Diseases

Candida

Image galley: Fig. 2.1c, d.
Organisms

- Candida albicans (the most common organism), *Candida glabrata, Candida tropicalis, Candida parapsilosis*

Clinical features

- Usually women with reproductive age period
- Repeated episodes of infection
- Erythema
- Pruritus
- Dysuria
- Vaginal discharge

Predisposing factors

- Diabetes mellitus
- Use of steroid, oral contraceptives, antibiotic
- Immunosuppressive conditions

Cytology and histopathology

- Histopathological examination is rarely done in candida infection
- Histopathology: Hyperkeratotic epithelium with underlying chronic inflammation
- Cytology: fungal pseudohyphae, spores

Treatment: Topical antifungal agent.

Trichomonas Vaginalis

Image galley: Fig. 2.2a, b.
   Causative organism: Trichomonas vaginalis.
   Transmission: Always sexually transmitted.
   Clinical features

- Pruritus
- Dyspareunia
- Purulent vaginal discharge, yellowish green in colour
- Vagina and cervix: erythematous particularly cervix is fiery red known as "Strawberry cervix"

Cytology
Papanicolaou's smear of cervical smear shows:

- Pear shaped organism with pale nuclei
- Diameter 10 μm (approximately)

- Polar flagella
- Necrotic debris in the background

Histopathology

- Not suitable to identify the organism
- The biopsy shows epithelial hyperplasia, necrosis, acute inflammatory cells and organisms are not identified

Treatment

- Metronidazole
- Treatment of the male partner

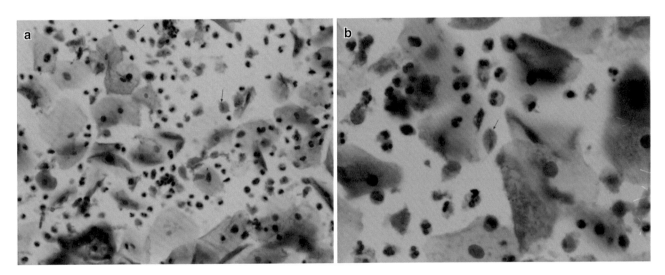

Fig. 2.2 (**a**) Trichomonas vaginalis: Abundant trichomonas vaginalis in the smear (see red arrows). (**b**) Trichomonas vaginalis: Pear shaped organisms are highlighted in higher magnification (see red arrow)

Bacterial Vaginosis

Image galley: Fig. 2.3a, b.
Synonyms:

- Nonspecific vaginitis, Gardnerella vaginitis

Causative organisms

- Gardnerella vaginalis, Prevotella bivia, Mobiluncus mulieris, Mycoplasma hominis, Bacteroides, Peptostreptococcus

Clinical features

- Foul smelling vaginal discharge
- Fishy smell
- Pruritus

Cytology

- Characteristic clue cells: Large cells with dot like bacilli
- Inflammatory changes in the cells may or may not be present

Diagnostic check points

- Clue cells in the cervical smear
- Foul smelling thin discharge
- Acidic pH of the discharge (4.5)
- Fishy smelling discharge if the discharge is made alkaline

Treatment

- Metronidazole
- Topical clindamycin application

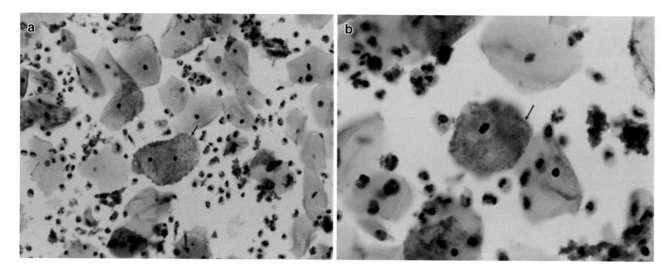

Fig. 2.3 (**a**) Bacterial vaginosis: Smear shows many clue cells (see arrow). (**b**) Bacterial vaginosis: Cells with many dot shaped bacilli in the cytoplasm (see arrow)

Actinomycosis

Image galley: Fig. 2.4.
Causative organisms:

- Actinomyces israelii, Actinomyces bovis, and Actinomyces naeslundii
- Gram positive filamentous bacteria

Clinical features

- Foul smelling vaginal discharge

Common sources

- Intra uterine contraceptive
- Pessaries
- Forgotten tampons

Cytology

- Clumps of bacteria radiating as filamentous structure from the central core
- Cotton ball or "wooly body" look
- Filamentous bacteria with acute angle delicate branching

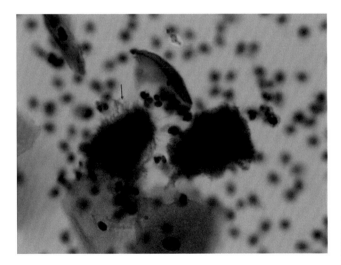

Fig. 2.4 Actinomycosis: Clusters of filamentous organisms (see *arrow*)

Benign Miscellaneous Lesions of Vagina

Vaginal Prolapse

Image galley: Fig. 2.5a, b.
Cause

- Multiple pregnancies may cause reduced support by the ligaments of vagina

Clinical features

- Sensation of fullness of the lower abdomen
- Low backache
- Vaginal discharge

Histopathology

- Squamous epithelium shows
  - Hyperkeratosis
  - Acanthosis
  - Parakeratosis

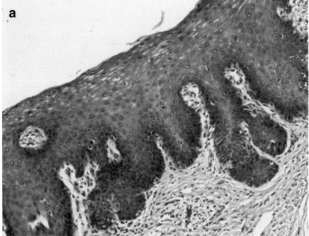

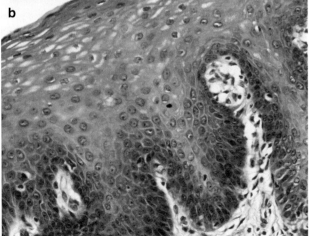

Fig. 2.5 (**a**) Vaginal prolapse: Hyperplastic squamous epithelium. (**b**) Vaginal prolapse: Higher magnification shows acanthosis

Atrophic Vaginitis

Image gallery: Fig. 2.6.
Common occurrence

- Post-menopausal woman due to loss of estrogenic support
- Postpartum period

Clinical features

- Dry vagina
- Pain in the vulva
- Itching

Histopathology

- Thin epithelial layer: only 4–5 cells layer
- No glycogen in the epithelial cells
- Occasionally ulcerated epithelial layer
- Chronic inflammation in the stroma

Differential diagnosis

- Vaginal intraepithelial neoplasia (VAIN): Rarely inflammation may cause atypia in the epithelial cells mimicking VAIN.

Treatment

- Hormone replacement therapy
- Local estrogenic hormone as tablet or cream

Fallopian Tube Prolapse

Image galley: Fig. 2.7a–c.
Common occurrence

- After hysterectomy when the tube is placed at the apex of the vagina

Clinical features

- Pain in abdomen
- Vaginal bleeding
- Red nodular mass

Histopathology

- Stroma is richly vascularized
- Oedematous
- Multiple tubules and gland like structures
- Ciliated columnar lining
- Nuclear overlapping of the epithelial cells and multilayering

Differential diagnosis

- Adenocarcinoma:
- Fibroepithelial polyp

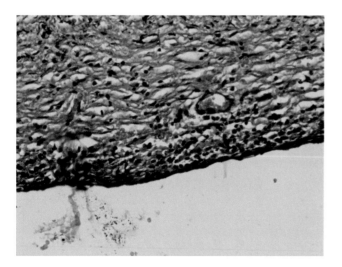

Fig. 2.6 Atrophic vaginitis: Thin epithelial layer

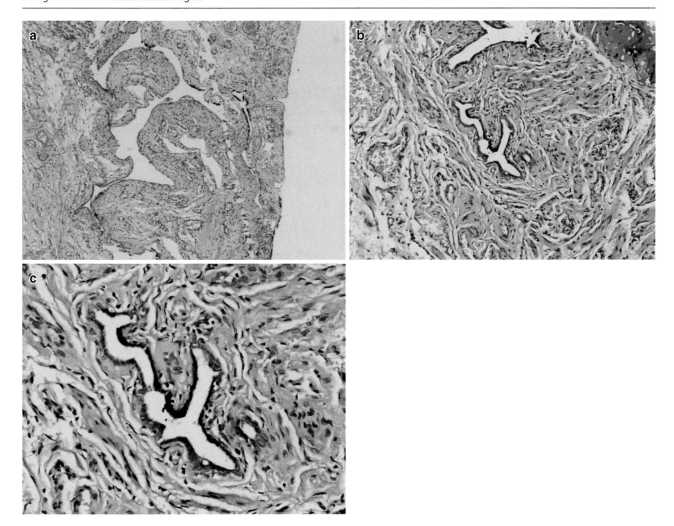

Fig. 2.7 (**a**) Fallopian tube prolapse: Multiple slit like spaces in the wall of vagina. (**b**) Fallopian tube prolapse: Multiple tubular structures. (**c**) Fallopian tube prolapse: The tubular structure is lined by tubal epithelial cells

Vaginal Vault Granulation Tissue

Image galley: Fig. 2.8a, b.

> *Incidence*: Usually seen in post-hysterectomy patient.
> *Gross*: Red, polypoid lesion.
> *Histopathology*: Multiple newly formed blood vessels and inflammatory cells.

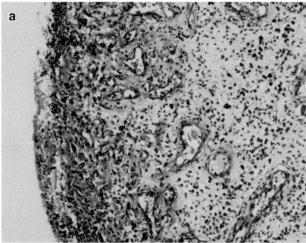

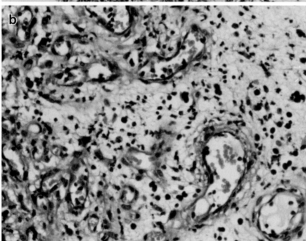

Fig. 2.8 (**a**) Vaginal vault granulation tissue: Ulcerated epithelium with multiple thin walled capillaries. (**b**) Vaginal vault granulation tissue: Abundant capillaries and inflammatory cells

Epithelial Tumours of Vagina

Squamous Intraepithelial Lesions

Low Grade Squamous Intraepithelial Lesion

Image galley: Fig. 2.9.

> *Synonym*: Mild squamous dysplasia, vaginal intraepithelial neoplasia grade 1.
> *Etiology*

- It is caused by HPV infection: Low and high risk group
- Immunosuppression
- History of diethylstilbestrol therapy

Clinical feature

- Asymptomatic
- Usually multifocal and multicentric
- Visible after application of 3.5% acetic acid or Lugol's iodine solution

Histopathology

- Mild nuclear pleomorphism of the nuclei of the squamous cells of the lower third of the epithelium
- Koilocytotic changes in the superficial cells

Prognosis

- Mostly regresses
- May progress when it is associated with high risk HPV

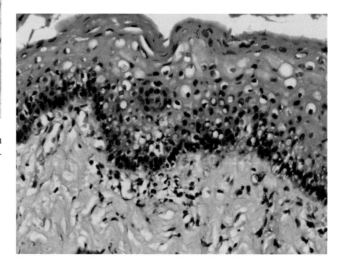

Fig. 2.9 Low grade squamous intraepithelial lesion: Mild nuclear pleomorphism of the nuclei of the squamous cells of the lower third of the epithelium

High Grade Squamous Intraepithelial Lesion

Image galley: Fig. 2.10a–d.
Synonym

- Moderate squamous dysplasia, Severe squamous dysplasia vaginal intraepithelial neoplasia grade 2, vaginal intraepithelial neoplasia grade 3,

Clinical feature

- Asymptomatic
- Usually multifocal and multicentric
- Visible after application of 3.5% acetic acid or Lugol's iodine solution
- Location: upper one third of vagina
- Often coexists with cervical intraepithelial neoplasia

Histopathology

- Cells show loss of polarity in the lower two third to full thickness of the squamous epithelium
- Moderate nuclear pleomorphism
- Hyperchromatic nuclei with high nucleocytoplasmic ratio
- Absence of maturation

Ancillary studies

- VAIN 1: Ki 67 positive basal cells
- VAIN 2/3: Ki 67 positive cells throughout the epithelium

Diagnostic key features: See Box 2.1.

Box 2.1 Diagnostic Key Features of Vaginal Intraepithelial Neoplasia

Low grade squamous intraepithelial lesion
- The squamous cells of the lower third of the epithelium involved
- Mild nuclear atypia
- Koilocytosis
- Ki 67 positivity in basal layer of cells

High grade squamous intraepithelial lesion
- The lower two third to full thickness of the squamous epithelium involved
- Moderate nuclear atypia
- Ki 67 positive cells throughout the epithelium

Prognosis

- Risk of progression to invasive carcinoma if untreated
- Chance of progression is more in multifocal lesion

Management

- Topical 5-Fluoruracil application
- Cryosurgery
- Loop electroexcision
- Laser therapy

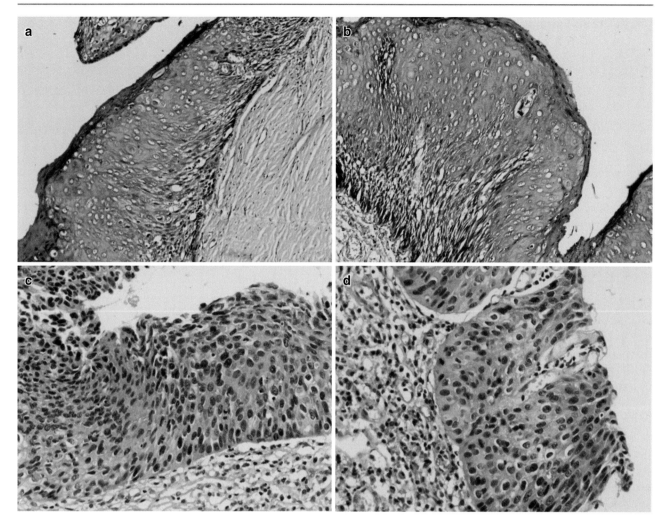

Fig. 2.10 (**a**) High grade squamous intraepithelial lesion: Loss of polarity of the epithelial cells. (**b**) High grade squamous intraepithelial lesion: Nuclei of the cells are enlarged and pleomorphic. (**c**) High grade squamous intraepithelial lesion: Pleomorphic and hyperchromatic cells. (**d**) High grade squamous intraepithelial lesion: Full thickness involvement by the dysplastic cells

Squamous Cell Carcinoma

Image galley: Fig. 2.11a–e.
Epidemiology

- Uncommon tumour
- Consists of 1% of all gynaecological cancer
- Median age 68 year

Etiology

- High risk HPV associated with HSIL
- HPV negative cases may occur

Risk factors

- HPV infection
- Poor socioeconomic condition
- Pelvic radiation
- Immunosuppression

Clinical features

- Vaginal bleeding
- Vaginal discharge
- Dyspareunia

Gross features

- Exophytic mass
- Ulcerated
- At times endophytic and constrictive annular lesion

Histopathology
Keratinizing squamous cell carcinoma

- Multiple keratin pearls
- Oval to polyhedral cells with intracellular keratinization
- Moderate nuclear pleomorphism

Non-Keratinizing squamous cell carcinoma

- No keratin pearls
- Nests of tumour cells
- Polyhedral cells with central pleomorphic nuclei

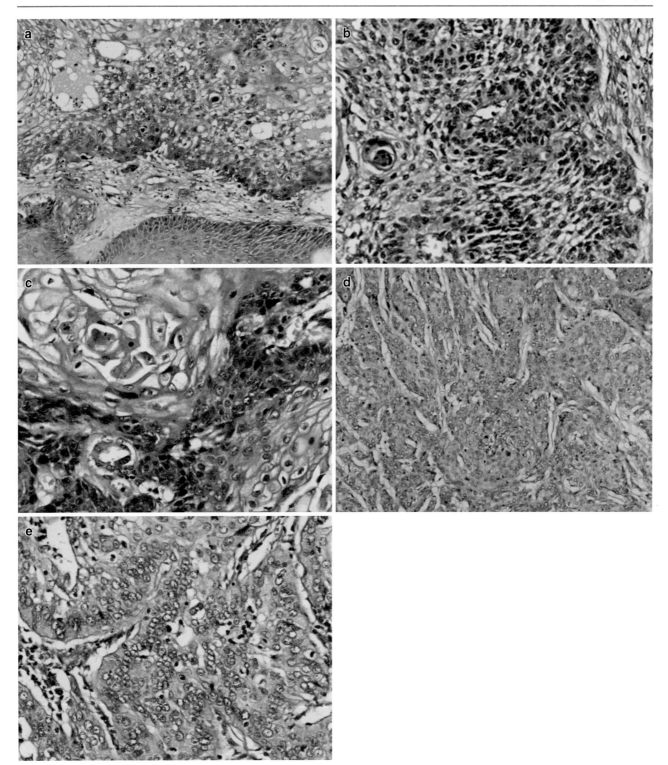

Fig. 2.11 (**a**) Keratinizing squamous cell carcinoma: Diffuse sheet of malignant squamous cells. (**b**) Keratinizing squamous cell carcinoma: Polyhedral cells with central nuclei. Cell to cell junction is present. (**c**) Keratinizing squamous cell carcinoma: Keratin pearl adjacent to malignant cells. (**d**) Non keratinizing squamous cell carcinoma: Multiple nests of tumour cells. (**e**) Non keratinizing squamous cell carcinoma: Cells with polyhedral shape. Nuclei are enlarged and pleomorphic

Other Variants of Squamous Cell Carcinoma

Verrucous Carcinoma

Image galley: Fig. 2.12a, b.
Incidence

- Rare tumour of the vagina

Synonyms

- Giant condyloma acuminatum, well differentiated squamous cell carcinoma, squamous papillomatosis

Histopathology

- Surface epithelium shows hyperkeratosis and acanthosis

- Characteristic broad based bull dozer like pushing margin of the tumour cells
- Relatively monomorphic tumour cell population

Differential diagnosis

- Large condyloma: Koilocytotic changes

Prognosis and treatment

- Frequent recurrence is common
- Wide local resection or radical surgery
- Radiation is prohibited as it may transform the tumour into traditional squamous cell carcinoma

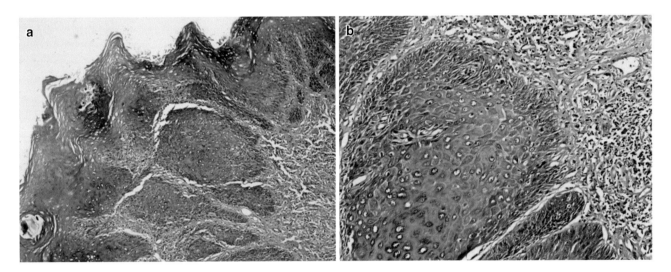

Fig. 2.12 (**a**) Verrucous carcinoma: Surface epithelium shows hyperkeratosis and acanthosis with bulbous epithelial projection. (**b**) Verrucous carcinoma: broad based bull dozer like pushing margin of the tumour cells. Note minimal atypia of the cells

Basaloid Carcinoma

Image galley: Fig. 2.13a.
Incidence

- Uncommon in vagina

Histopathology

- Palisading arrangement of basal cells invading the subepithelial tissue
- Relatively monomorphic cells with mild elongated nuclei

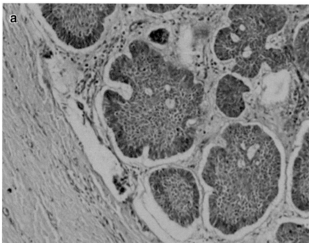

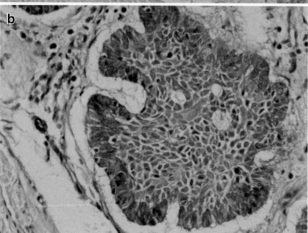

Fig. 2.13 (**a**) Basaloid carcinoma: Palisading arrangement of basal cells invading the subepithelial tissue. (**b**) Basaloid carcinoma: Higher magnification highlights the palisading arrangement of cells. Note the cells are monomorphic in appearance

Papillary Squamotransitional Carcinoma

Image galley: Fig. 2.14.
Incidence

- Rare occurrence

Synonym

- Transitional cell carcinoma, papillary squamous cell carcinoma, mixed squamous and transitional cell carcinoma

Gross features

- Papillary growth

Histopathology

- Papillae with central fibrovascular core
- Lining cells look like transitional cells: Oval to elongated nuclei
- Nuclear grooves present

Immunostaining

- CK 7 positive
- CK 20 negative

Differential diagnosis

- Transitional cell carcinoma of urinary bladder: Typically positive for both CK 7 and CK 20

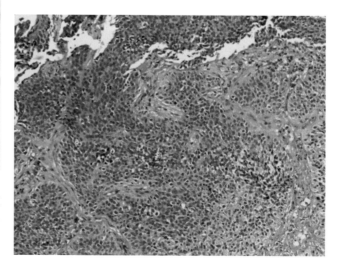

Fig. 2.14 Papillary Squamotransitional carcinoma: Papillary arrangement of cells. Look the transitional appearance of the cells

Benign Squamous Lesions

Condyloma Accuminatum

Image galley: Fig. 2.15a–c.
Synonym: Vaginal wart.
Etiology

- HPV 6/11

Gross feature

- Papillary growth

Histopathology

- Multiple papillae
- Hyperkeratosis, acanthosis and parakeratosis
- Koilocytotic cells present

Prognosis and treatment

- Spontaneous regression
- Surgical resection

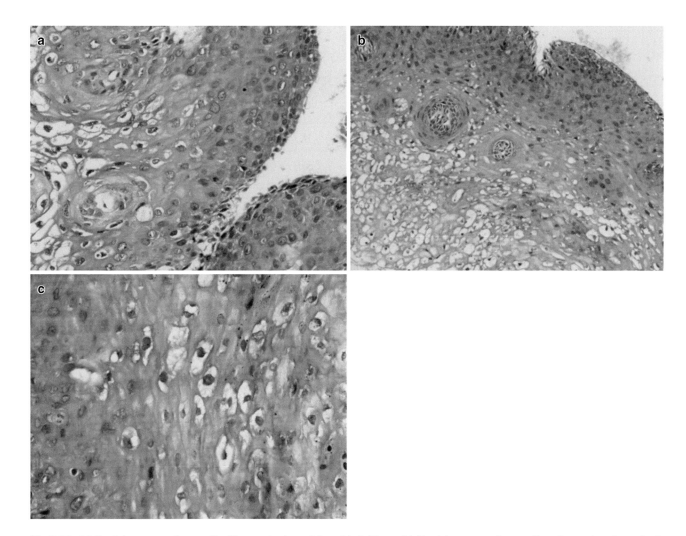

Fig. 2.15 (**a**) Condyloma accuminatum: Papillary projections of the epithelial layer. (**b**) Condyloma accuminatum: Hyperkeratosis and acanthosis of the lining epithelium. (**c**) Condyloma accuminatum: Koilocytotic changes in the epithelium

Squamous Papilloma

Image galley: Fig. 2.16a, b.
Synonym

- Squamous papillomatosis

Clinical features

- Itching
- Vaginal discharge

Gross feature

- Papillary growth: Single or multiple

Histopathology

- Multiple papillary projections
- Central fibrovascular core
- Parakeratosis and acanthosis

Differential diagnosis

- Condyloma accuminatum: Characterized by koilocytosis and mild nuclear atypia

Treatment

- Excision

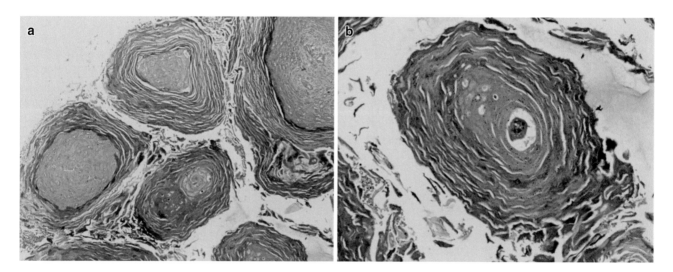

Fig. 2.16 (**a**) Squamous papilloma: Multiple papillary projections with central fibrovascular core. (**b**) Squamous papilloma: the epithelium shows parakeratosis and acanthosis. The cells do not show any atypia or koilocytotic changes

Fibroepithelial Polyp

Image gallery: Fig. 2.17a, b.
Synonym

- Mesodermal stromal polyp

Gross

- Single polypoid lesion
- No stalk

Histopathology

- Polyp covered with squamous epithelium
- Stroma contains fibroblasts
- Occasional multinucleated cells

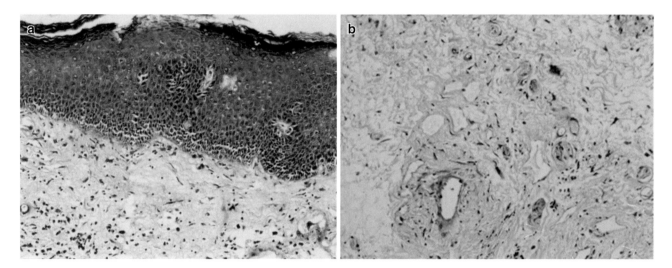

Fig. 2.17 (**a**) Fibroepithelial polyp: The polyp is covered with squamous epithelium. (**b**) Fibroepithelial polyp: The stroma shows thin walled vessels and fibroblasts

Glandular Tumours

Clear Cell Adenocarcinoma

Image gallery: Fig. 2.18a–c.
Synonym

- Mesonephroma

Risk factors

- Commonly associated with maternal exposure of diethylstilbestrol (DES)

Clinical features

- Peak age: 19 years
- Common complaints: Vaginal bleeding, dyspareunia
- Location: 2/3rd of the cases in anterior wall of the upper third part of vagina and 1/3rd cases in cervix

Gross

- Polypoid or ulcerated growth

Histopathology

- Mainly tubulocystic pattern, occasionally solid and papillary pattern
- Cells with clear cytoplasm and central nuclei
- Pleomorphic nuclei with prominent nucleoli
- Hobnail cells
- Many mitotic figures

Immunohistochemistry

- Positive: CK 7, CD 15

Molecular genetics

- High frequency of microsatellite instability

Key diagnostic features: Box 2.2.

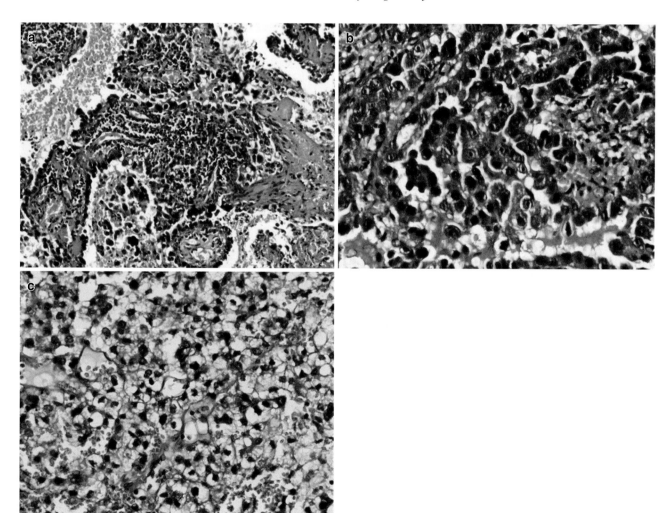

Fig. 2.18 (**a**) Clear cell adenocarcinoma. Multiple papillary structures. (**b**) Clear cell adenocarcinoma: Papillae with fibrovascular core. (**c**) Clear cell adenocarcinoma: Diffuse sheet of cells. Individual cells have abundant clear cytoplasm and central moderately pleomorphic nuclei

> **Box 2.2 Key Diagnostic Features of Clear Cell Adenocarcinoma**
> - History of diethylstilbestrol exposure
> - Solid and tubulocystic pattern
> - Cells with clear cytoplasm and central moderately pleomorphic nuclei
> - PAS positive and diastase sensitive
> - Prominent hobnail appearance
> - Positive for CK 7, CD 15

Differential diagnosis

- Microglandular hyperplasia of cervix: Presence of squamous metaplasia, monomorphic cells

- Metastatic clear cell carcinoma: Sloid sheets of clear cell, no hobnail pattern, typical history of kidney tumour
- Arias Stella reaction: Usually present in pregnant woman, no hobnail cells

Prognosis and treatment

- Frequently the tumour spreads outside the pelvis
- Good prognosis: Five year survival in FIGO stage I tumour is 93%.
- Recurrence may be seen in 1/4th cases

Endometrioid Carcinoma

Image gallery: Fig. 2.19a, b.
Occurrence

- Rare tumour
- May arise from vaginal adenosis
- Associated with vaginal endometriosis

Histopathology

- Morphology resembles uterine endometrioid carcinoma

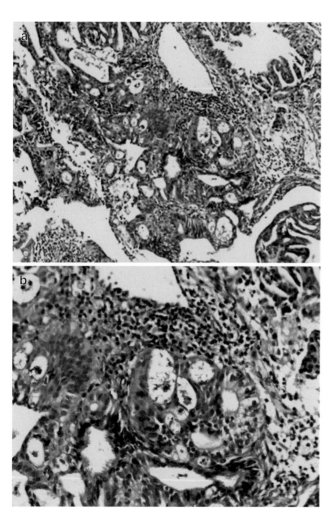

Fig. 2.19 (**a**) Endometrioid carcinoma: Multiple endometrial type of glands. (**b**) Endometrioid carcinoma: The glandular lining cells show moderate nuclear pleomorphism. Foci of squamous differentiation is also seen

Benign Glandular Lesions

Adenosis

Image gallery: Fig. 2.20a, c.
Synonym

- Adenomatosis vaginae

Epidemiology

- Commonly seen in DES exposure cases

Clinical features

- Reddish granular patches in vagina

Histopathology

- Multiple glands underneath the squamous epithelium
- Endocervical type: Lined by mucus secreting columnar cell
- Tubo-endometrial type: Small cuboidal cells often ciliated
- Infrequently the glands are lined by embryonic type small cells

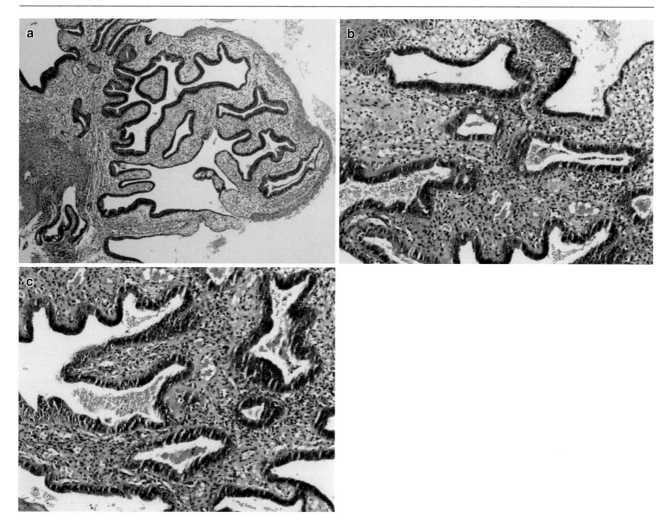

Fig. 2.20 (**a**) Adenosis: Multiple glands underneath the epithelial lining. (**b**) Adenosis: The dilated glands lined by columnar epithelial cells. (**c**) Adenosis: Higher magnification shows tall mucus secreting columnar epithelial lining of the glands

Endometriosis

Image gallery: Fig. 2.21a, b.
Incidence

- Infrequent, only 10% cases of pelvic endometriosis

Mode of occurrence

- Implantation: directly
- Retrograde lymphatic spread
- Metaplasia of the epithelium

Clinical features

- Vaginal bleeding
- Reddish elevated lesion or cystic structure

Histopathology

- Multiple endometrial glands embedded in stroma
- Pigment laden macrophages

Differential diagnosis

- Carcinosarcoma
- Adenosarcoma

Treatment

- Large lesion: Excision
- Small lesion: Laser ablation

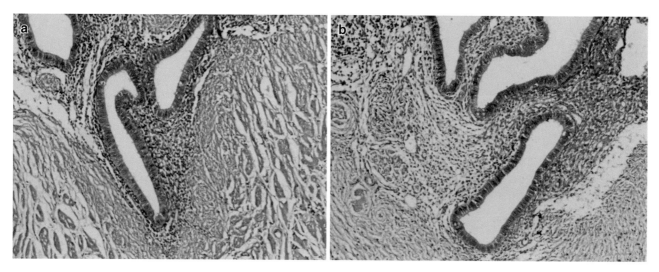

Fig. 2.21 (**a**) Endometriosis: Endometrial glands and stroma in the vaginal wall. (**b**) Endometriosis: Endometrial glands lined by cuboidal cells

Cysts of Vagina

Müllerian Cyst

Image gallery: Fig. 2.22.
Incidence

- The commonest cyst of vagina

Size

- 1–5 cm in diameter

Lining of cyst

- Müllerian duct lining:
  – Endocervical: Mucus secreting columnar
  – Endometrial: Cuboidal
  – Tubal: Ciliated columnar

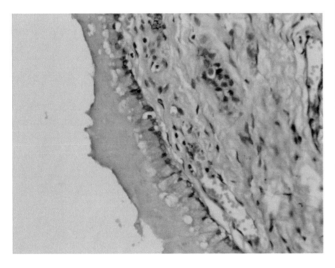

Fig. 2.22 Müllerian cyst: The cyst is lined by mucus secreting columnar epithelial cells

Bartholin Cyst

Image gallery: Fig. 2.23a, b.
Location

- Vestibule

Lining of cyst: Squamous, columnar or transitional epithelium.

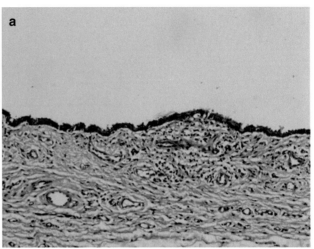

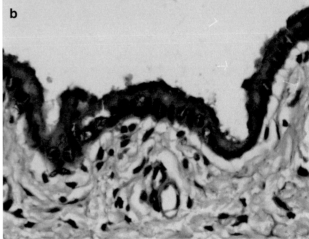

Fig. 2.23 (**a**) Bartholin cyst: The cyst wall is lined by columnar cells. (**b**) Bartholin cyst: The higher magnification shows better morphology of the tall mucus secreting columnar cells

Epithelial Inclusion Cyst of Vagina

Image gallery: Fig. 2.24.
  Incidence: Commonest vaginal cyst.
  Lining of cyst

- Squamous epithelium
- Cyst contains keratin flakes

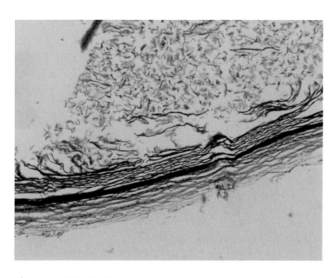

Fig. 2.24 Epithelial inclusion cyst of vagina: The cyst wall is lined by the squamous epithelial cell. The cyst contains keratin flakes

Soft Tissue Tumour

Leiomyoma

Image gallery: Fig. 2.25a, b.
Incidence: The commonest soft tissue tumours of vagina.
Clinical features

- Any age group, commonly around 40 years
- Vaginal pain, dyspareunia

Gross features

- Soft to firm
- 2–4 cm diameter

Histopathology

- Multiple fascicles of spindle cells with blunt ended nuclei

Treatment

- Surgical excision

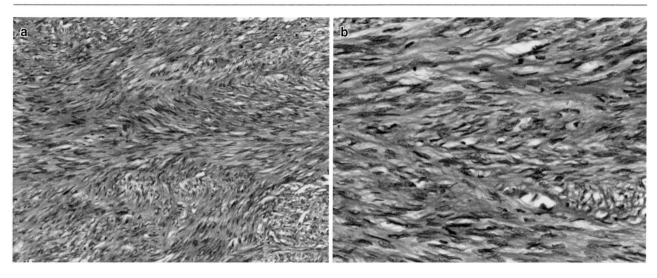

Fig. 2.25 (**a**) Leiomyoma: The cells are arranged in interlacing fascicles. (**b**) Leiomyoma: The cells with oval to spindle shaped nuclei having blunt ends

Leiomyosarcoma

Image gallery: Fig. 2.26a, b.
Occurrence

- The commonest sarcoma of vagina

Clinical features

- Commonest around 47 years
- Vaginal pain and bleeding

Histopathology.
Criteria of malignancy: Three or more of these features

- Size: More than 5 cm in diameter
- Margin: Infiltrating
- Mitosis: More than 5/ 10 high power field
- Atypia: Significant

Immunohistochemistry

- Positive for desmin, h-caldesmon, smooth muscle actin

Prognosis and treatment

- Aggressive tumour: Five year survival rate is 43%
- Surgical resection followed by radiotherapy

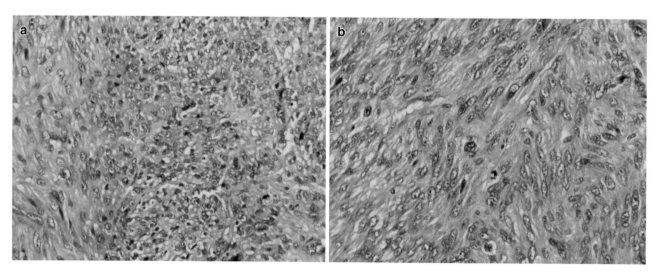

Fig. 2.26 (**a**) Leiomyosarcoma: Oval to spindle cells arranged in short fascicle. (**b**) Leiomyosarcoma: Cells with moderately pleomorphic nuclei showing high mitotic activity

Embryonal Rhabdomyosarcoma

Image gallery: Fig. 2.27a–d.
Synonym

- Sarcoma botryoides

Epidemiology

- Commonest malignant tumour of vagina in infant and child

Clinical features

- Mean age 2 year
- Mass in vagina and vaginal bleeding

Gross features

- Grape like bulky, polyp like mass
- Nodular mass with intact overlying epithelium

Histopathology

- Cambium layer: Thick dense collection of tumour cells underneath the subepithelium
- Small round cells with scanty cytoplasm
- Nuclei have open chromatin and inconspicuous nucleoli
- High mitosis
- Rarely cells with cytoplasmic cross striations present

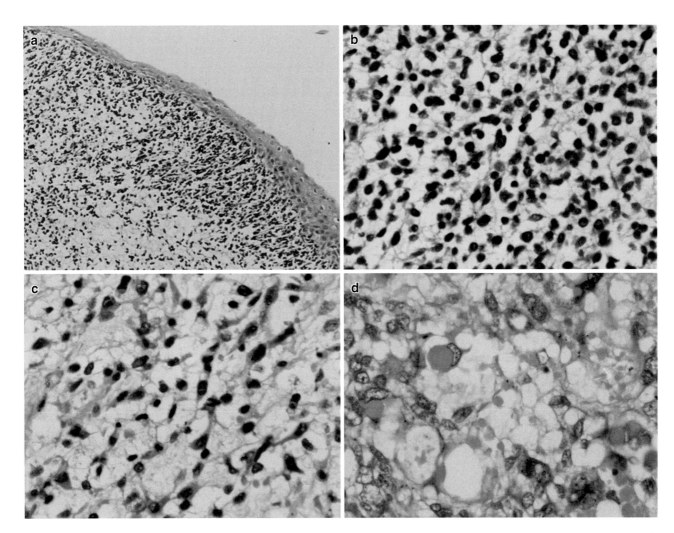

Fig. 2.27 (**a**) Embryonal rhabdomyosarcoma: Dense collection of tumour cells underneath the subepithelium. (**b**) Embryonal rhabdomyosarcoma: Round to oval cells in loose stroma. (**c**) Embryonal rhabdo-myosarcoma: The tumour cells show mildly pleomorphic hyperchromatic nuclei. (**d**) Embryonal rhabdomyosarcoma: Rhabdoid cells showing deep pink cytoplasm and eccentric nuclei

Immunohistochemistry

- Positive for desmin, h-caldesmon, myogenin

Key diagnostic features: Box 2.3.
Differential diagnosis

Box 2.3 Key Diagnostic Features of Embryonal Rhabdomyosarcoma
- The presence of cambium layer of tumour cells: The densely aggregated tumour cells under the epithelium with a gap of loose connective tissue
- Small round cells with scanty cytoplasm and nuclei show open chromatin
- Infrequently cytoplasmic cross striations
- Tumour cells are positive for desmin, h-caldesmon, myogenin

---

- Fibroepithelial polyps: Absent cambium layer
- Rhabdomyomas: Differentiated muscle cells present

Prognosis

- The known prognostic factors are
    - Histology: Alveolar sarcoma has worse prognosis
    - Higher stage
    - Marked atypia
- Five year survival: 90% in botryoides tumour

Treatment: Radical surgery followed by chemotherapy.

Melanoma

Image gallery: Fig. 2.28a–d.
Incidence

- Rare: less than 3% of vaginal tumours

Histogenesis

- Aberrant melanocytes

Clinical features

- Mean age: 60 year
- Vaginal bleeding, mass
- Location: lower 1/3rd of vagina

Gross features

- Nodular or polypoid
- Ulcerated
- Blackish

Histopathology

- Pattern: Sheets, nest, trabeculae
- Junctional activity present

- Cells: oval to elongated spindle shaped
- Moderate to marked nuclear pleomorphism
- Prominent nucleoli
- Intracellular melanin pigment

Immunohistochemistry

- Positive: Melan A, HMB 45, S-100

Differential diagnosis

- Poorly differentiated squamous cell carcinoma
- Nevus
- Metastatic melanoma

Prognosis

- Poor prognosis
- Five year survival rate: 20%

Treatment

- Radical surgery
- Pelvic exenteration if there deep invasion present

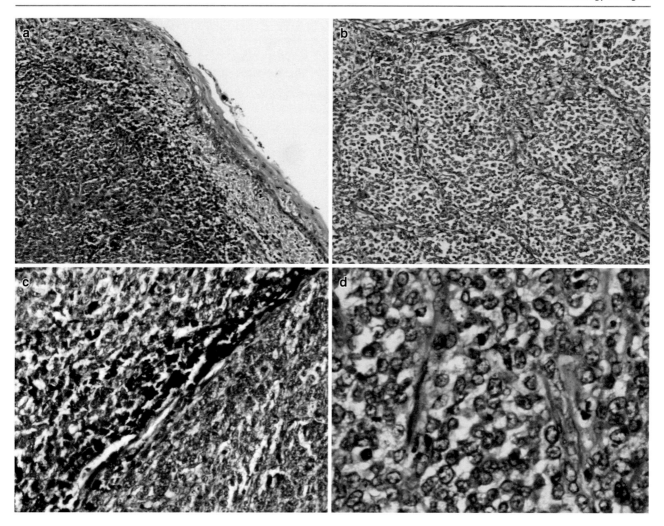

Fig. 2.28 (**a**) Melanoma: Diffuse sheet of tumour cell underneath the epithelium. (**b**) Melanoma: Nests of tumour cells. (**c**) Melanoma: The tumour cells show melanin pigment. (**d**) Melanoma: The individual tumour cells with scanty cytoplasm and large nuclei with prominent nucleoli

Lymphoid Neoplasms

Non-Hodgkin's Lymphoma

Image gallery: Fig. 2.29.
Incidence

- Primary tumour is very rare

Clinical features

- Bleeding, pain and discharge from vagina

Histopathology

- The types of lymphomas are: Diffuse large B cell lymphoma, marzinal zone lymphoma and follicular lymphoma

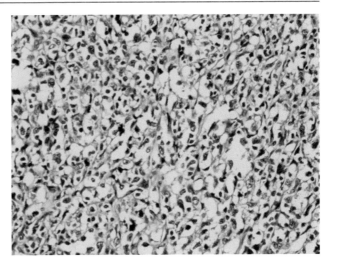

Fig. 2.29 Non-Hodgkin's lymphoma: Discrete lymphoid cells in a case of diffuse large cell lymphoma

Miscellaneous Tumours

Germ Cell Tumours

Endodermal Sinus Tumour
Image gallery: Fig. 2.30a, b.
Incidence: Extremely uncommon.
Histogenesis: Possibly from aberrant germ cells.
Clinical features

- Vaginal bleeding
- Discharge per vagina

Gross features

- Polypoid mass
- 4–10 cm diameter

Histopathology

- Morphology is similar to ovarian endodermal sinus tumour
- Microcystic pattern, papillary structure or solid sheet
- Schiller Duval bodies

Differential diagnosis

- Clear cell carcinoma
- Sarcoma botryoides

Prognosis and treatment

- Aggressive tumours
- Combination chemotherapy: bleomycin, cisplatin, etoposide
- Surgery: Complete or partial vaginectomy along with chemotherapy

Monitoring

- Alpha fetoprotein level in serum

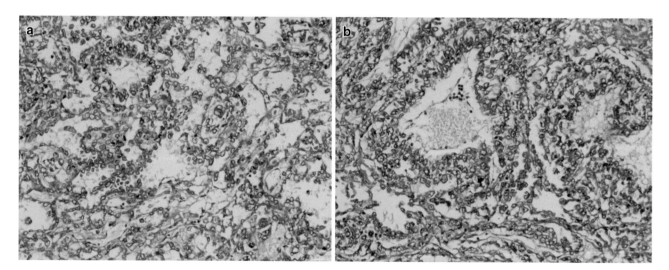

Fig. 2.30 (**a**) Endodermal sinus tumour: Tumour cells are arranged as microcytic spaces. Many pinkish hyaline globules are seen in the background. (**b**) Endodermal sinus tumour: The cystic spaces are lined by tumour cells having large nuclei with prominent nucleoli

Paraganglioma

Image gallery: Fig. 2.31a–d.

Definition: This is a tumour that derives from the neural crest cells of the autonomic paraganglia.

Incidence: Extremely uncommon in vagina.

Clinical features

- Predominantly occurs in adult female
- Patient presents with mass in vagina
- Irregular bleeding per vagina

Gross features

- Well circumscribed
- Grey white

Histopathology

- Small nest or trabecular appearance
- Zellballen pattern: Small nests of cells surrounded by delicate fibrovascular stroma
- Cells have abundant eosinophilic cytoplasm with central round nuclei

Immunohistochemistry

Positive: Chromogranin, synaptophysin, CD56, with surrounding S100 protein–positive.

Prognosis and treatment

- Surgical resection
- Benign in behaviour

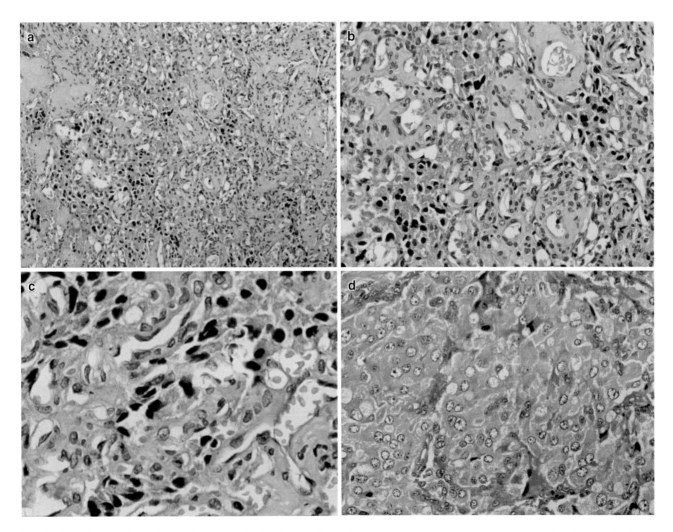

Fig. 2.31 (**a**) Paraganglioma: Nests of tumour cells. (**b**) Paraganglioma: Zellballen pattern is seen. (**c**) Paraganglioma: Small nests of cells are separated by thin walled vessels. (**d**) Paraganglioma: The individual cells show abundant cytoplasm with central large round nuclei

Metastatic Tumours

Metastatic Granulosa Cell Tumour in Vaginal Wall

Image gallery: Fig. 2.32.
Occurrence: Metastatic from the ovary.

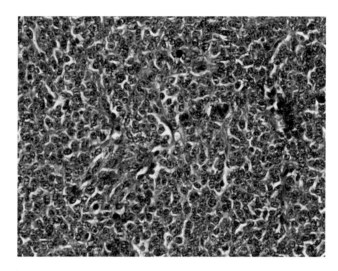

Fig. 2.32 Metastatic granulosa cell tumour in vaginal wall: Diffuse sheet of tumour cells with scanty cytoplasm and single prominent nucleoli

Metastatic Endometrioid Carcinoma

Image gallery: Fig. 2.33.
Occurrence: Metastatic from the endometrium.

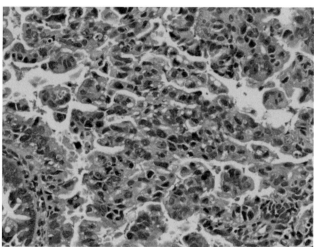

Fig. 2.33 Metastatic endometrioid carcinoma in vaginal wall in a known case of endometrioid carcinoma of uterus

Metastatic Carcinosarcoma

Image gallery: Fig. 2.34a, b.
Occurrence: Metastatic from the uterine corpus.

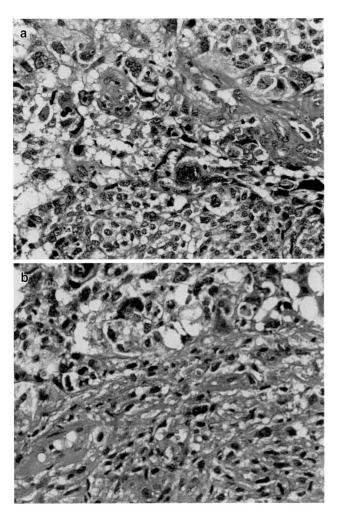

Fig. 2.34 (**a**) Metastatic carcinosarcoma in vaginal wall from a known case of carcinosarcoma of uterus. Both carcinoma and sarcoma elements are present. (**b**) Metastatic carcinosarcoma: The carcinoma cells show moderately vacuolated cytoplasm and pleomorphic round nuclei. The sarcoma elements displaying oval to spindle shaped nuclei

Reference

1. Kurman RJ, Carcangiu ML, Herrington S, Young RH. Tumours of vagina. In: WHO classification of tumours of female genital reproductive organs. 4th ed. Lyon: International Agency for Research on Cancer; 2014.

Suggested Reading

Aho M, Vesterinen E, Meyer B, Purola E, Paavonen J. Natural history of vaginal intraepithelial neoplasia. Cancer. 1991;68(1):195–7.

Cai T, Li Y, Jiang Q, Wang D, Huang Y. Paraganglioma of the vagina: a case report and review of the literature. Onco Targets Ther. 2014;7:965–8.

Chauhan S, Nigam JS, Singh P, Misra V, Thakur B. Endodermal sinus tumour of vagina in infants. Rare Tumours. 2013;5(2):83–4.

Coleman JS, Gaydos CA, Witter F. Trichomonas vaginalis vaginitis in obstetrics and gynecology practice: new concepts and controversies. Obstet Gynecol Surv. 2013;68(1):43–50.

Crowther ME, Lowe DG, Shepherd JH. Verrucous carcinoma of the female genital tract: a review. Obstet Gynecol Surv. 1988;43(5):263–80.

Curtis EM, Pine L. Actinomyces in the vaginas of women with and without intrauterine contraceptive devices. Am J Obstet Gynecol. 1981;140(8):880–4.

Dhanasekharan A, Cherian AG, Emmanuel P, Patel K. Endodermal sinus tumour of the vagina in a child. J Obstet Gynaecol India. 2012;62(Suppl 1):81–2.

Evans DT. Actinomyces israelii in the female genital tract: a review. Genitourin Med. 1993;69(1):54–9.

Gadducci A, Fabrini MG, Lanfredini N, Sergiampietri C. Squamous cell carcinoma of the vagina: natural history, treatment modalities and prognostic factors. Crit Rev. Oncol Hematol. 2015;93(3):211–24.

Guastafierro S, Tedeschi A, Criscuolo C, Celentano M, Cobellis L, Rossiello R, Falcone U. Primary extranodal non-Hodgkin's lymphoma of the vagina: a case report and a review of the literature. Acta Haematol. 2012;128(1):33–8.

Gupta D, Malpica A, Deavers MT, Silva EG. Vaginal melanoma: a clinicopathologic and immunohistochemical study of 26 cases. Am J Surg Pathol. 2002;26(11):1450–7.

Gupta D, Neto AG, Deavers MT, Silva EG, Malpica A. Metastatic melanoma to the vagina: clinicopathologic and immunohistochemical study of three cases and literature review. Int J Gynecol Pathol. 2003;22(2):136–40.

Hilgers RD, Malkasian GD Jr, Soule EH. Embryonal rhabdomyosarcoma (botryoid type) of the vagina. A Clinicopathologic review. Am J Obstet Gynecol. 1970;107(3):484–502.

Hiniker SM, Roux A, Murphy JD, Harris JP, Tran PT, Kapp DS, Kidd EA. Primary squamous cell carcinoma of the vagina: prognostic factors, treatment patterns, and outcomes. Gynecol Oncol. 2013;131(2):380–5.

Hwang JH, Oh MJ, Lee NW, Hur JY, Lee KW, Lee JK. Multiple vaginal mullerian cysts: a case report and review of literature. Arch Gynecol Obstet. 2009;280(1):137–9.

Jentschke M, Hoffmeister V, Soergel P, Hillemanns P. Clinical presentation, treatment and outcome of vaginal intraepithelial neoplasia. Arch Gynecol Obstet. 2016;293(2):415–9.

Khosla D, Patel FD, Kumar R, Gowda KK, Nijhawan R, Sharma SC. Leiomyosarcoma of the vagina: a rare entity with comprehensive review of the literature. Int J Appl Basic Med Res. 2014;4(2):128–30.

Kranl C, Zelger B, Kofler H, Heim K, Sepp N, Fritsch P. Vulval and vaginal adenosis. Br J Dermatol. 1998;139(1):128–31.

Lossick JG, Kent HL. Trichomoniasis: trends in diagnosis and management. Am J Obstet Gynecol. 1991;165:1217–22.

Matias-Guiu X, Lerma E, Prat J. Clear cell tumours of the female genital tract. Semin Diagn Pathol. 1997;14(4):233–9.

Nordqvist SR, Fidler WJ Jr, Woodruff JM, Lewis JL Jr. Clear cell adenocarcinoma of the cervix and vagina. A clinicopathologic study of 21 cases with and without a history of maternal ingestion of estrogens. Cancer. 1976;37(2):858–71.

Ramin SM, Ramin KD, Hemsell DL. Fallopian tube prolapse after hysterectomy. South Med J. 1999;92(10):963–6.

Rose PG, Stoler MH, Abdul-Karim FW. Papillary squamotransitional cell carcinoma of the vagina. Int J Gynecol Pathol. 1998;17(4):372–5.

Shen JG, Chen YX, Xu DY, Feng YF, Tong ZH. Vaginal paraganglioma presenting as a gynecologic mass: case report. Eur J Gynaecol Oncol. 2008;29(2):184–5.

Silverberg SG, Frable WJ. Prolapse of fallopian tube into vaginal vault after hysterectomy. Histopathology, cytopathology, and differential diagnosis. Arch Pathol. 1974;97(2):100–3.

Spiegel CA, Amsel R, Eschenbach D, Schoenknecht F, Holmes KK. Anaerobic bacteria in nonspecific vaginitis. N Engl J Med. 1980;303(11):601–7.

Suh MJ, Park DC. Leiomyosarcoma of the vagina: a case report and review from the literature. J Gynecol Oncol. 2008;19(4):261–4.

Tsokos M, Webber BL, Parham DM, Wesley RA, Miser A, Miser JS, Etcubanas E, Kinsella T, Grayson J, Glatstein E, et al. Rhabdomyosarcoma. A new classification scheme related to prognosis. Arch Pathol Lab Med. 1992;116(8):847–55.

Vang R, Medeiros LJ, Fuller GN, Sarris AH, Deavers M. Non-Hodgkin's lymphoma involving the gynecologic tract: a review of 88 cases. Adv Anat Pathol. 2001;8(4):200–17.

Verstraelen H, Verhelst R. Bacterial vaginosis: an update on diagnosis and treatment. Expert Rev. Anti-Infect Ther. 2009;7(9):1109–24.

Classification of tumours of the uterine cervix according to World Health Organization is highlighted in Fig. 3.1a, b [1].

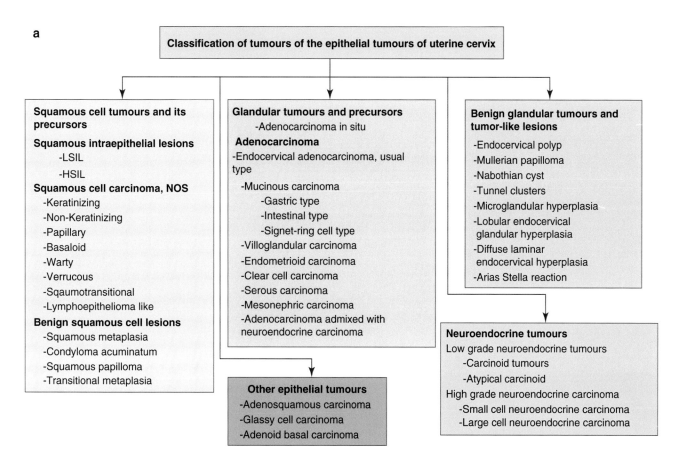

a

Classification of tumours of the epithelial tumours of uterine cervix

Squamous cell tumours and its precursors

Squamous intraepithelial lesions
- LSIL
- HSIL

Squamous cell carcinoma, NOS
- Keratinizing
- Non-Keratinizing
- Papillary
- Basaloid
- Warty
- Verrucous
- Sqaumotransitional
- Lymphoepithelioma like

Benign squamous cell lesions
- Squamous metaplasia
- Condyloma acuminatum
- Squamous papilloma
- Transitional metaplasia

Glandular tumours and precursors
- Adenocarcinoma in situ

Adenocarcinoma
- Endocervical adenocarcinoma, usual type
  - Mucinous carcinoma
    - Gastric type
    - Intestinal type
    - Signet-ring cell type
  - Villoglandular carcinoma
  - Endometrioid carcinoma
  - Clear cell carcinoma
  - Serous carcinoma
  - Mesonephric carcinoma
  - Adenocarcinoma admixed with neuroendocrine carcinoma

Other epithelial tumours
- Adenosquamous carcinoma
- Glassy cell carcinoma
- Adenoid basal carcinoma

Benign glandular tumours and tumor-like lesions
- Endocervical polyp
- Mullerian papilloma
- Nabothian cyst
- Tunnel clusters
- Microglandular hyperplasia
- Lobular endocervical glandular hyperplasia
- Diffuse laminar endocervical hyperplasia
- Arias Stella reaction

Neuroendocrine tumours
Low grade neuroendocrine tumours
- Carcinoid tumours
- Atypical carcinoid
High grade neuroendocrine carcinoma
- Small cell neuroendocrine carcinoma
- Large cell neuroendocrine carcinoma

Fig. 3.1 (**a**) Classification of the epithelial tumours of cervix. (*LSIL* Low grade squamous intraepithelial lesion, *HSIL* High grade squamous intraepithelial lesion). (**b**) Classification of the non-epithelial tumours of cervix. (**c**) Normal squamous epithelium: normal squamous lining of the ectocervix. (**d**) Lymphoid follicles underneath the squamous epithelium. (**e**) Endocervical lining: tall columnar mucus secreting cells with basally placed nuclei resembling a "picket fence" appearance. (**f**) Squamocolumnar junction: junction of the squamous and columnar epithelium

© Springer Nature Singapore Pte Ltd. 2019
P. Dey, *Color Atlas of Female Genital Tract Pathology*, https://doi.org/10.1007/978-981-13-1029-4_3

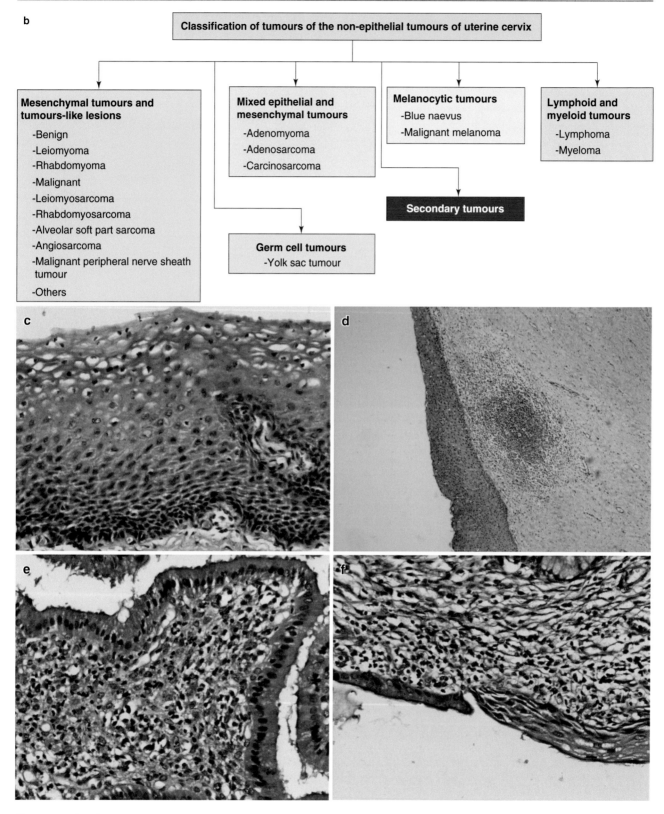

Fig. 3.1 (continued)

Normal Epithelial Layer of Cervix

Image gallery: Fig. 3.1c–f
Squamous epithelium

- The ectocervix is lined by the squamous epithelium
- The squamous epithelial layer has three zones
  - *Basal/parabasal cell layer*:
    The basal cells are located over the basement membrane.
    The cells are relatively small with scanty cytoplasm and round nuclei.
    The parabasal cells lie just over the basal cells
  - *Intermediate cell layer*: Intermediate cells make this layer. These cells are polyhedral in shape and have abundant cytoplasm with central vesicular nuclei
  - *Superficial zone (Superficial cell layer)*: This layer contains superficial cells with abundant cytoplasm and central pyknotic nuclei.

Columnar epithelium

- The mucus secreting columnar epithelium covers the endocervix
- The cells are tall columnar with abundant granular cytoplasm
- Nuclei are basally placed and round monomorphic in appearance

Squamocolumnar junction
Definition: Squamocolumnar junction indicates the junctional area between the ectocervical squamous epithelium and endocervical columnar epithelium.

Transformation zone
Image gallery: Fig. 3.2
Definition: The migrated endocervical epithelium is replaced by the metaplastic squamous epithelium and a new squamocolumnar junction is formed over the course of time. This zone of metaplastic endocervical region is known as transformation zone.

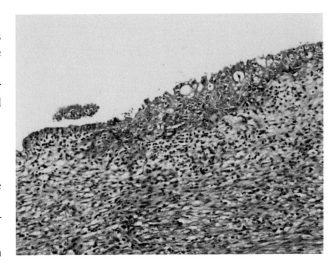

Fig. 3.2 Transformation zone: the metaplastic endocervical epithelium makes the transformation zone

Normal Cervical Smear

Image gallery: Fig. 3.3a–e
  Superficial squamous cell:

- Polygonal cells

- Abundant orangeophilic cytoplasm
- Central small pyknotic nuclei

Intermediate squamous cell:

- Polygonal cells

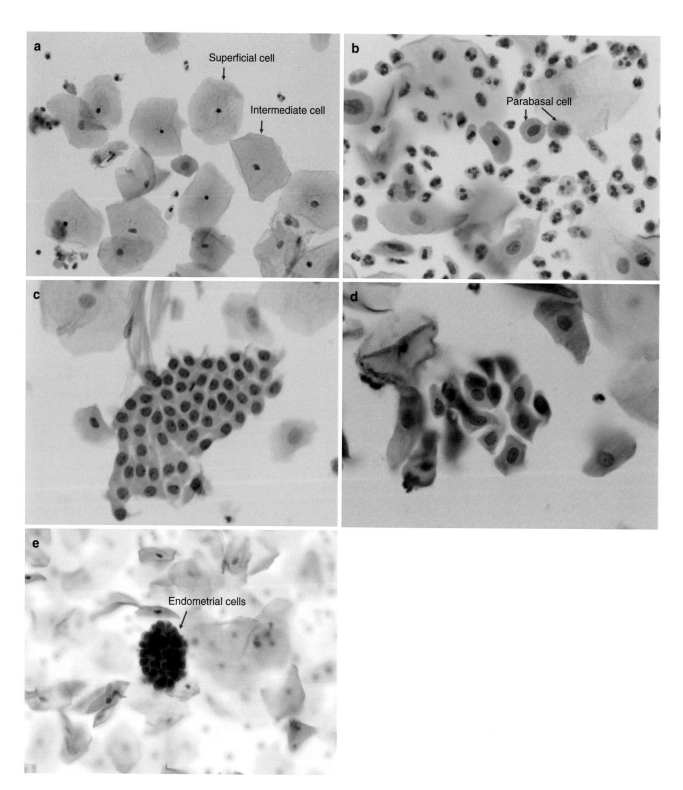

Fig. 3.3 (**a**) Cervical smear: superficial and intermediate cells. (**b**) Cervical smear: parabasal cells. (**c**) Cervical smear: Endocervical cells showing honeycomb appearance. (**d**) Cervical smear: metaplastic cells. (**e**) Cervical smear: endometrial cells

- Greenish abundant cytoplasm
- Relatively larger vesicular nucleus

Parabasal cells

- Small round cells
- Thick cytoplasm
- Large nuclei occupying 2/3rd of the cytoplasm

Endocervical cells

- Monolayer sheets of cells
- Honeycomb appearance
- Small cells with moderate cytoplasm
- Small round monomorphic nuclei

Metaplastic cells

- Oval to polygonal cells

- Geometrically extended cytoplasm
- Relatively smaller cell superficial squamous cells
- Large nuclei

Immature squamous metaplastic cells

- Metaplastic cells
- Large nuclei with pleomorphism
- No chromatin abnormality

Tubal metaplasia

- The cells with basal plate and tufts of cilia

Endometrial cell

- Tight cohesive cells
- Cells with scanty cytoplasm
- Round monomorphic nuclei

Inflammatory Lesions

Cervicitis

Image gallery: Fig. 3.4a–d

- Cause: Nonspecific infection, trauma, intrauterine contraceptive devices
- Histopathology: Neutrophilic infiltration in the subepithelium in acute cervicitis and chronic inflammatory cells in chronic cervicitis.

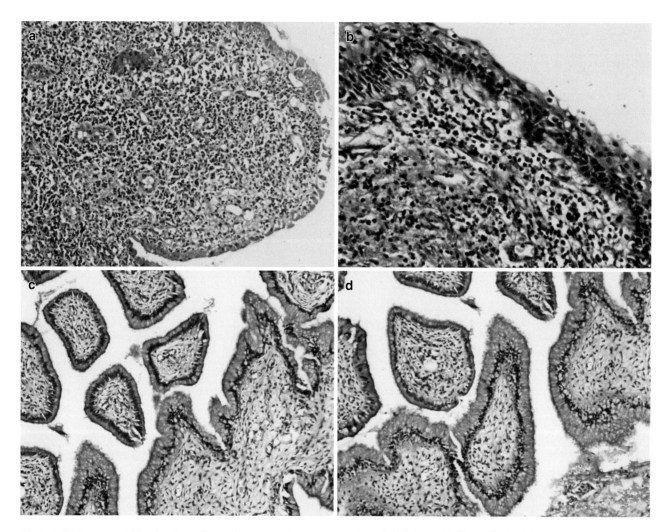

Fig. 3.4 (**a**) Acute cervicitis: abundant polymorphs underneath the epithelial layer. (**b**) Chronic cervicitis: chronic inflammatory cell infiltration in the subepithelium. (**c**) Cervicitis: papillary projections of the endocervical lining epithelium. (**d**) Cervicitis: papillae with the core containing vessels and lymphocytes

Specific Infections

Herpes Simplex
Image gallery: Fig. 3.5a, b

- *Causative agent*
    - Herpes simplex virus—2 subtype 90% of the genital herpes simplex infection.
    - HSV-1: 10–15% of genital herpes simplex infection
- *Symptoms*: Fever, itching sensation, dysuria and inguinal lymphadenopathy

- *Gross features*: Ulceration of the cervix, rarely fungating mass like lesion
- *Histopathology and cytology*
    - Ulceration of the lining epithelium
    - Suprabasal vesicles
    - Parabasal and endocervical cells show intranuclear owl eye like inclusion, ground glass like nuclei and multinucleated giant cells with faceted nuclei.

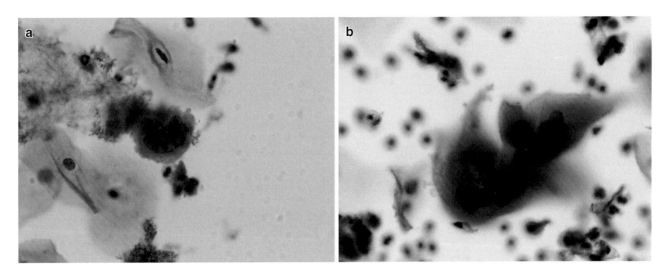

Fig. 3.5 (**a**) Herpes simplex: cervical smear shows multinucleated giant cells with ground glass nuclei. (**b**) Herpes simplex: cervical smear shows typical multinucleated cells with compressed nuclei

Tuberculosis of Cervix

Image gallery: Fig. 3.6

    Causative agent: Mycobacterium tuberculosis

    Epidemiology:

- Secondary to tuberculosis in other genital region such as fallopian tube or endometrium
- It represents 24% of female genital tract tuberculosis

    Symptoms: Asymptomatic or irregular friable growth that bleeds on touch

    Gross features: Either normal looking cervix or ulcerated lesion that may mimic carcinoma

Histopathology

- Often ulcerated lining epithelium
- Multiple epithelioid cell granulomas in the stroma
- Multinucleated giant cells, epithelioid cells and lymphocytes
- Necrosis

    Ancillary tests to confirm: Ziehl Neelsen stain for acid fast bacilli, bacterial culture, polymerase chain reaction

    Treatment: Anti tubercular therapy

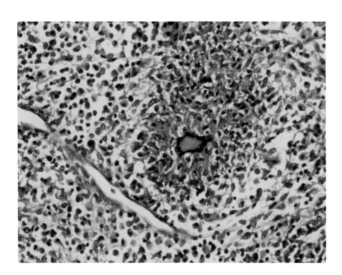

Fig. 3.6 Tuberculosis of cervix: epithelioid cell granulomas in cervix

Epithelial Tumours

Precursors of Squamous Cell Tumours

Terminology: See Fig. 3.7

- At first the cervical preneoplastic lesions were classified as mild dysplasia, moderate dysplasia, severe dysplasia and carcinoma in situ.
- Later on, the cervical preneoplastic lesions were considered as a single disease entity and the name was given as "cervical intraepithelial lesion" (CIN). The CIN was classified as CIN 1, CIN 2 and CIN 3. Here, severe dysplasia and carcinoma in situ were clubbed together as CIN 3
- The Bethesda system classified the lesion as Low grade squamous intraepithelial lesion (LSIL) and high grade squamous intraepithelial lesion (HSIL)

Causative organism: See Fig. 3.8

- Human Papilloma virus is the causative organism of cervical SIL and carcinoma

Life cycle of HPV: See Fig. 3.9

- *Entry*: HPV enters in the cervical squamous epithelium through micro abrasions during sexual intercourse
- *Latent phase*
  - HPVs stay as latent phase within the nucleus of the cervical epithelium. It does not incorporate within the genome (DNA) of the host.
  - No morphological abnormality seen
- *Productive phase*
  - Viral DNA is incorporated within the DNA of the host and the virus proliferates independently
  - Cytological abnormality seen

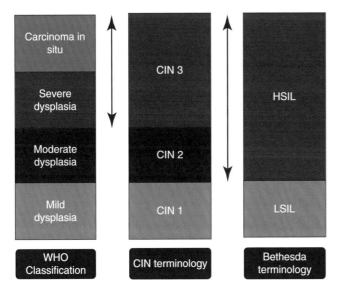

Fig. 3.7 Comparison of different terminologies used in cervical squamous intraepithelial lesions. (*WHO* World health organization, *CIN* Cervical intraepithelial neoplasia, *HSIL* High grade squamous intraepithelial lesion, *LSIL* Low grade squamous intraepithelial lesion)

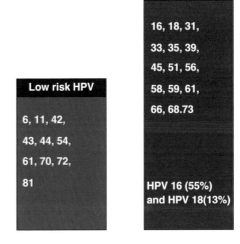

Fig. 3.8 HPV types and risk potential for carcinoma of cervix

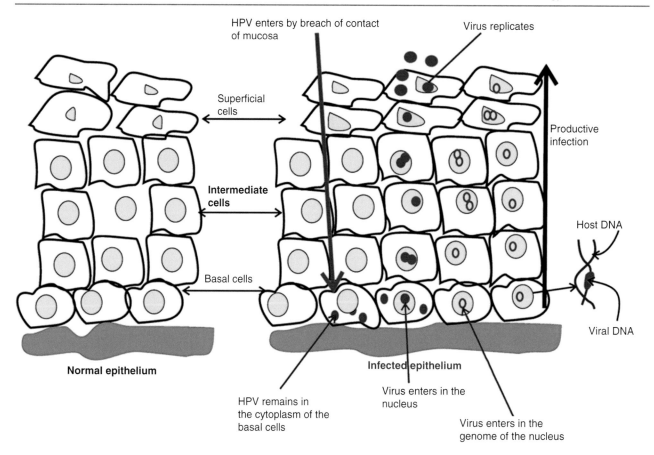

Fig. 3.9 HPV life cycle in the cervical epithelium

Low Grade Squamous Intraepithelial Lesion (LSIL)

Image gallery: Figs. 3.10 and 3.11
Synonym

- Mild squamous dysplasia
- Cervical intraepithelial neoplasia grade 1

Epidemiology

- Predominantly related with HPV 6 and 11
- Caused by high risk HPV (mainly 16 and 18)

Clinical features

- Usually young patients

- Asymptomatic
- Detected by routine cervical cytology screening

Colposcopy examination

- Aceto-white area

Cytology

- Discrete superficial and intermediate squamous cells
- Nucleus is enlarged and occupying more than 1/3rd of the cytoplasmic area
- Nuclear size is more than three times of the normal looking intermediate cells.
- Moderately pleomorphic nuclei
- Irregular nuclear margin
- Finely granular chromatin

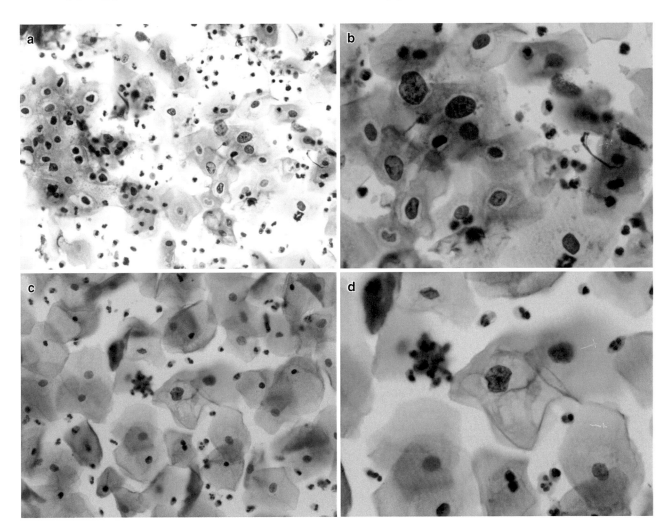

Fig. 3.10 (**a**) Cervical smear of low grade squamous intraepithelial lesion: epithelial cells show mild enlargement of nuclei. (**b**) Cervical smear of low grade squamous intraepithelial lesion: the cells have high nucleocytoplasmic ratio. Nuclei are mildly hyperchromatic. (**c**) Cervical smear of low grade squamous intraepithelial lesion: the epithelial cell showing koilocytotic change. (**d**) Cervical smear of low grade squamous intraepithelial lesion: the koilocytotic cell have enlarged nuclei and perinuclear cytoplasmic halo. (**e**) Cervical smear of low grade squamous intraepithelial lesion: the epithelial cells showing nuclear enlargement. (**f**) Cervical smear of low grade squamous intraepithelial lesion: many koilocytotic cells present. (**g**) Colposcopy of low grade squamous intraepithelial lesion: thin aceto-white area. (Courtesy Dr P Saha, Department of Gynecology and Obstetrics, PGIMER, Chandigarh)

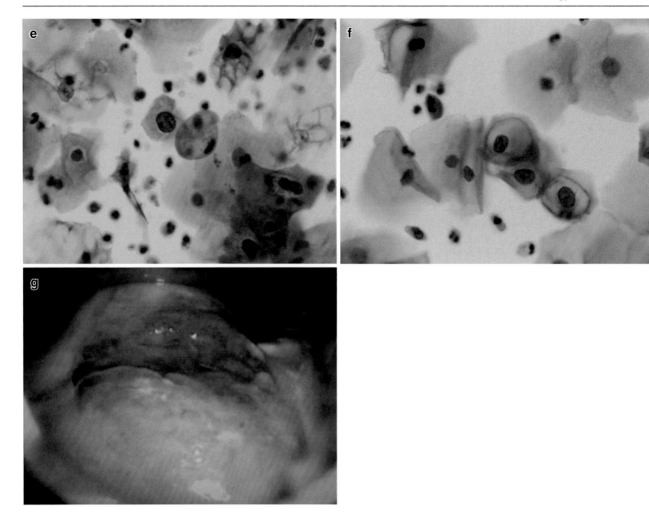

Fig. 3.10 (continued)

- Inconspicuous nucleoli
- Koilocyosis: Centrally placed enlarged nuclei with perinuclear halo. Sharply condensed cytoplasmic margin.

Histopathology

- Thickened epithelium
- The epithelium may show acanthosis and parakeratosis
- Only lower 1/3rd of the epithelium shows proliferation and atypia
- Upper 2/3rd shows normal maturation
- Nuclei of the cells show mild enlargement, pleomorphism and hyperchromasia
- Coarse granular chromatin
- Irregular nuclear membrane
- Koilocytes present
- Mitosis: Present in the basal 1/3rd of the epithelium

Differential diagnosis

- Nonspecific perinuclear halos : In trichomonas vaginalis infection

- Reactive inflammatory changes: Metaplastic cells may mimic LSIL
- HSIL

Ancillary studies

- P16 immunostaining: p16 is the indirect marker of HPV infection and p16 immunostaining is strongly positive in the basal 1/3rd of the epithelial cells. Therefore p16 immunostaining helps to differentiate reparative atypia or squamous metaplasia from LSIL.
- Ki 67: LSIL cases show increased Ki67 positive cells. This reflects the increased cell proliferation in this lesion.

Progression

- Vast majority of the cases regress within 10 year period (88%)
- Only 10–12 progress to carcinoma in 10 year

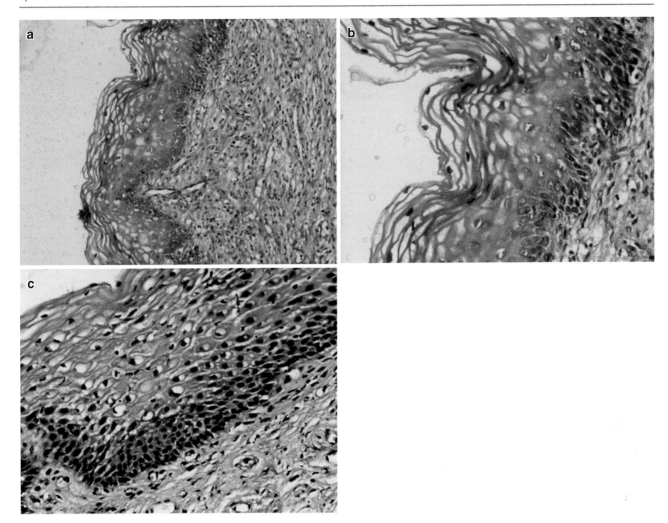

Fig. 3.11 (a) Low grade squamous intraepithelial lesion: only the basal one third of the epithelium showing dysplastic cells. (b) Low grade squamous intraepithelial lesion: loss of polarity in the epithelial cells. (c) Low grade squamous intraepithelial lesion: lower third of the epithelial cells show mild nuclear enlargement and pleomorphism

High Grade Squamous Intraepithelial Lesion (HSIL)

Image gallery: Figs. 3.12a–f and 3.13a–g)
Abbreviation: High grade squamous intraepithelial lesion: HSIL
Synonym

- Moderate dysplasia
- Severe dysplasia
- Cervical intraepithelial neoplasia grade 2
- Cervical intraepithelial neoplasia grade 3

Epidemiology:

- HSIL is caused by HPV 16, 18, 31, 33, 35, 39, 45, 51, 52, 56
- HPV 16, 18 together are responsible for 50% HSIL
- Incidence is 31.5 per 100,000 Caucasian American
- In cervical smear screening : 0.5–0.8% Papanicolaou's smear

Clinical features

- Asymptomatic and recognized by routine cervical cancer screening

Colposcopy

- Acetowhite area present. It may have irregular surface, with sharp outer margin. The intensity of the color is variable
- Small vessels have hairpin like U turn that may give rise to coarse punctuation
- The small vessels anastomose and produces mosaic like pattern which is known as mosaicism
- Coarse mosaicism and punctuation may overlap to produce umbilication

Cytology

- Discrete and loose clusters of cells
- Cells are relatively smaller in size and predominant cell population is parabasal
- Moderately pleomorphic nuclei
- Nuclei show:
  - Moderate pleomorphism
  - Moderate enlargement
  - High nucleo-cytoplasmic ratio
  - Significantly irregular margin
  - Nuclear chromatin shows irregular clumping
  - Usually absent nucleoli
  - Glandular involvement by dysplastic cells give rise to prominent nucleoli

Histology of HSIL

- Thickened epithelium

- Dysplastic cells occupy more than lower 1/3rd of the epithelium to full thickness
- Nuclei show: Moderate pleomorphism, moderate to marked enlargement, irregular membrane with focal thickening and coarsely granular chromatin
- Mitotic activity is present throughout the epithelial layer
- Abnormal mitosis present
- Koilocytosis may also be present in variable number
  - *Koilocytotic HSIL*
    Large number of Koilocytotic cells are present
    Atypical cells are also seen in the entire epithelial layer
  - *Keratinizing HSIL*
    HSIL shows superficial keratinization and parakeratosis
  - *HSILs with immature metaplastic differentiation*
    It simulates reactive squamous metaplasia
    The lesion shows immature cells with high nucleocytoplasmic ratio and hyperchromatic nuclei in the superficial layer.

Ancillary studies

- P16 immunostaining: It is strongly positive in HSIL. Positive p16 immunostaining helps to differentiate the lesion from reactive atypia.
- Ki 67: This cell proliferation marker is higher in HSIL than LSIL
- Cyclin D: No expression in high risk HPV infection
- DNA aneuploidy: HSIL cases frequently show DNA aneuploidy

Differential diagnosis (Fig. 3.13h)

- Immature squamous metaplasia: Characterized by (Table 3.1)
  - No nuclear pleomorphism
  - Maintained cell polarity
  - Mature superficial cells
  - Fine chromatin
- Reactive hyperplasia: Characterized by
  - Maintained cell polarity
  - Lack of pleomorphism
  - Regular nuclear margin
  - Fine chromatin
- Atrophic epithelium
  - Bland looking nuclei
  - No nuclear atypia
  - No loss of polarity
- LSIL: Characterized by (Table 3.2)
  - Abnormal cells remain predominantly in basal third
  - Degree of nuclear atypia is less than HSIL
  - Atypical mitotic figure absent
  - Frequent koilocyosis

Progression (see Fig. 3.13i)

- Progression rate of HSIL to carcinoma is higher than LSIL
- Near about 17–21% of HSIL cases progress to invasive carcinoma in 10 years period whereas 12% of LSIL cases progress to invasive carcinoma
- No biomarker can predict which case will proceed to invasive carcinoma

Management
Removal of the lesion by:

- Cone biopsy
- Loop electrosurgical excision
- Cold knife conization

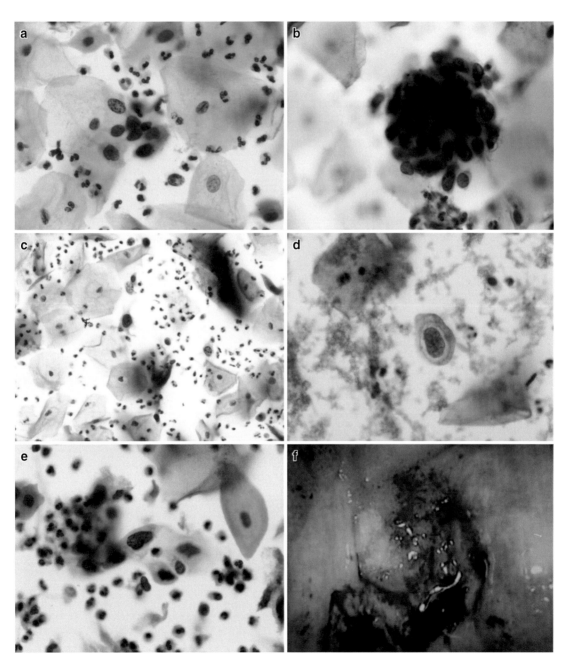

Fig. 3.12 (a) Cervical smear of high grade squamous intraepithelial lesion: loose cluster of epithelial cells. (b) Cervical smear of high grade squamous intraepithelial lesion: tight cohesive cluster of epithelial cells (hyperchromatic crowded group) with scanty cytoplasm and hyperchromatic nuclei. (c) Cervical smear of high grade squamous intraepithelial lesion: discrete epithelial cell with hyperchromatic round nuclei. (d) Cervical smear of high grade squamous intraepithelial lesion: nuclei is hyperchromatic and occupying more than 2/3rd of the cytoplasm. (e) Cervical smear of high grade squamous intraepithelial lesion: nuclei show irregular outer margin. (f) Colposcopy picture of high grade squamous intraepithelial lesion: thick acetowhite area. (Courtesy Dr P Saha, Department of Gynecology and Obstetrics, PGIMER, Chandigarh)

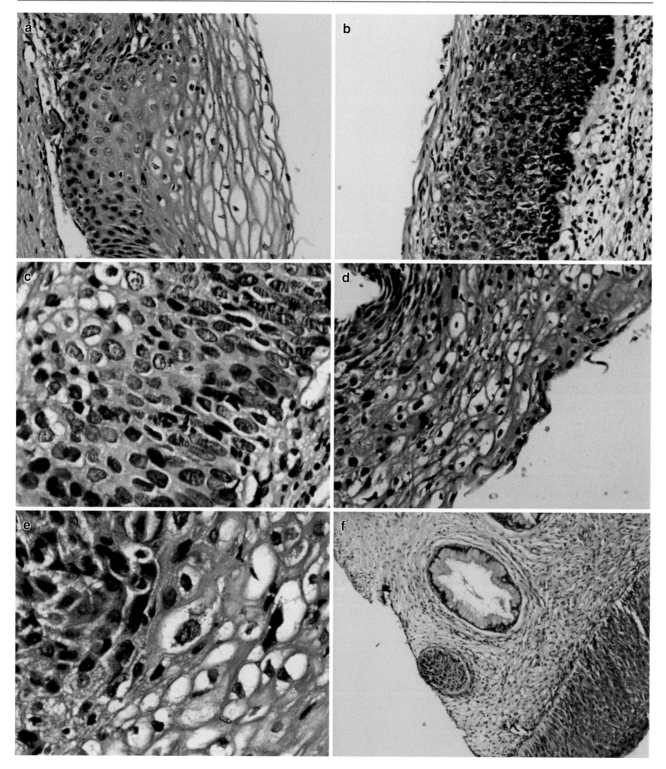

Fig. 3.13 (**a**) High grade squamous intraepithelial lesion: this can also be labelled as cervical intraepithelial neoplasia 2. Note that only lower 2/3rd of the epithelium is involved. (**b**) High grade squamous intraepithelial lesion: this can also be labelled as cervical intraepithelial neoplasia 3. Note that more than lower 2/3rd of the epithelium is involved. (**c**) High grade squamous intraepithelial lesion (CIN 3): the cells show loss of polarity. The nuclei of the cells are enlarged, moderately pleomorphic and hyperchromatic. (**d**) High grade squamous intraepithelial lesion: marked koilocytotic changes in the epithelium. (**e**) High grade squamous intraepithelial lesion: koilocytotic cells showing nuclear enlargement and perinuclear halo. (**f**) High grade squamous intraepithelial lesion (CIN 3): note the involvement of the gland by the dysplastic cells. (**g**) High grade squamous intraepithelial lesion (CIN 3): glandular involvement by the dysplastic cells. Note the maintained basement membrane of the gland. (**h**) Differential diagnosis of high grade squamous intraepithelial lesion (HSIL). (**i**) Progression of cervical intraepithelial neoplasia (CIN)

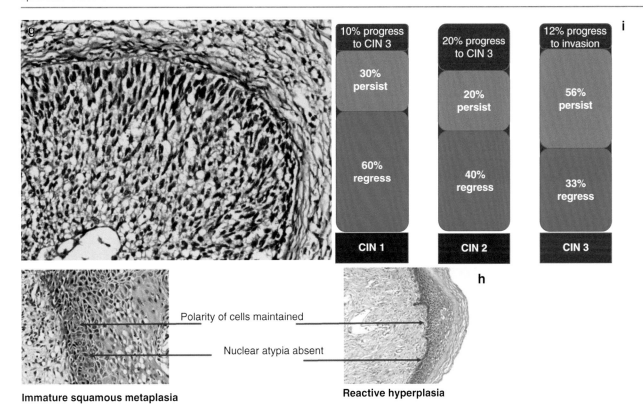

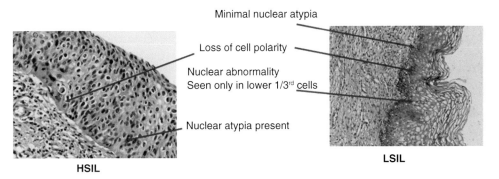

Immature squamous metaplasia

Reactive hyperplasia

HSIL

LSIL

Fig. 3.13 (continued)

Table 3.1 Immature metaplasia versus HSIL

Features	Immature metaplasia	HSIL
Polarity of the cells	Maintained	Not maintained
Cell differentiation	Not affected and superficial mature cells seen	Markedly affected
Mitotic activity	Only present in lower 1/3rd	Throughout the epithelial layer
Chromatin pattern	Fine	Coarse
Nuclear pleomorphism	Mild	Significant
P16 immunostaining	Negative or patchy positive	Strong positivity

Table 3.2 LSIL versus HSIL

Features	LSIL	HSIL
HPV types	Low risk HPV (6,11)	High risk HPV (16,18)
Involved epithelium	Only basal 1/3rd	More than basal 1/3rd
Mitotic activity	Only basal 1/3rd	Whole epithelial layer
Atypical mitosis	Absent	Frequent
Koilocytosis	Frequent	Infrequent
DNA Ploidy	Diploid	Aneuploid
Ki 67	Low index	High index

Squamous Cell Carcinoma

Image gallery: Figs. 3.14 and 3.15
  Epidemiology

- Second most common cancer in the world
- Higher incidence in the poor nations
- Incidence is going low in the screened population and in developed countries
- Annual death rate near about 230,000

Etiology

- HPV infection is the most important etiological factor
- Other factors:Multiple sex partner, early sexual exposure, cigarette smoking, multiparity, poor hygiene, HIV infection

Clinical features

- Commonly seen in fifth decade
- Post coital bleeding
- Vaginal bleeding
- Advanced stage: Anuria, hydroureter

Gross features

- Commonly: Reddish, friable polypoid mass
- Occasionally: Endophytic ulcerated, bleeds to touch

Cytology

- Discrete and loose clusters of cells
- Cells are large and oval to polyhedral in shape

- Nuclei are enlarged with high nucleo cytoplasmic ratio
- Hyperchromatic and moderately pleomorphic nuclei
- Irregular coarsely clumped chromatin
- Tadpole cells present: cells with extended tail like cytoplasm and one sided nuclei
- Fibre cell: Elongated spindle shaped cells
- Tumour diathesis: Necrotic tissue fragments with entangled RBCs and polymorphs and tumour cells

Histopathology
Non-keratinizing squamous cell carcinoma

- Solid sheet, nest, trabeculae or cords of cells
- Polygonal cells with deep eosinophilic cytoplasm
- Moderate to severe pleomorphism depending on the grade of tumour
- Coarsely granular chromatin
- Intracellular bridge
- No keratin pearl
- Cells may be small with scanty cytoplasm resembling small cell carcinoma

Keratinizing squamous cell carcinoma

- Characterized by multiple keratin pearls
- Solid sheet, cords, nests of cells
- Polygonal cells with moderately pleomorphic and hyperchromatic nuclei
- Irregular coarse chromatin
- Abundant keratohyalin granules in the cytoplasm

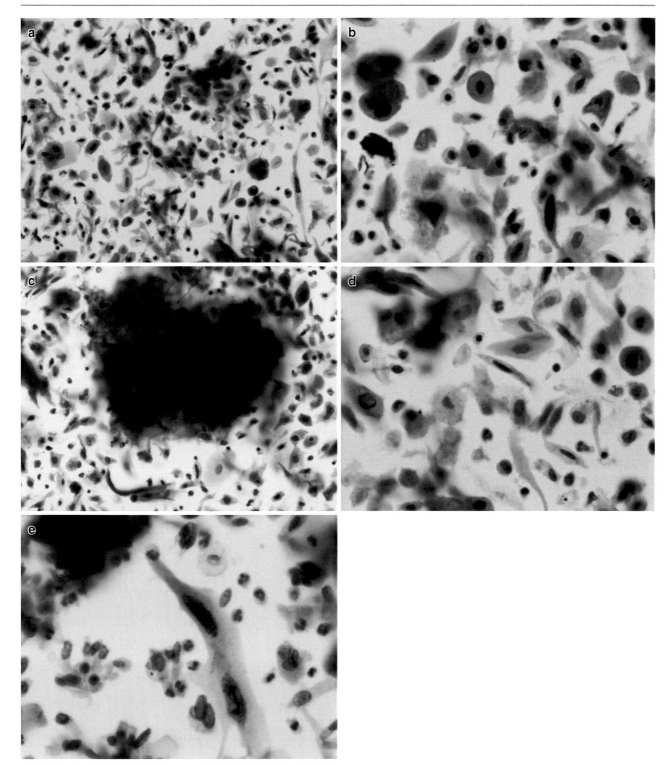

Fig. 3.14 (a) Cervical smear of squamous cell carcinoma: discrete oval to polyhedral cells with enlarged hyperchromatic nuclei. (b) Cervical smear of squamous cell carcinoma: cells with orangeophilic cytoplasm and hyperchromatic nuclei. (c) Cervical smear of squamous cell carcinoma: tumour diathesis. (d) Cervical smear of squamous cell carcinoma: many fibre cells are present. (e) Cervical smear of squamous cell carcinoma: higher magnification of the fibre cells

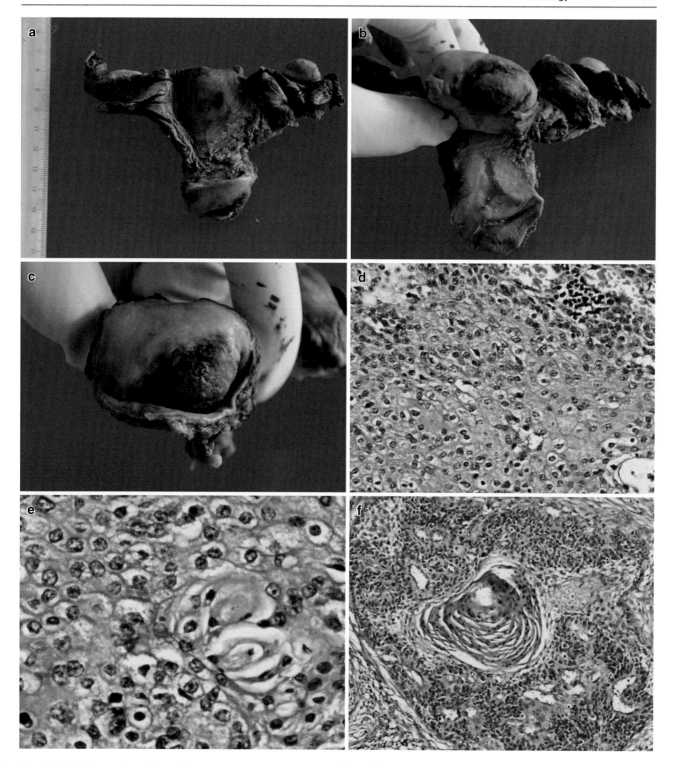

Fig. 3.15 (**a**) Resected specimen of a case of squamous cell carcinoma: note the enlarged cervix. (**b**) Resected specimen of a case of squamous cell carcinoma: growth in the anterior lip of cervix. (**c**) Resected specimen of a cases of squamous cell carcinoma: the growth shows irregular ulcerated surface. (**d**) Keratinizing squamous cell carcinoma: sheets of polygonal tumour cells with central hyperchromatic nuclei. (**e**) Keratinizing squamous cell carcinoma: polygonal cells with intercellular bridge. (**f**) Keratinizing squamous cell carcinoma: squamous pearl. (**g**) Keratinizing squamous cell carcinoma: giant cell reaction around the squamous pearl. (**h**) Non-keratinizing squamous cell carcinoma: diffuse sheet of round to oval tumour cells. (**i**) Non-keratinizing squamous cell carcinoma: round cells with scanty cytoplasm having dark hyperchromatic nuclei

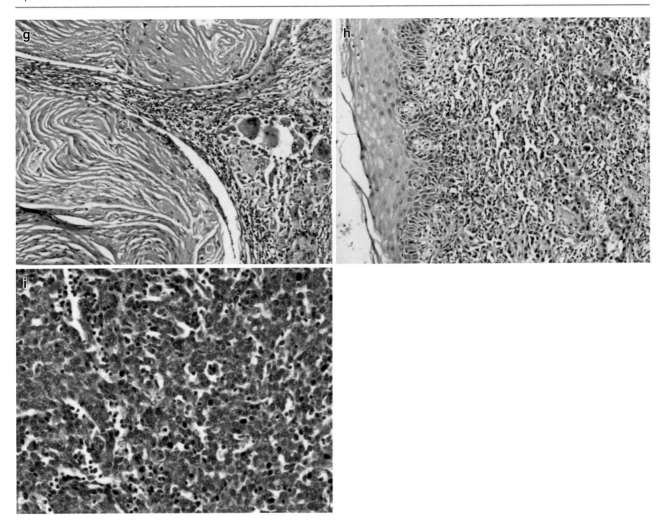

Fig. 3.15 (continued)

Minimally Invasive (Early Invasive) Carcinoma

Image gallery: Fig. 3.16a–c

Synonym: Early invasive carcinoma, Stage IA1

Definition: Stromal invasion is less than 3 mm in depth and less than 7 mm in width. There should not be any lymphovascular invasion present.

Epidemiology:

- Common in 35–45 year age
- About 4% cases are in association with SIL cases
- It represents 20% cervical carcinoma cases

Clinical feature: Usually asymptomatic and mostly detected during histopathological examination of SIL cases.

Gross features: Grossly it looks like normal

Histopathology:

- Squamous epithelium shows intraepithelial neoplasia of varying degrees
- Breach of basement membrane
- Nests of infiltrating cells in the stroma with irregular margin
- Infiltration of lymphocytes around the tumour cells

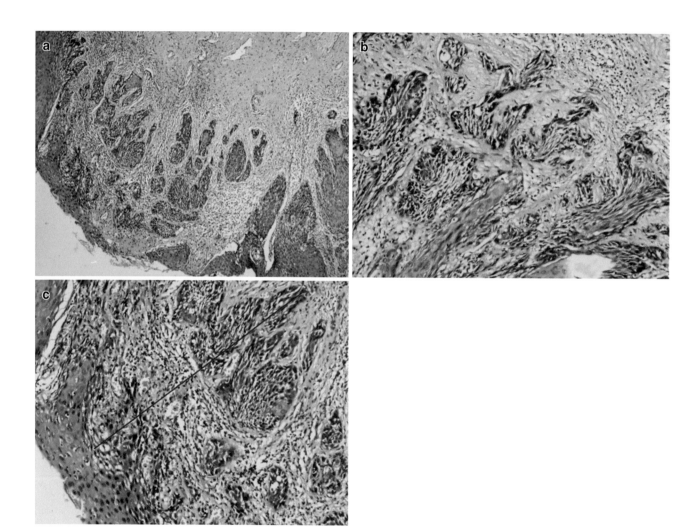

Fig. 3.16 (**a**) Minimally invasive carcinoma: the tumour cells have infiltrated in the adjacent stroma with lymphocytic infiltration around them. (**b**) Minimally invasive carcinoma: the irregular contour of the clusters of infiltrating tumour cells. (**c**) Minimally invasive carcinoma: the depth of invasion is measured from the basement membrane of the surface epithelium or crypt of the gland to the distant most tumour cell

Features of Invasion

Image gallery: Fig. 3.17a–c
Histopathological features

- Complete loss of polarity and maturation along with stromal desmoplasia

- Epithelial stromal interface becomes indistinct or blurred
- Focal maturation of the tumour forming epithelial cells
- Scalloping margin in the junction of the tumour and stroma
- Pseudo-gland formation

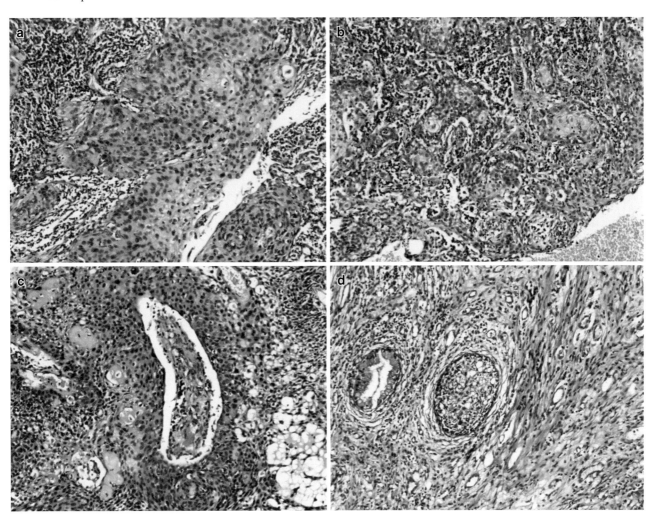

Fig. 3.17 (**a**) Features of invasion of squamous cell carcinoma in small biopsy: blurred epithelial and stromal interface. (**b**) Features of invasion of squamous cell carcinoma in small biopsy: focal maturation of the tumour forming epithelial cells. (**c**) Features of invasion of squamous cell carcinoma in small biopsy: focal maturation and retraction of spaces. (**d**) Mimicker of invasion: crypt involvement by dysplastic cells mimicking invasion. (**e**) Mimicker of invasion: higher magnification showing the intact basement membrane of the endocervical gland. (**f**) Mimicker of invasion: tangential cutting simulating invasion. (**g**) Mimicker of invasion: dense inflammation underneath the epithelium of HSIL may mimic invasion. (**h**) Mimicker of invasion: large aggregate of lymphoid cells and endothelial cells may mimic malignancy

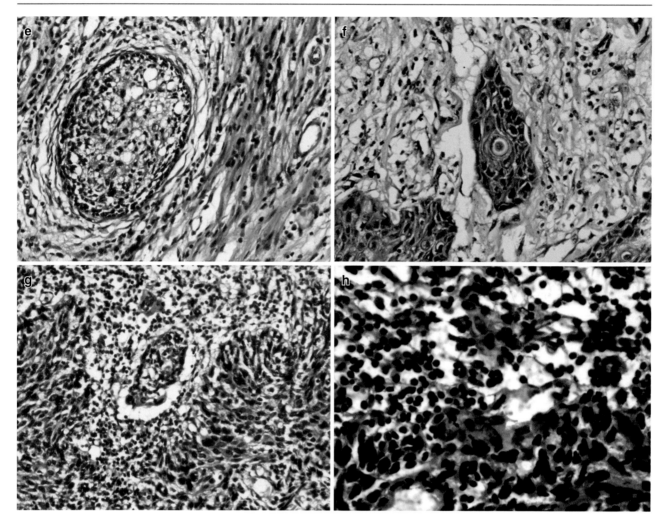

Fig. 3.17 (continued)

Mimickers of invasion (Fig. 3.17d–h)

- Crypt involvement by dysplastic cells
- Tangential cutting
- Large aggregates of lymphoid cells and endothelial cells

Papillary Squamous Cell Carcinoma

Image gallery: Fig. 3.18a, b

Histopathology

- Many papillary structure with central fibrovascular core
- Individual cells of the lining of papillae show squamoid cells
- Cells are oval to polyhedral with hyperchromatic nuclei
- Invasion present at the base of the papillary tissue
- High mitosis

Immunocytochemistry

- CK 7 positive and CK 20 negative

Differential diagnosis

- Warty carcinoma: No keratinization or koilocytes
- Condyloma accuminatum with atypia: Koilocytes and no stromal invasion

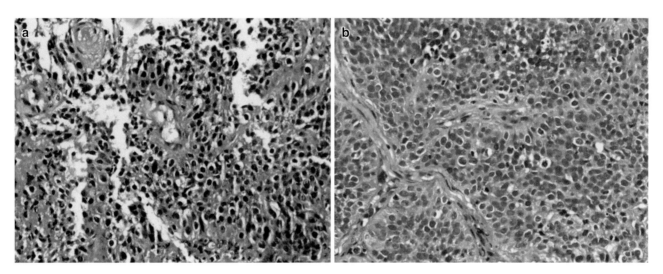

Fig. 3.18 (**a**) Papillary squamous cell carcinoma: papillary structures with central fibrovascular core. (**b**) Papillary squamous cell carcinoma: the cells showing oval to polyhedral squamoid cells

Basal Cell Carcinoma

Image gallery: Fig. 3.19a–c

> *Histopathology*

- Nests and cords of tumour cells
- Cells simulate basal cells having scanty cytoplasm

- Brisk mitotic activity
- Rarely keratin pearls are present

Behaviour: Aggressive tumour

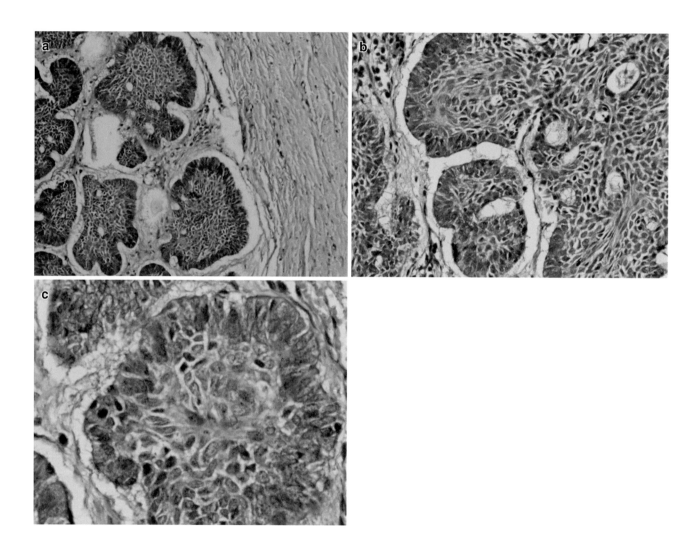

Fig. 3.19 (**a**) Basal cell carcinoma: nests of tumour cells infiltrating in the stroma. (**b**) Basal cell carcinoma: the peripheral tumour cells show palisading arrangement. (**c**) Basal cell carcinoma: the cells are oval to round and simulate basal cells

Lymphoepithelioma Like Carcinoma

Image gallery: Fig. 3.20a, b

Histopathology

- Resembles nasopharyngeal carcinoma
- Nests and sheets of tumour cells
- Lymphocytes in between the tumour cells

- Syncytial like cells as the border of the cells are indistinct
- Cells have moderate amount of cytoplasm
- Vesicular nuclei having single prominent nucleoli

Comments: No relation with EBV

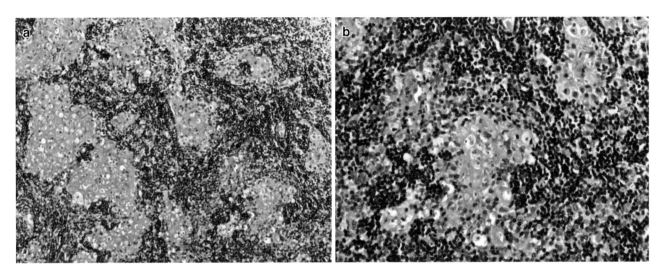

Fig. 3.20 (**a**) Lymphoepithelioma like carcinoma: diffuse sheet of tumour cells with infiltrating lymphocytes. (**b**) Lymphoepithelioma like carcinoma: syncytial cluster of tumour cells with pale cytoplasm

Glassy Cell Carcinoma

Image gallery: Fig. 3.21a–c

It is a type of poorly differentiated adenosquamous cell carcinoma

Incidence: Less than 1% of cervical carcinoma

Histopathology:

- Large cells with abundant eosinophilic cytoplasm
- Centrally placed nuclei with prominent nucleoli
- No intercellular bridges
- High mitotic activity
- Infrequently keratin pearls are seen
- Glandular lumen may also be present

Differential diagnosis

- Lymphoepithelioma like carcinoma: Unlike this tumour, the glassy cell carcinoma has abundant glassy eosinophilic cytoplasm, distinct cell margin and has prominent nucleoli

Prognosis: Aggressive behaviour

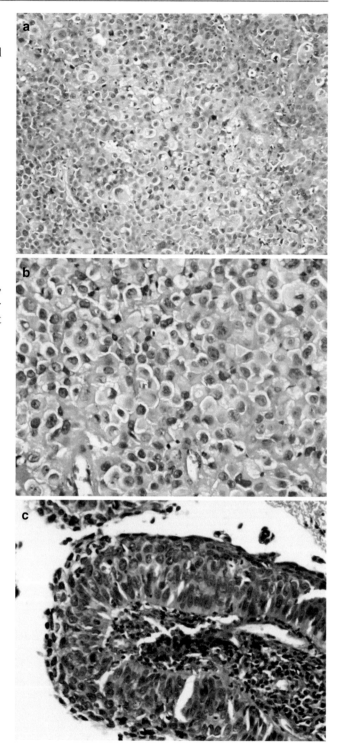

Fig. 3.21 (**a**) Glassy cell carcinoma: diffuse sheet of tumour cells. (**b**) Glassy cell carcinoma: cell with abundant glassy cytoplasm. (**c**) Glassy cell carcinoma: papillary structure with central fibrovascular core

Benign Squamous Cell Lesions

Squamous Metaplasia

Image gallery: Fig. 3.22a–c

Definition: The replacement of endocervical columnar epithelial cells by squamous epithelium

Location: It is usually located in squamocolumnar junction

Epidemiology: It is a common physiological phenomenon

Mechanism

- Mature ectocervical squamous epithelial cells extend towards the endocervical canal and replacing the endocervical columnar cells
- Reserve cells underneath the endocervical cells proliferate and differentiate into mature squamous cells

Causes: Trauma, inflammation, chronic irritation

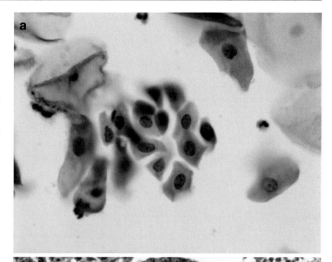
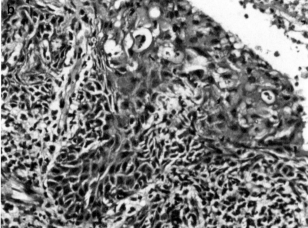
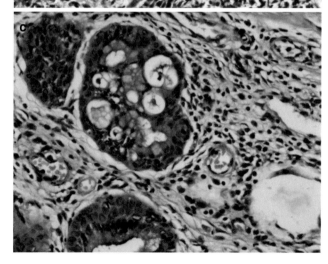

Fig. 3.22 (**a**) Cervical smear: metaplastic cells. (**b**) Squamous metaplasia: the endocervical lining is replaced by squamous epithelial cells. (**c**) Squamous metaplasia: the endocervical glands show squamous metaplasia

Immature Squamous Metaplasia

Image gallery: Fig. 3.23a–e
Characteristic features:

- No surface maturation

- Immature looking cells with enlarged nuclei
- Nuclear atypia is absent

Differential diagnosis

- Squamous intraepithelial lesion

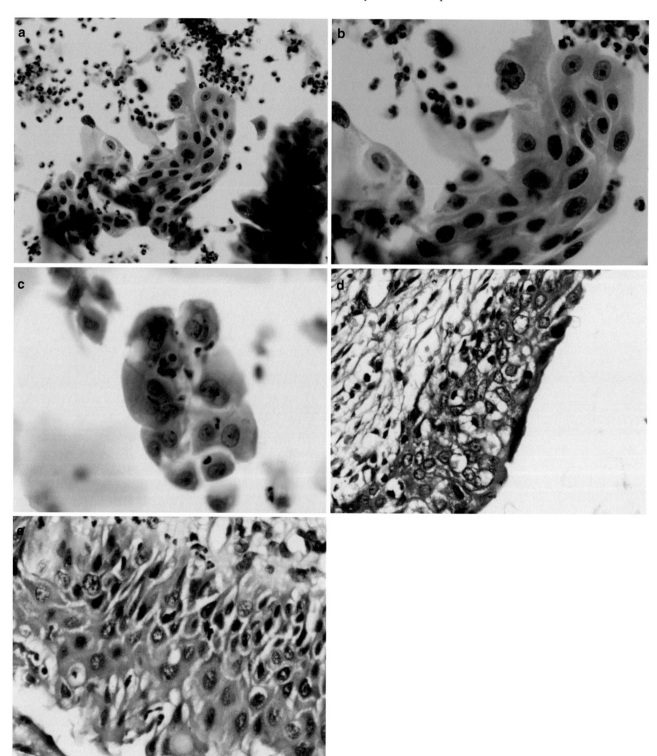

Fig. 3.23 (**a**) Immature squamous metaplasia: metaplastic cells in cluster showing nuclear enlargement. (**b**) Immature squamous metaplasia: higher magnification showing nuclear pleomorphism. (**c**) Cervical smear: immature squamous metaplastic cells: nuclear enlargement and pleomorphism present. However, nucleo-cytoplasmic ratio is not much altered. (**d**) Immature metaplasia: epithelium is replaced by immature looking metaplastic cells. (**e**) Immature metaplasia: note the immature looking cells in higher magnification

Tubal Metaplasia

Image gallery: Fig. 3.24a–c

Definition: Here the endocervical coluumnar epithelium is replaced by Müllerian type of epithelium with cillia on the luminal side

Location: Upper part of the cervical canal adjacent to internal oss.

Histopathology

- The mucus secreting columnar epithelium is replaced by tubal type ciliated columnar cells

Differential diagnosis

- Extensivetubal metaplasia of cervix may be mistaken as adenocarcinoma

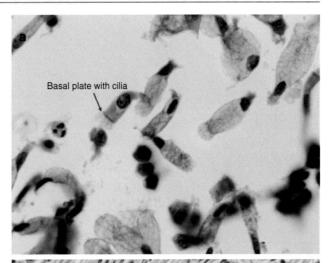
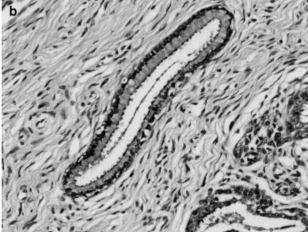
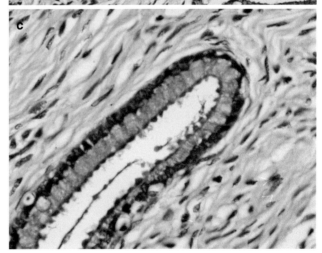

Fig. 3.24 (**a**) Cervical smear: tubal metaplasia. The columnar cells showing bunch of cilia. (**b**) Tubal metaplasia: endocervical cells are replaced by ciliated columnar cell. (**c**) Tubal metaplasia: note the cilia in the luminal side of the cells

Squamous Papilloma

Image gallery: Fig. 3.25a, b
  Definition

- This is a benign exophytic lesion covered with squamous epithelial cells along with central fibrovascular core

Incidence

- Uncommon in cervix but more frequent in vulva and vagina

Histopathology

- Multiple papillary structure
- Outer layer : benign squamous cells
- No koilocytotic cells
- Inner fibrovascular core

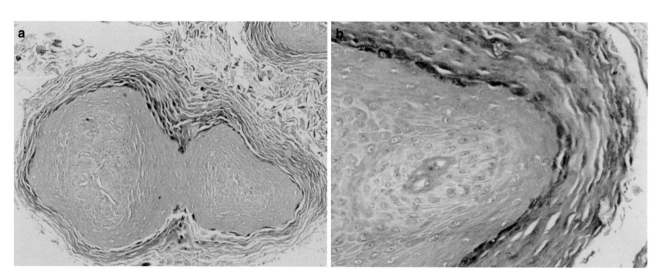

Fig. 3.25 (**a**) Squamous papilloma: papillary structure lined by squamous cells. (**b**) Squamous papilloma: higher magnification of the papillary structure

Condyloma Accuminatum

Image gallery: Fig. 3.26a–c
   Synonym: LSIL, CIN 1
   Common association: Low risk HPV: HPV 6 and 11
   Clinical features:

- Wart like lesion

Histopathology

- Epithelium shows hyperkeratosis, acanthosis and papillimatosis
- Marked koiocytosis

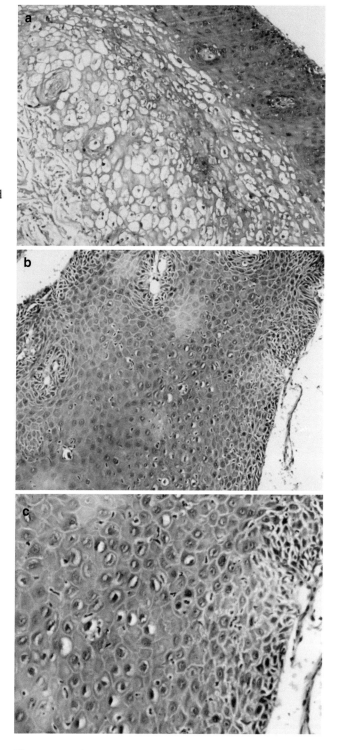

Fig. 3.26 (**a**) Condyloma accuminatum: hyperkeratotic epithelial cell layer. (**b**) Condyloma accuminatum: many koilocytotic cells present. Cells show minimal nuclear pleomorphism. (**c**) Condyloma accuminatum: koilocytotic cells showing enlarged nuclei and perinuclear halo

Glandular Tumours

Atypical Glandular Cells

Image gallery: Fig. 3.27a–d
  Cytology

- Cells are arranged in small clusters with overlapping nuclei and also discretely
- The individual cells have abundant, vacuolated cytoplasm with well-defined margin

- Nuclei are mildly enlarged (3–5 times of normal endocervical cells), pleomorphic with a small nucleoli
- Rare mitotic figures

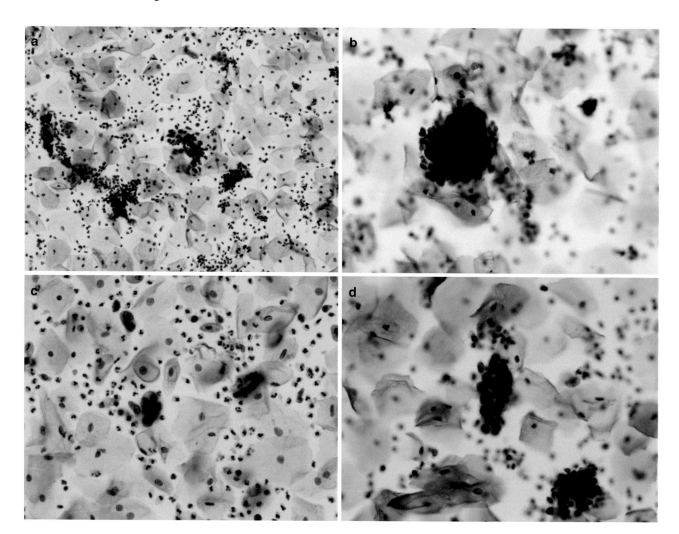

Fig. 3.27 (**a**) Cervical smear of atypical glandular cell of undetermined significance: small clusters of cells with overlapping nuclei. (**b**) Cervical smear of atypical glandular cell of undetermined significance: hyperchromatic crowded group of cells. Cells have scanty cytoplasm and round hyperchromatic nuclei. (**c**) Cervical smear of atypical glandular cell of undetermined significance: note the cluster of cells with vacuolated cytoplasm. (**d**) Cervical smear of atypical glandular cell of undetermined significance: clusters of cells with round nuclei and high nucleo cytoplasmic ratio

Adenocarcinoma In Situ

Image gallary: Figs. 3.28 and 3.29
  Incidence

- Uncommon tumour and exact prevalence not known

  Clinical features

- Mean age 29 year
- Common in 4th decade
- Asymptomatic
- Detected at the time of cervical screening

  Cytology

- Cells are in tight cohesive groups (hyperchromatic crowded groups), rosettes/gland and also discrete
- Feathering appearance: The nuclei and cytoplasm appear to be coming out in the periphery of the cluster
- The cells are columnar in appearance
- Nuclei: Enlarged, hyperchromatic with large irregular chromatin.
- Nucleoli: Small to inconspicuous
- Characteristically tumour diathesis is absent

  The most important feature: Absent tumour diathesis
  Histopathology (Table 3.3)

- Normal architecture of the gland is preserved
- Interglandular papillary projections or cribriform appearance may be seen
- Pseudostratification of the cells forming two to multiple rows
- Nuclei show:
  - Enlargement
  - Elongated nuclei give cigar shaped appearance
  - Coarse chromatin
  - Nucleolar prominence
  - Granular eosinophilic cytoplasm with mucin production

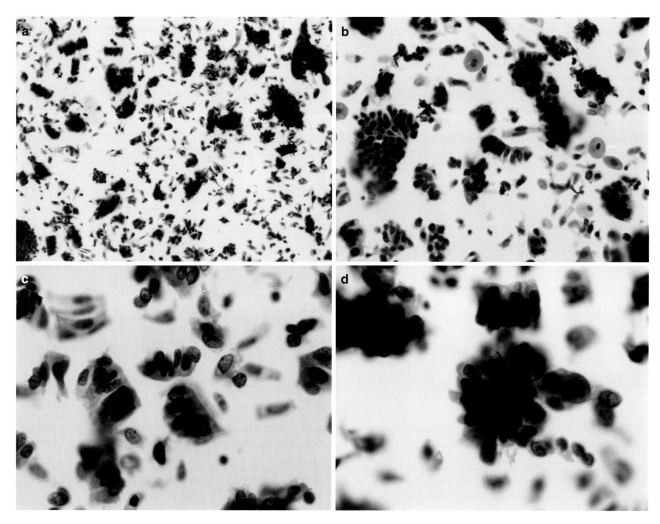

Fig. 3.28 (**a**) Cervical smear of adenocarcinoma in situ: abundant discrete and cohesive clusters of cells. No tumour diathesis is present in such case. (**b**) Cervical smear of adenocarcinoma in situ: strips of cells in a row and discrete columnar cells. (**c**) Cervical smear of adenocarci- noma in situ: the cells have columnar appearance. Nuclei are enlarged and pleomorphic. Nucleoli are small. (**d**) Cervical smear of adenocarci- noma in situ: the cluster of cells with moderate nuclear pleomorphism

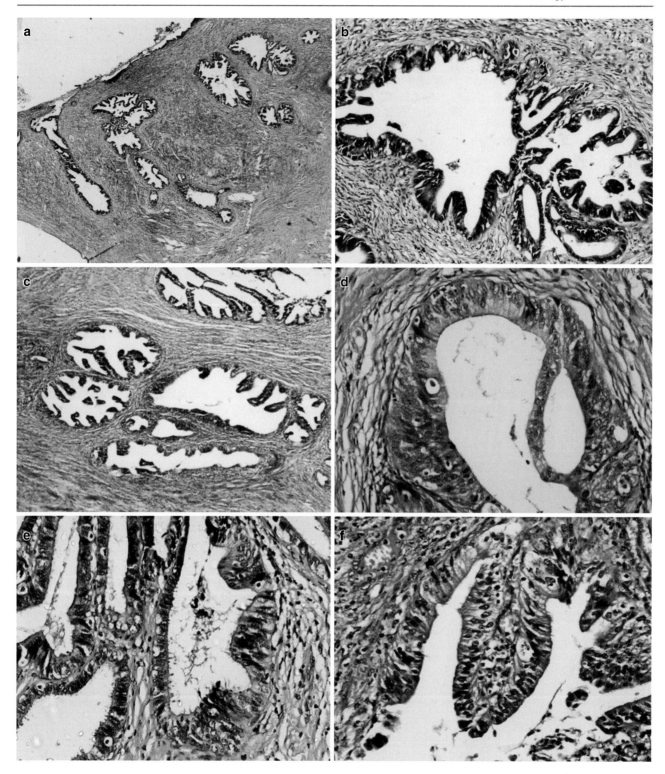

Fig. 3.29 (**a**) Adenocarcinoma in situ: the abnormal glands with pre-served normal architecture. (**b**) Adenocarcinoma in situ: the glands are lined by the cells with moderate nuclear atypia. (**c**) Adenocarcinoma in situ: multiple glands with intact basement membrane. The lining of the gland is multi-layered and shows papillary projections. (**d**) Adenocarcinoma in situ: note the multi-layered epithelial cells. (**e**) Adenocarcinoma in situ: focal crowding of the glandular epithelial cells. (**f**) Adenocarcinoma in situ: the papillary infolding of the lining cells of the glands. (**g**) Adenocarcinoma in situ: small papillary projec-tions by the lining epithelial cells. Note the nuclear atypia. (**h**) Differential diagnosis of adenocarcinoma in situ of cervix

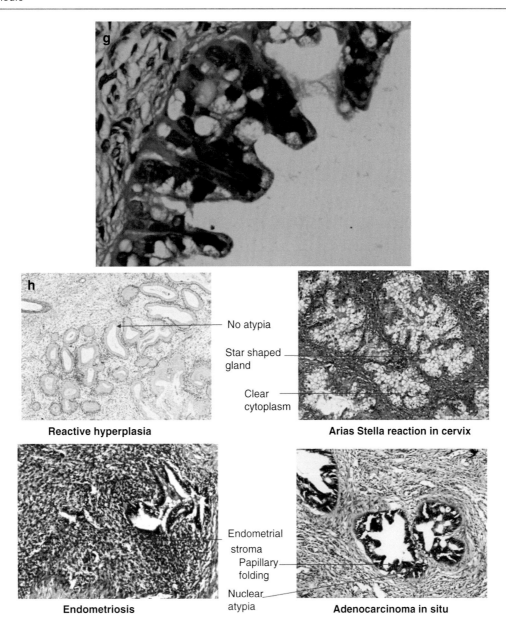

Reactive hyperplasia

Arias Stella reaction in cervix

No atypia

Star shaped gland

Clear cytoplasm

Endometriosis

Adenocarcinoma in situ

Endometrial stroma

Papillary folding

Nuclear atypia

Fig. 3.29 (continued)

- Frequent mitosis

Immunohistochemistry

- Positive for p53, p21 and CEA
- High Ki 67 index

Differential diagnosis (Fig. 3.30h)

- Reactive/reparative atypia: No mitosis, N/C ratio maintained, chromatin pattern normal
- Arias–Stella reaction; Hobnail appearance, abundant clear cytoplasm, no mitosis

- Mitotically active endocervical glands: Lack of nuclear stratification and atypia
- Radiation atypia: Maintained N/C ratio, no stratification, no mitosis
- Endometriosis: Endometrial stroma, hemosiderin laden macrophages, negative for p16, CEA and low Ki 67 index.
- Tubal metaplasia: Lack of nuclear atypia, mitosis, nuclear stratification

Treatment

- Conization with close follow up by cervical smear
- Hysterectomy if family is completed

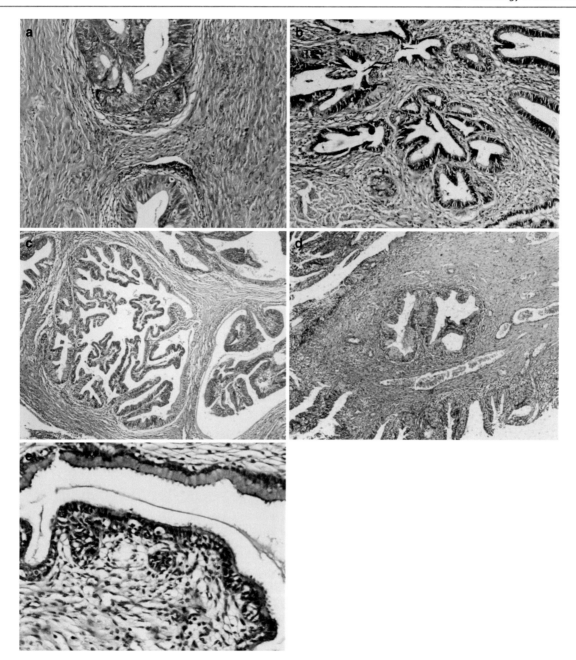

Fig. 3.30 (**a**) Microinvasive carcinoma: cribriform appearance of the glands. (**b**) Microinvasive carcinoma: complex branching pattern of the glands. (**c**) Microinvasive carcinoma: closely spaced glands with archi-tectural disarray. (**d**) Desmoplastic stromal reaction around the glands indicating invasion in the stroma. (**e**) Small islands of cells with periph-eral lymphocytic infiltration indicating microinvasion

Table 3.3   Essential histopathological criteria for adenocarcinoma in situ

Features	Description
Architectural pattern	• Maintained normal architecture of the gland • Papillary infoding of the inner lining of gland
Crowding of cells	• Nuclear true stratification
Nuclear and cytoplasmic abnormality	• Moderately enlarged • Prominent nucleoli • Coarse chromatin • Eosinophilic cytoplasm
Mitosis	• Freuent mitosis
Stromal response	• No desmoplasa • No periglandular lymphocytic infiltration

Microinvasive Carcinoma

Image gallary: Fig. 3.30a–e

Definition: This is the glandular tumour with distortion of the normal architecture and stromal invasion is less than 5 mm from the base of the surface epithelium or the volume of the tumour is less than 500 mm³.

Synonym: Early invasive carcinoma, FIGO stage IA adenocarcinoma

Epidemiology: Approximately 12% of all microinvasive carcinoma (squamous and glandular)

Clinical feature:

- Age: Around 40 years
- Asymptomatic patient
- The patients are initially detected by cervical smear screening and is initially detected as atypical glandular cells
- It is usually confirmed in cone biopsy specimen

Histopathology

- Architecturally abnormal glands
- Cribriform arrangement
- Crab like irregular infiltration of the glandular epithelium in the stroma

- The tumour cells show moderate nuclear pleomorphism
- Villoglandular papillary pattern shows exophytic growth

Features of invasion

- Desmoplastic stromal reaction around the gland
- Isolated small cluster of tumour cells or fragmented glands within the cervical stroma

Criteria of microinvasion: Box 3.1

Box 3.1 FIGO criteria of microinvasion
- Stromal invasion is less than 5 mm in depth
- Horizontal spread or width of the tumour is less than 7 mm

Prognosis and treatment

- Hysterectomy is the treatment of choice
- Conization of cervix can be done if the patient wants family to complete
- Excellent prognosis

Adenocarcinoma

Usual Type of Endocervical Adenocarcinoma

Image gallery: Figs. 3.31a–d and 3.32a–j
  Epidemiology

- Constitutes 70–90% of all the cervical adenocarcinomas

  Association

- High risk HPV

  Clinical features

- Mean age 55 year
- Vaginal bleeding

Gross features

- Commonly polypoid fungating mass/ ulcerated lesion

Cytology

- Cellular smear
- Multiple three dimensional tight cohesive clusters of cells
- Cells arranged as tail of the bird and wings of the bird
- Cells are columnar in look
- Cytoplasmic vacuoles present
- Nuclei show
    - Moderate enlargement
    - Pleomorphism
    - Prominent nucleoli
    - Coarse granular or fine chromatin
- Thin watery tumour diathesis

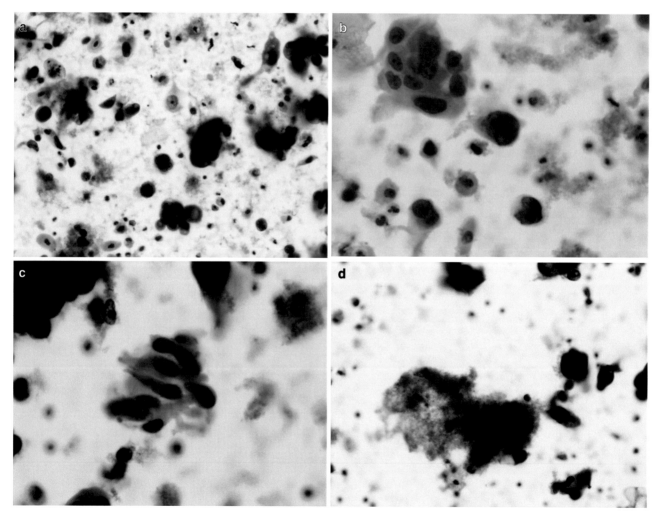

Fig. 3.31 (**a**) Cervical cytology smear of invasive adenocarcinoma: multiple three dimensional tight cohesive clusters of cells along with many discrete cells. (**b**) Cervical cytology smear of invasive adenocarcinoma: cells are round with coarse chromatin and prominent nucleoli.

(**c**) Cervical cytology smear of invasive adenocarcinoma: linear strip of tall columnar cells. (**d**) Cervical cytology smear of invasive adenocarcinoma: tumour diathesis indicates invasive carcinoma

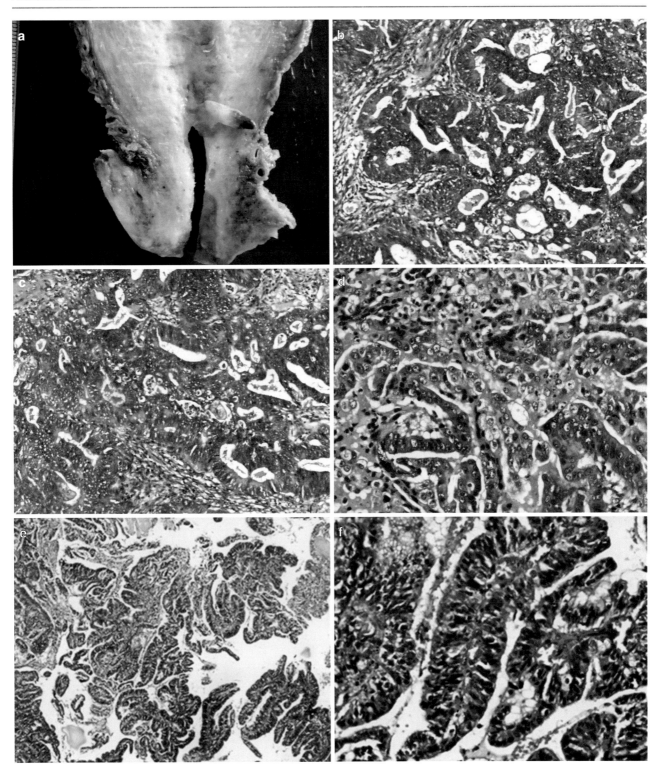

Fig. 3.32 (**a**) Gross picture of endocervical adenocarcinoma: ill defined greyish black lesion in the cervix. (**b**) Usual type of endocervical adenocarcinoma: complex architectural pattern of the glands. Note the cribriform appearance. (**c**) Usual type of endocervical adenocarcinoma: the lining epithelium showing pseudostratification and a mixed character of endometrial and mucinous feature. (**d**) Usual type of endocervical adenocarcinoma: the glandular lining cells are columnar in appearance with large pleomorphic nuclei having a prominent nucleoli. (**e**) Usual type of endocervical adenocarcinoma: multiple papillary con-figuration of the glands. (**f**) Usual type of endocervical adenocarcinoma: higher magnification of the papillae. (**g**) Usual type of endocervical adenocarcinoma: moderately differentiated type. Here the solid component is more than 11–50% area. (**h**) Usual type of endocervical adenocarcinoma: large areas of solid component in a poorly differentiated adenocarcinoma. (**i**) Usual type of endocervical adenocarcinoma: strong p16 expression in tumour cells. (**j**) Usual type of endocervical adenocarcinoma: tumour cells are negative for estragon receptors

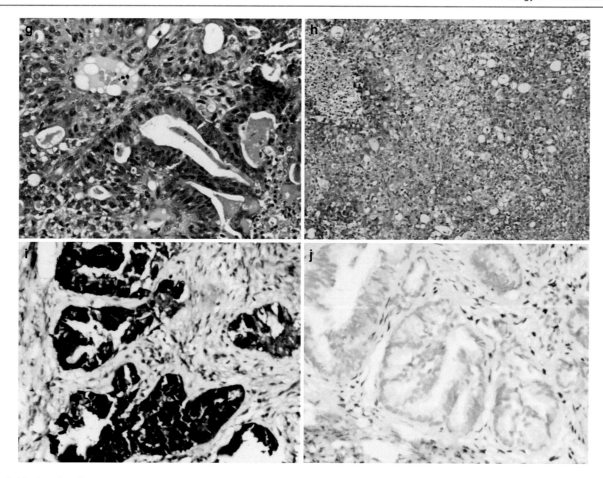

Fig. 3.32 (continued)

Histopathology

- Cribriform appearance or complex architectural pattern
- Desmoplastic reaction around gland
- Glands resemble mixture of endometrioid and endocervical type
- Tall columnar cells with abundant cytoplasm
- Basally placed nuclei with moderate pleomorphism
- Prominent nucleoli
- High mitotic activities

Immunohistochemistry

- Positive for p16 and ProEXC
- High Ki 67 index
- ER and PR negative

Differentiation:

Grade 1: Less than 10% solid component and more than 90% tumour is composed of glands

Grade 2: Solid component is 11–50 % tumour and remaining part is glandular component

Grade 3: More than 50% solid component

Differential diagnosis

- Endometrial adenocarcinoma: In small biopsies it is often difficult to distinguish endocervical and endometrial adenocarcinoma. The following features suggest endocervical adenocarcinoma (Table 3.4)
  - Absence of squamous morules
  - Adenocarcinoma in situ changes
  - Squamous dysplasia of the overlying epithelium
  - Strong p16 positivity
  - Negative ER/PR

Table 3.4 Endocervical versus endometrial adenocarcinoma

Features	Endocervical adenocarcinoma	Endometrial adenocarcinoma
Squamous morules	Usually absent	Often present
Atypical hyperplasia	Absent	Present
Squamous dysplasia of the overlying epithelium	Often present	Absent
Desmoplastic reaction in the stroma	Often present	Absent
Foamy histiocytes	Absent	Present
p16	Strongly positive	Negative
Pro Exc	Strongly positive	Negative
ER/PR	Negative	Positive
Vimentin	Negative	Positive

Mucinous Carcinoma, Not Otherwise Specified

Image gallery: Fig. 3.33a–c

Definition: This is a type of cervical mucinous adenocarcinoma that is difficult to categorize as gastric or intestinal type.

Histopathology

- Invasive adenocarcinoma
- Glands are lined by mucinous epithelium

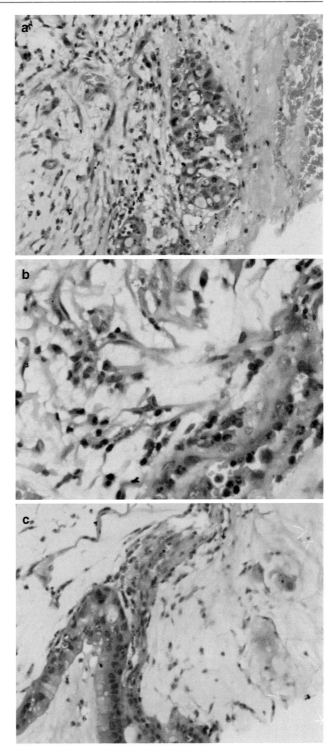

Fig. 3.33 (**a**) Mucinous carcinoma, not otherwise specified: the clusters and discrete tumour cells within the mucus pool. (**b**) Mucinous carcinoma, not otherwise specified: the tumour cells are floating in the pool of mucin. (**c**) Mucinous carcinoma, not otherwise specified: the glands are lined by tall mucus secreting epithelial cells

Mucinous Carcinoma of Gastric Type (Minimal Deviation Adenocarcinoma)

Image gallery: Fig. 3.34a–g

Definition: This is a type of adenocarcinoma that shows differentiation of gastric types

Synonym: Well differentiated variety is also known as minimal deviation adenocarcinoma (MDA) and adenoma malignum

Incidence

- Common type of gastric mucinous adenocarcinoma consists of nearly 25% of cervical adenocarcinoma.
- However, MDA represents only 1–3% of adenocarcinoma of cervix
- Strongly related with Peutz–Jeghers syndrome
- Not related with high risk HPV infection

Clinical features

- Mean age 40 year
- Menorrhagia and mucoid discharge from the vagina

Gross features

- Firm, friable and indurated mass
- At times grossly no abnormality

Histopathology

- Variable sized irregular shaped glands
- Angular projections of the gland
- Cystic dilatation of the gland
- Desmoplastic stroma
- Gland lining: Tall mucous secreting columnar cells often resemble normal endocervical cell

- Occasional foci show cells with enlarged, pleomorphic nuclei

Immunocytochemistry

- Negative: ER and PR, p16 (as it is unrelated with HPV infection)
- Positive: CEA, p53, CK 7
- Often positive for HIK1083, antibody against gastric gland mucin

Differential diagnosis

- Normal endocervical glands: Regular gland architecture, absent in deeper stroma and mostly superficial
- Lobular endocervical hyperplasia: Present in the inner half of cervical wall, lobular architecture
- Tunnel clusters: Uniform architectural pattern, no nuclear atypia or mitosis
- Adenomyoma of endocervical type: Composed of dilated endocervical glands, and smooth muscle. Usually maintains lobular architecture and does not show any desmoplastic reaction.

Essential diagnostic key points: See Box 3.2

Box 3.2 Essential key points in diagnosing MDA
- Irregular chaotic arrangement of the endocervical glands deep in the stroma
- Evidence of mitosis of the glandular lining cells
- Stromal desmoplasia around the gland
- Large variable sized irregular angular outpouching of the gland

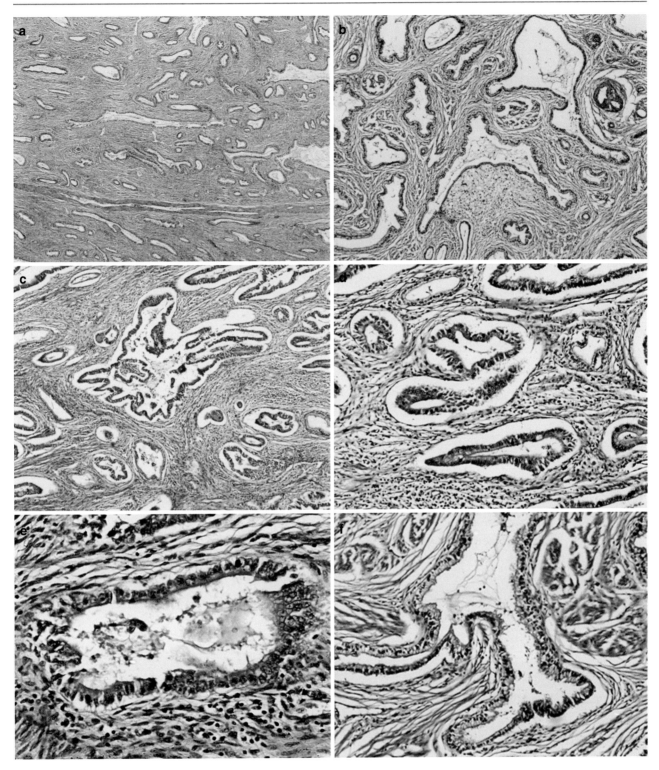

Fig. 3.34 (**a**) Minimal deviation adenocarcinoma: the glands are infiltrated deep in the cervical stroma. (**b**) Minimal deviation adenocarcinoma: the glands apparently look normal, however they are showing architectural abnormality. Note the irregular margin and angulated projections of the margin of the glands. (**c**) Minimal deviation adenocarcinoma: the glandular architecture is abnormal. Note the variable size and branching pattern of the glands. (**d**) Minimal deviation adenocarci-noma: the glandular lining cells are tall mucin secreting columnar cells with mild nuclear pleomorphism. (**e**) Minimal deviation adenocarcinoma: the lining cells of the glands show mild pleomorphism. (**f**) Minimal deviation adenocarcinoma: at places the glandular lining cells are almost normal looking in an architecturally abnormal gland. (**g**) Differential diagnosis of minimal deviation adenocarcinoma of cervix

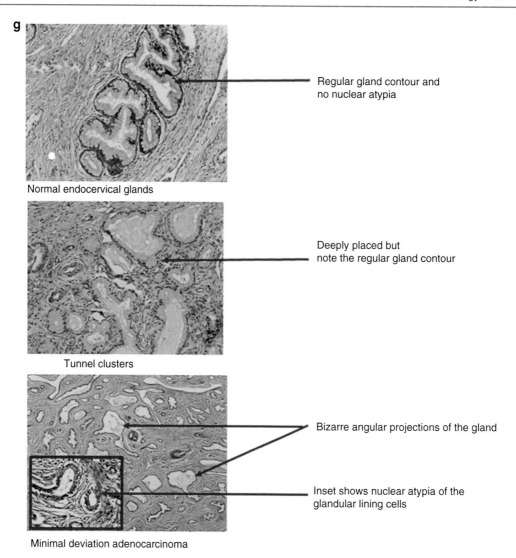

g

Normal endocervical glands

Regular gland contour and
no nuclear atypia

Tunnel clusters

Deeply placed but
note the regular gland contour

Minimal deviation adenocarcinoma

Bizarre angular projections of the gland

Inset shows nuclear atypia of the
glandular lining cells

Fig. 3.34 (continued)

Endometrioid Adenocarcinoma of Cervix

Image gallery: Fig. 3.35a–g
  Incidence: About 30–50% of adenocarcinoma of cervix
  Histopathology

- Cribriform and complex papillary arrangement
- Stratified epithelial cells
- Relatively small cell size with scanty cytoplasm
- Lack of mucin production

  Immunocytochemistry

- Strong diffuse p16 positivity
- CEA positive
- Negative for ER and PR

  Differential diagnosis (Box 3.3)

Box 3.3 Diagnostic clues to differentiate endometrioid cervical versus endometrioid uterine carcinoma

- Note for any atypical glandular hyperplasia elements: Favors uterine origin
- Note for superficial squamous lining with dysplastic changes: Favors cervical origin
- Note the gross findings:
    - Bulky uterus: Favors uterine origin
    - Cervical enlargement in absence enlarged uterus: Favors cervical origin
- P16 immunostaining
    - Strong diffuse: Favors cervical origin
    - Patchy: Favors uterine origin

- *Endometrioid adenocarcinoma of uterus*: Bulky uterus, and immunocytochemistry pattern of patchy p16 positivity, and ER/PR positivity are helpful in diagnosis.

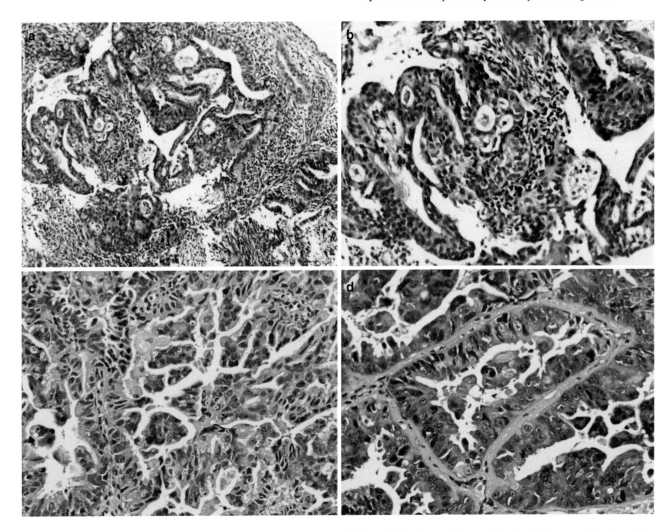

Fig. 3.35 (**a**) Endometrioid type adenocarcinoma of cervix: glands are closely spaced with little intervening stroma. (**b**) Endometrioid adenocarcinoma of cervix: the carcinoma resembles endometrial adenocarcinoma. (**c**) Endometrioid type adenocarcinoma of cervix: the glands are lined by cuboidal epithelial cells with moderate nuclear atypia. (**d**) Endometrioid adenocarcinoma of cervix: higher magnification of the same. (**e**) Endometrioid type adenocarcinoma of cervix: strong p16 positive cells. (**f**) Endometrioid type adenocarcinoma of cervix: ER positive stroma but tumour cells are negative for ER. (**g**) Endometrioid type adenocarcinoma of cervix: CK 7 positive tumour cells

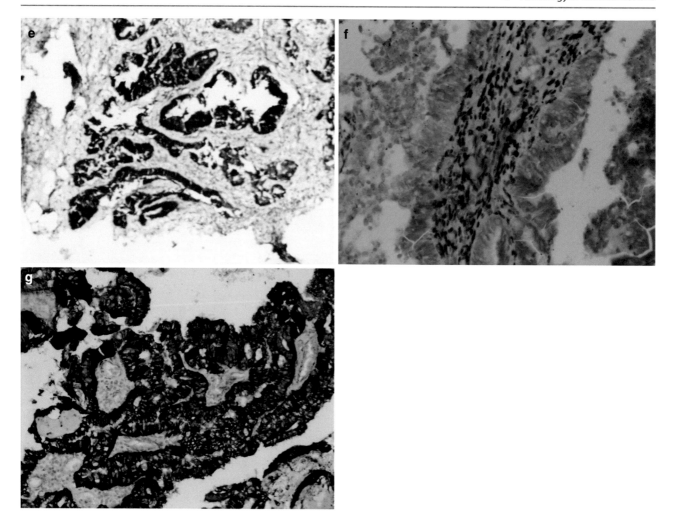

Fig. 3.35 (continued)

Clear Cell Carcinoma

Image gallery: Fig. 3.36a–e

Epidemiology

- Rare in cervix. Only 4% of cervical adenocarcinoma
- Previously it was related with diethylstilbestrol exposure (presently not seen)

Clinical feature

- Mean age of the DES exposed patient is 19 year

Histopathology

- Tubulocystic common, other patterns are solid and papillary
- Prominent hobnail appearance
- Cell with clear vacuolated cytoplasm
- Hyaline globules that are PAS positive

Differential diagnosis

- Microglandular hyperplasia: No mitosis, no atypia
- Arias Stella reaction: Absent of cytological atypia

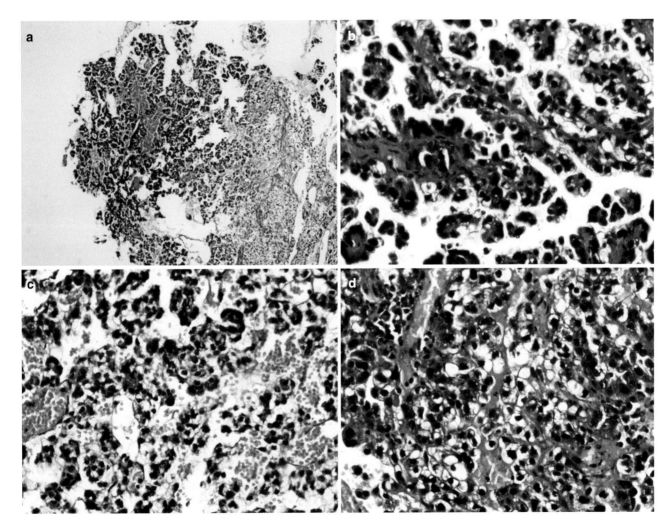

Fig. 3.36 (**a**) Clear cell carcinoma of cervix: papillary structures. (**b**) Clear cell carcinoma of cervix: papillae with fibrovascular core. Note hobnail appearance. (**c**) Clear cell carcinoma of cervix: small groups of tumour cells. (**d**) Clear cell carcinoma of cervix: solid sheet of cells with abundant vacuolated cytoplasm and central nuclei. (**e**) Differential diagnosis of clear cell carcinoma of cervix

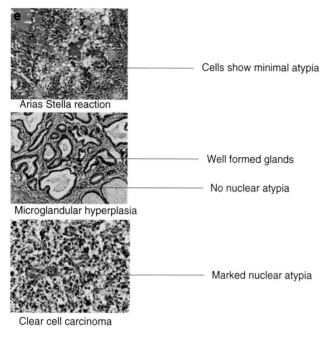

Arias Stella reaction — Cells show minimal atypia

Microglandular hyperplasia — Well formed glands — No nuclear atypia

Clear cell carcinoma — Marked nuclear atypia

Fig. 3.36 (continued)

Serous Carcinoma

Image gallery: Fig. 3.37a–e
Epidemiology

- Rare tumour of cervix and represents less than 1% of cervical adenocarcinoma.
- In young patients it is associated with HPV infection
- Bimodal age distribution
- Metastasis should be excluded

Histopathology

- Multiple complex papillae
- Glands and solid areas
- Cells show enlarged nuclei with prominent nucleoli
- High mitotic activities

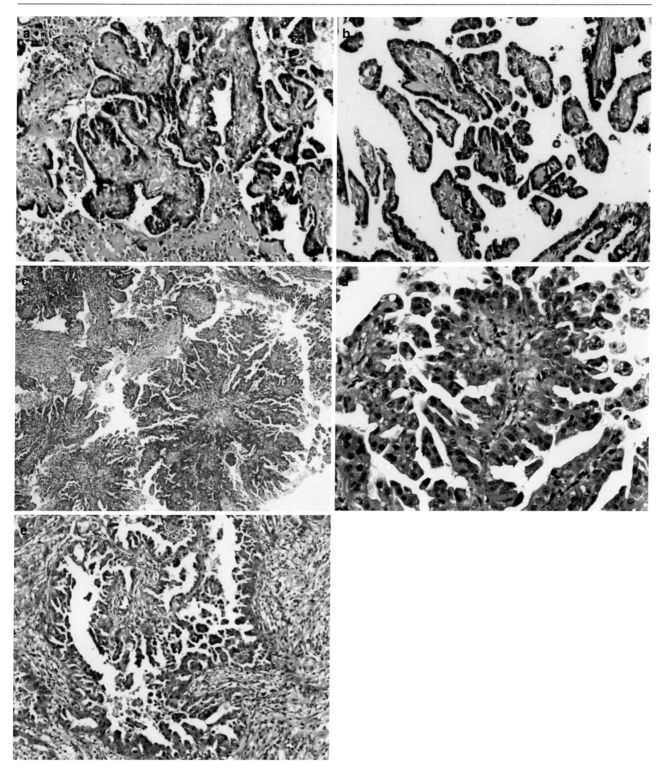

Fig. 3.37 (**a**) Serous carcinoma: multiple complex papillae. (**b**) Serous carcinoma: papillae with fibrovascular core. (**c**) Serous carcinoma: complex papillary configuration. (**d**) Serous carcinoma: higher magnification of papillae. The small microclusters detached from the tip of the papillae. (**e**) Serous carcinoma: small clusters of shredded out cells from the tip of papillae

Mesonephric Carcinoma

Image gallery: Fig. 3.38a, b
    Incidence: Exceedingly rare tumour
    Association: HPV related (high risk type)
    Clinical features

- Mean age 53 year
- Complaints vaginal bleeding

Histopathology

- Abundant irregular tubules
- Gland like structures, slit like channels and papillae
- Crowded glands and tubules
- The tubules are lined by columnar cells with mild nuclear pleomorphism

Immunohistochemistry

- Positive for CK and EMA
- Often shows calretinin and CD 10 positivity

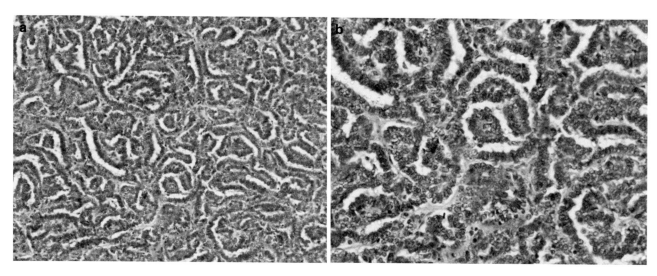

Fig. 3.38 (**a**) Mesonephric carcinoma: tubules and gland like structures. (**b**) Mesonephric carcinoma: multiple tubular structures lined by cuboidal cells

Villoglandular Carcinoma

Image gallery: Fig. 3.39a–e
Epidemiology

- Uncommon tumour of cervix
- HPV related: HPV 16/18/45
- Oral contraceptive related

Clinical features

- Mean age 35 year
- Exophytic growth

Histopathology

- Finger like papillary structures
- Thin central fibrovascular stroma within villi

- Spindle shaped stromal cells in the fibrovascular tissue
- Villus structure is lined by tall columnar cells resemble endocervical or endometrioid type
- Mild nuclear atypia
- Pseudostratification present
- Mitosis frequent

Prognosis

- Excellent prognosis if only superficially invasive
- Conservative surgery: Conization

Differential diagnosis

- Serous carcinoma of cervix:
  - Short and stout papillae
  - Detached tufts of cells
  - Significant nuclear atypia

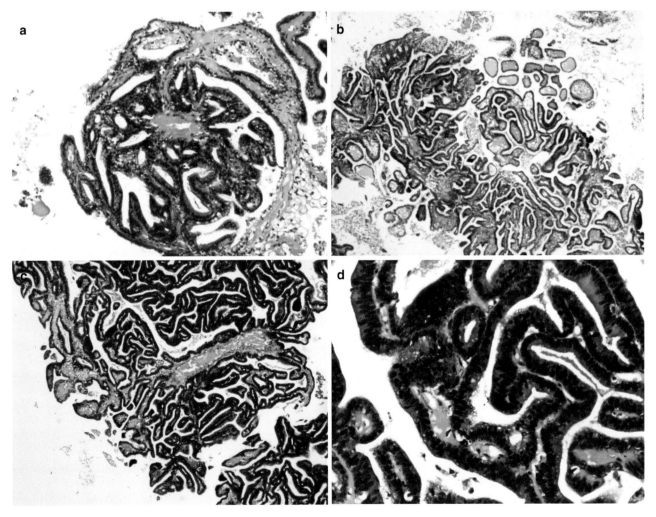

Fig. 3.39 (**a**) Villoglandular carcinoma: tubular and finger like papillary structures. (**b**) Villoglandular carcinoma: multiple villi with fibrovascular core. (**c**) Villoglandular carcinoma: the villi have central thin fibrovascular core. (**d**) Villoglandular carcinoma: higher magnification of the same. The lining cells of the villi are tall columnar with basally placed nuclei. (**e**) Distinguishing features between serous carcinoma and villoglandular carcinoma

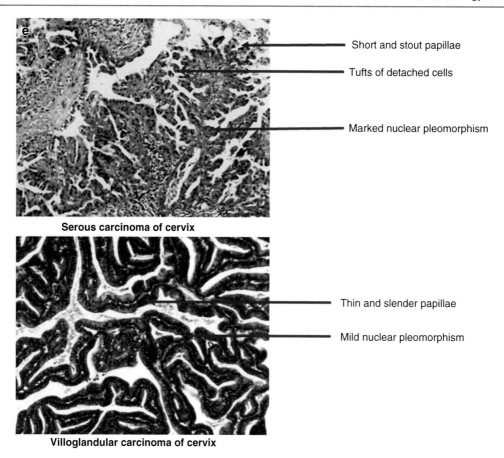

Serous carcinoma of cervix

— Short and stout papillae

— Tufts of detached cells

— Marked nuclear pleomorphism

Villoglandular carcinoma of cervix

— Thin and slender papillae

— Mild nuclear pleomorphism

Fig. 3.39 (continued)

Other Epithelial Tumours

Adenosquamous Carcinoma

Image gallery: Fig. 3.40a, b

Definition: This is a malignant neoplasm consisting of both adenocarcinoma and squamous cell carcinoma

Epidemiology

- About 0.5–2 per 100,000 women
- The incidence varies from 25 to 50% depending on the defining criteria of squamous elements
- If only definitely recognizable squamous element is considered then the tumour represents approximately 28% of adenocarcinomas
- HPV related: HPV 16 and HPV 18

Clinical features

- Mean age is 57 years
- Vaginal bleeding
- Located near the transformation zone

Histopathology

- Malignant glands are either mucus secreting or endometrioid type
- Clearly recognizable squamous cell carcinoma with evidence of either intercellular bridging or keratinization
- Poorly differentiated component show solid sheets of cells with abundant glassy eosinophilic cytoplasm

Differential diagnosis

- Poorly differentiated squamous cell carcinoma: Occasionally the tumour may show discrete mucus producing cells
- Endometrioid adenocarcinomas: This tumour may show foci of squamous differentiation and should not be considered as adenosquamous carcinoma. In case of adenosquamous carcinoma, the glandular epithelial cells are endocervical type

Prognosis

- No difference in prognosis when compared with squamous cell carcinoma of same stage
- Possibly poor prognostic outcome in advanced stage

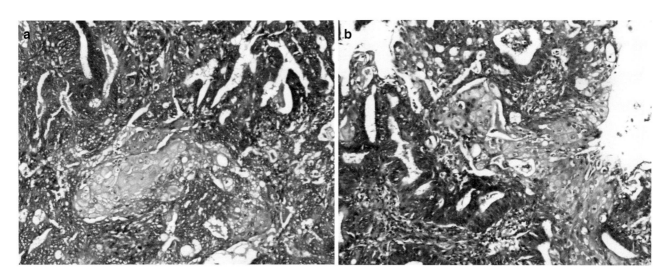

Fig. 3.40 (**a**) Adenosquamous carcinoma: adenocarcinoma with foci of squamous component. (**b**) Adenosquamous carcinoma: note the adenocarcinoma and also squamous area. The squamous component shows features of malignancy

Adenoid Cystic Carcinoma

Image gallery: Fig. 3.41a, b
  Epidemiology

- Rare tumour, represents less than 1% of cervical carcinomas
- Mean age 60 years
- Associated with HPV infection

  Clinical features

- Post-menopausal bleeding
- Exophytic growth in cervix

Histopathology

- Resembles adenoid cystic carcinoma of salivary gland
- Cribriform, tubular, nests or solid pattern
- Basaloid cells with scanty cytoplasm and round mildly pleomorphic hyperchromatic nuclei having inconspicuous nucleoli
- Eosinophilic hyaline material within the gland like structure or cyst that represents basal lamina
- Frequent mitotic activity

  Immunohistochemistry

- Positive: EMA, CEA and also S-100 protein

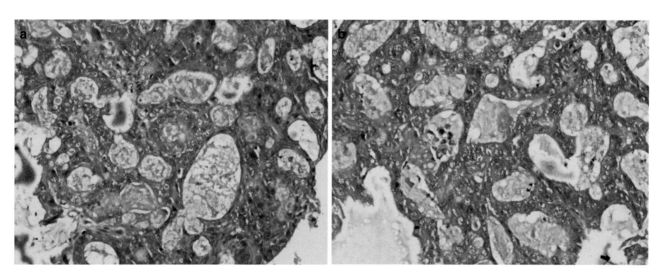

Fig. 3.41 (**a**) Adenoid cystic carcinoma: cribriform pattern of tumour. (**b**) Adenoid cystic carcinoma: note the relatively monomorphic basaloid cells with scanty cytoplasm and round mildly pleomorphic hyperchromatic nuclei

- Negative: Unlike salivary gland adenoid cystic carcinoma the cervical one is negative for various myoepithelial markers such as calponin, smooth muscle actin etc

Differential diagnosis

Adenoid basal cell carcinoma: Almost similar morphology, however it does not show any stromal desmoplasia or hyaline globules, and lacks mitosis. It has better prognosis than ADC.

Prognosis

- Aggressive
- Metastasis and frequent local recurrence are common

Reporting cervical carcinoma

The reporting of cervical carcinoma is highlighted in the Box 3.4 and Fig. 3.42

Box 3.4 Reporting cervical carcinoma
- Microscopic appearance
- Histological type
- Grade of tumour
- Depth of tumour invasion in the wall: Measure from the basement membrane to the innermost depth of invasion
- Thickness of the lateral wall of the cervix and extension of the tumour in the lateral wall
- Lymphovascular involvement
- Any associated changes in the epithelium (intraepithelial neoplasm or adenocarcinoma in situ)
- Status of the margins
- Involvement of the other organs: uterus, vagina, pelvic wall, and bladder
- Vaginal cuff
- Lymph node status
- Ancillary investigations: HPV status, Ploidy of the tumour etc.

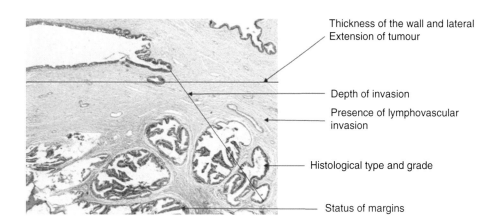

Thickness of the wall and lateral Extension of tumour

Depth of invasion

Presence of lymphovascular invasion

Histological type and grade

Status of margins

Fig. 3.42 Reporting cervical carcinoma

Neuroendocrine Tumours

Large Cell Neuroendocrine Tumours

Image gallery: Fig. 3.43a–c
   Synonym: Neuroendocrine carcinoma
   Histopathology

- Organoid, trabecular, ribbon like pattern
- Large cells with moderate amount of cytoplasm
- Enlarged nuclei with prominent nucleoli
- Frequent mitosis

Immunohistochemistry

- Positive: NSE, chromogranin, and synaptophysin

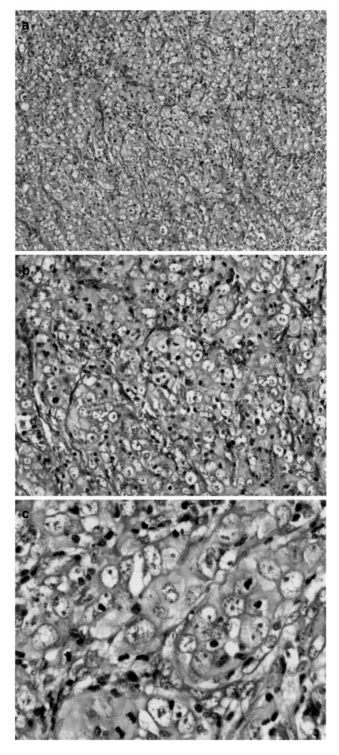

Fig. 3.43 (**a**) Large cell neuroendocrine tumours of cervix: organoid pattern of tumour cells. (**b**) Large cell neuroendocrine tumours of cervix: nest of cells separated by thin fibrous septa. (**c**) Large cell neuroendocrine tumours of cervix: large cells with moderate amount of cytoplasm having enlarged nuclei with prominent nucleoli

Small Cell Carcinoma

Image gallery: Fig. 3.44a–f
  Epidemiology

- Consists of 6% of carcinoma of cervix
- Frequently (80%) related with HPV infection

Clinical feature

- Mean age 36 year
- Vaginal bleeding
- Paraneoplastic syndrome such as Cushing's disease

Macroscopy

- Ulcerated lesion
- Exophytic mass

Histopathology

- Nests, insular or trabecular arrangement
- Small cells with scanty cytoplasm
- Round nuclei with fine stippled chromatin
- Inconspicuous nucleoli
- Nuclear smudging and artifact present

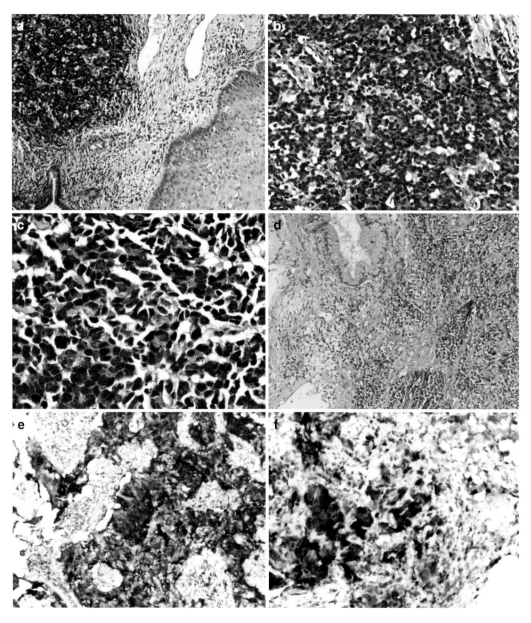

Fig. 3.44 (**a**) Small cell neuroendocrine tumours of cervix: solid sheets of tumour cells with intact squamous epithelial lining. (**b**) Small cell neuroendocrine tumours of cervix: small cells with scanty cytoplasm having hyperchromatic nuclei. (**c**) Small cell neuroendocrine tumours of cervix: higher magnification shows compressed oval to elongated nuclei. (**d**) Small cell neuroendocrine tumours of cervix: tumour infiltrates in the deeper stroma with intact endocervical gland. (**e**) Small cell neuroendocrine tumours of cervix: strong synaptophysin positive tumour cells. (**f**) Small cell neuroendocrine tumours of cervix: strong neurone specific enolase positive tumour cells. (**g**) Differential diagnosis of small cell neuroendocrine tumour of Cervix

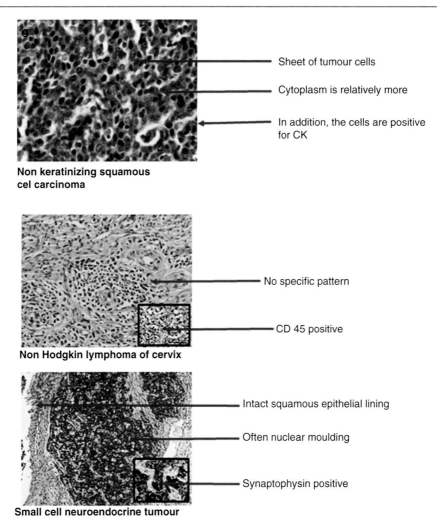

Non keratinizing squamous cel carcinoma — Sheet of tumour cells; Cytoplasm is relatively more; In addition, the cells are positive for CK

Non Hodgkin lymphoma of cervix — No specific pattern; CD 45 positive

Small cell neuroendocrine tumour — Intact squamous epithelial lining; Often nuclear moulding; Synaptophysin positive

Fig. 3.44 (continued)

Immunohistochemistry

- Positive: NSE, chromogranin, synaptophysin, low-molecular-weight keratin, EMA, and CEA

Differential diagnosis (Fig. 3.44g)

- Non keratinizing squamous cell carcinoma: Usually present in solid sheet and positive for neuroendocrine markers (Box 3.5)
- Non Hodgkin lymphoma: Positive for CD 45

Prognosis

- Aggressive malignancy
- Patient dies within one year

Treatment
Surgery and adjuvant chemotherapy

Box 3.5 Diagnostic clues of small cell carcinoma of cervix to distinguish it from squamous cell carcinoma
Morphology

- Note for favorable points of small cell carcinoma:
  - Any specific pattern: Trabecular, nest or insular
  - Normal overlying epithelium
  - Any crushing artefact or nuclear moulding: Favors small cell carcinoma
  - Absence of cell to cell junction

Immunohistochemistry

- Strongly positive for p16 as they are HPV related
- Negative for p63 (squamous cell carcinomas are positive for p63)
- Overlapping neuroendocrine markers may be confusing
- TTF 1 positivity may not be helpful to eliminate the metastasis from the lung

Benign Glandular Tumours and Tumour Like Lesions

Endocervical Polyp

Image gallery: Fig. 3.45a, b
   Epidemiology

- The commonest lesion of cervix
- It is seen in 5th decade of life
- May occur at any age

   Clinical features

- Bleeding per vagina
- Vaginal discharge

Gross

- Usually single
- Sessile or pedunculated
- Variable sized

Histopathology

- Fibroepithelial tissue
- Outer lining by endocervical mucus secreting cells or squamous metaplastic cell
- Stroma shows capillaries and loose connective tissue
- Dilated endocervical glands may be seen in the stroma

Prognosis and treatment

- Benign lesion and simple polypectomy is the treatment of choice

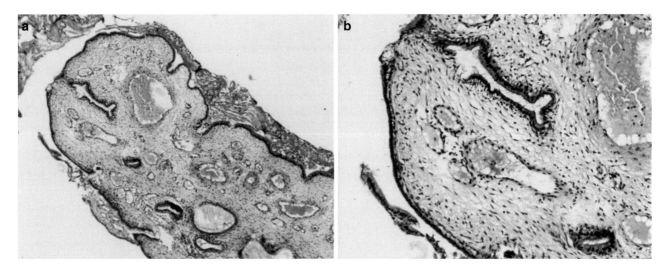

Fig. 3.45 (**a**) Endocervical polyp: fibroepithelial tissue lined by endocervical epithelium in all three sides. (**b**) Endocervical polyp: the stroma shows capillaries and loose connective tissue along with dilated endocervical glands

Nabothian Cyst

Image gallery: Fig. 3.46a, b
  Epidemiology

- The commonest acquired cyst

  Location

- Within the transformation zone

Cause

- Blockage of the crypt of the endocervical gland and accumulation of secretion

Histopathology

- Cystically dilated gland
- Lining of the cyst is tall columnar epithelium that may be flattened

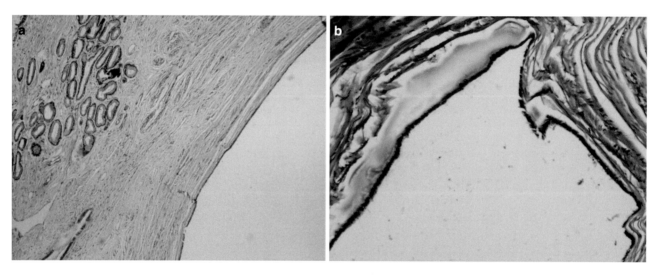

Fig. 3.46 (**a**) Nabothian cyst: cystically dilated gland. (**b**) Nabothian cyst: the cyst is lined by cuboidal to flattened endocervical cells

Tunnel Clusters

Image gallery: Fig. 3.47a, b

Definition: Collection of benign endocervical glands within the wall of cervix

Epidemiology

- Commonly present in multiparous women
- Approximately 8% adult women shows tunnel cluster

- Incidental finding in resected specimen of cervix

Histopathology

- Aggregates of closely spaced endocervical glands
- Glands are of variable sized
- Occasionally the glands are dilated
- Lining of the gland is mucus secreting cuboidal to columnar cells

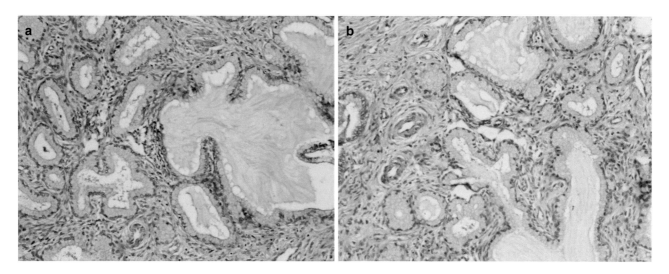

Fig. 3.47 (**a**) Tunnel clusters: aggregates of closely spaced endocervical glands deep within the stroma. (**b**) Tunnel clusters: variable sized glands lined by mucus secreting columnar cells

Endocervical Glandular Hyperplasia (Lobular)

Image gallery: Fig. 3.48a–c
Clinical features

- Incidental finding
- Asymptomatic
- Occasionally mucus or watery discharge
- Often associated with Peutz Jeghers syndrome

Histopathology

- Proliferation of the endocervical glands
- Lobular architectural pattern
- Gland lining: Mucus secreting columnar epithelial cells

Differential diagnosis

- Well differentiated adenocarcinoma: Stromal invasion, desmoplastic reaction, nuclear atypia and mitosis are present

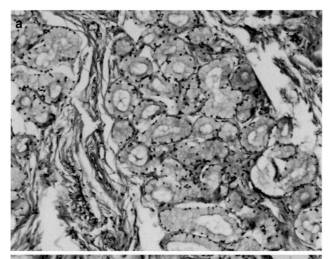
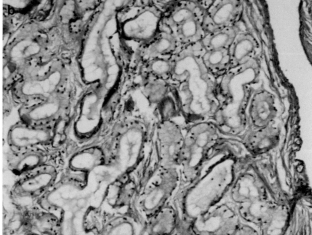
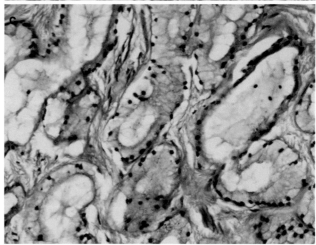

Fig. 3.48 (**a**) Endocervical glandular hyperplasia (lobular): proliferation of the endocervical glands. (**b**) Endocervical glandular hyperplasia (lobular): lobular architectural pattern of the aggregated glands. (**c**) Endocervical glandular hyperplasia (lobular): glands are lined by mucus secreting columnar epithelial cells

Microglandular Hyperplasia

Image gallery: Fig. 3.49a–c
  Epidemiology

- Commonly seen in reproductive age period
- Often associated with pregnancy or oral contraceptive use

  Clinical features

- Usually asymptomatic, incidental finding
- Post coital bleeding

  Histopathology

- Multiple closely packed variable sized glands
- Cystically dilated
- Glands lined by cuboidal to columnar mucus secreting cells

- Minimal nuclear atypia
- Signet ring cell may be present
- Squamous metaplasia is seen
- Stroma may have inflammatory cells

Differential diagnosis (Box 3.6) (Fig. 3.49d)

- Well differentiated adenocarcinoma: Lack of stromal invasion and bland looking epithelial cells along with low mitotic count exclude adenocarcinoma
- Clear cell carcinoma: Papillary structure, stromal invasion, nuclear atypia are features of clear cell carcinoma.

Prognosis

- Benign
- No malignant potential

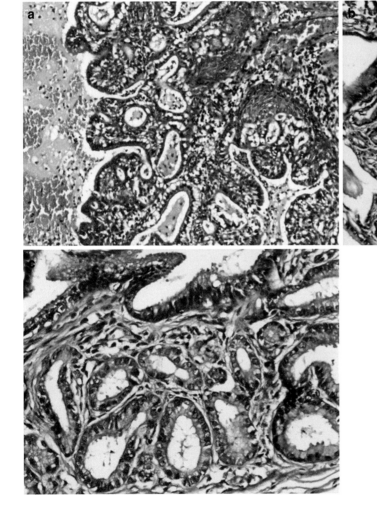

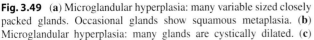

Fig. 3.49 (**a**) Microglandular hyperplasia: many variable sized closely packed glands. Occasional glands show squamous metaplasia. (**b**) Microglandular hyperplasia: many glands are cystically dilated. (**c**) Microglandular hyperplasia: glands lined by cuboidal to columnar mucus secreting cells. (**d**) Differential diagnosis of microglandular hyperplasia

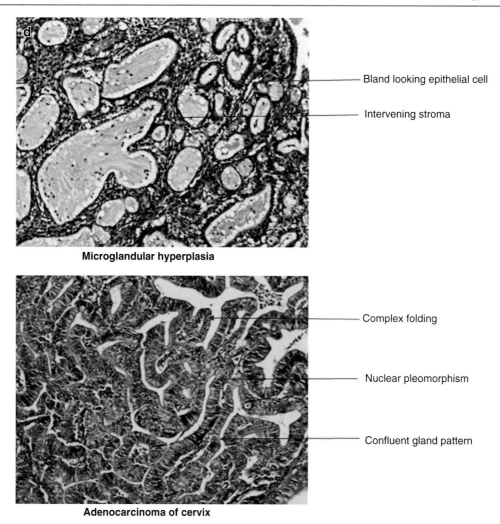

Microglandular hyperplasia

Bland looking epithelial cell

Intervening stroma

Complex folding

Nuclear pleomorphism

Confluent gland pattern

Adenocarcinoma of cervix

Fig. 3.49 (continued)

Box 3.6 Diagnostic key points to differentiate from adenocarcinoma
- Intervening stroma in between glands
- No stromal invasion: The most important feature
- Bland looking epithelium
- Focal squamous metaplasia
- Low mitotic count

Arias Stella Reaction

Image gallery: Fig. 3.50a–c
Epidemiology

- Occasionally present in the pregnant patient
- Usually located in proximal part of cervix
- Incidental finding

Histopathology

- Multiple star shaped dilated glands
- Pseudostratification
- Papilla formation of the lining epithelium
- Hobnail appearance
- Lining cells of the glands have abundant clear cytoplasm
- Hyperchromatic nuclei

Differential diagnosis

- Clear cell adenocarcinoma: Mass like lesion, stromal invasion, significant atypia and mitosis

Prognosis

- Benign
- No malignant potential

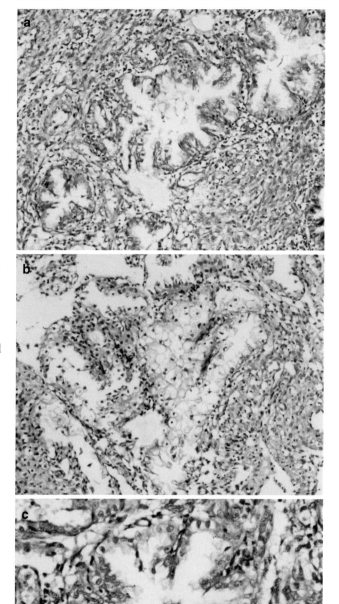

Fig. 3.50 (**a**) Arias Stella reaction: multiple star shaped dilated glands. (**b**) Arias Stella reaction: the glands are lined by cells with abundant clear cytoplasm and central monomorphic nuclei. (**c**) Arias Stella reaction: higher magnification of the glands

Endometriosis

Image gallery: Fig. 3.51a, b
  Epidemiology

- Present in reproductive age period
- Incidental

Mechanism

- Unknown
- Possibly implantation after surgical trauma in cervix such as after cone biopsy

Clinical features

- Usually asymptomatic

Gross features

- Small reddish nodular lesion
- Occasionally small cystic

Histopathology

- Endometrial glands
- Endometrial stroma
- Pigment laden macrophages

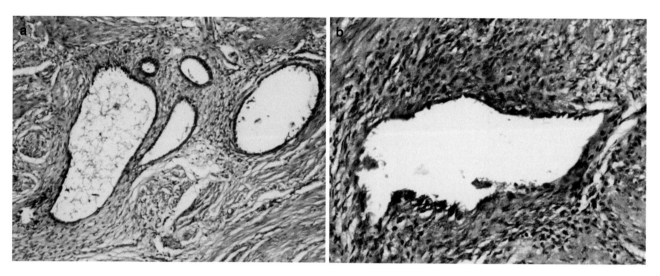

Fig. 3.51 (**a**) Endometriosis: endometrial glands embedded in the endometrial stroma. (**b**) Endometriosis: endometrial gland lined by cuboidal cells. Note the characteristic endometrial stroma

Mesenchymal Tumours and Tumour Like Lesions

Leiomyoma

Image gallery: Fig. 3.52a, b
  Incidence

- Relatively uncommon in cervix compared to uterus
- Represents only 8% of total leiomyoma of uterus

  Histogenesis

- Discrete smooth muscle cells of the uterus

  Clinical features

- Vaginal bleeding
- Dyspaerunia

Gross

- Grey white mass
- Cut surface whorled

Histopathology

- Same as uterine leiomyoma
- Bundles of oval to spindle cells with elongated blunt ended nuclei

Criteria of malignancy

- Same as mentioned in uterus

Prognosis

- Benign tumour and simple surgical resection is enough

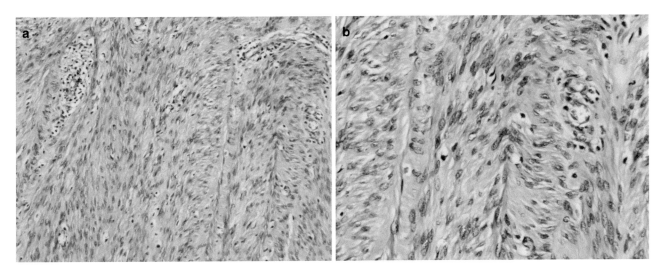

Fig. 3.52 (**a**) Leiomyoma: long fascicles of smooth muscle. (**b**) Leiomyoma: higher magnification of the same showing spindle cells with blunt ended nuclei

Malignant

Leiomyosarcoma

Image gallery: Fig. 3.53a, c
    Epidemiology

- The commonest sarcoma of cervix
- Sarcoma represents less than 1% of cancer cervix

    Histogenesis

- Occasional smooth muscle cells present in the cervix

    Clinical features

- Polyp like mass in cervix
- Vaginal bleeding

    Gross features

- Polypoid growth
- Protruding from the cervical canal
- Fleshy
- Grey white appearance

    Histopathology

- Interlacing fascicles of spindle cells with high mitotic activity
- Foci of coagulative necrosis

    Criteria of malignancy (at least two criteria should be present)

- Moderate nuclear pleomorphism
- Coagulative necrosis
- Mitosis: more than 10/10 high power field

    Immunocytochemistry

- Positive for desmin, h-caldesmon and SMA

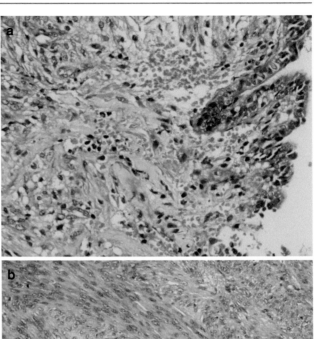
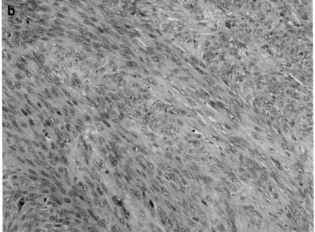
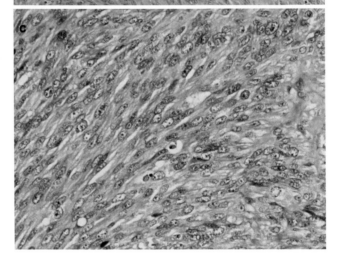

Fig. 3.53 (**a**) Leiomyosarcoma: the tumour underneath the endocervical lining epithelium. (**b**) Leiomyosarcoma: interlacing fascicles of spindle cells with high mitotic activity. (**c**) Leiomyosarcoma: higher magnification of the same

Rhabdomyosarcoma

Image gallery: Fig. 3.54a–d
  Synonym: Sarcoma botryoides
  Epidemiology

- Overall a rare tumour
- In adult population the cervix is the commonest site in female genital tract

Clinical feature

- Bleeding per vagina
- Protruding polypoid lesion

Gross findings

- Polypoid mass, soft and fleshy
- Hemorrhage and necrosis

Histopathology

- Prominent cambium layer: Subepithelial dense collection of tumour cells
- Oval to spindle tumour cells
- Skeletal muscle differentiation
- Occasionally cartilage present

Immunohistochemistry

- Positive: Desmin, myogenin

Prognosis and treatment

- Cervical rhabdomyosarcoma has relatively better prognosis than vaginal one
- Surgery followed by chemotherapy

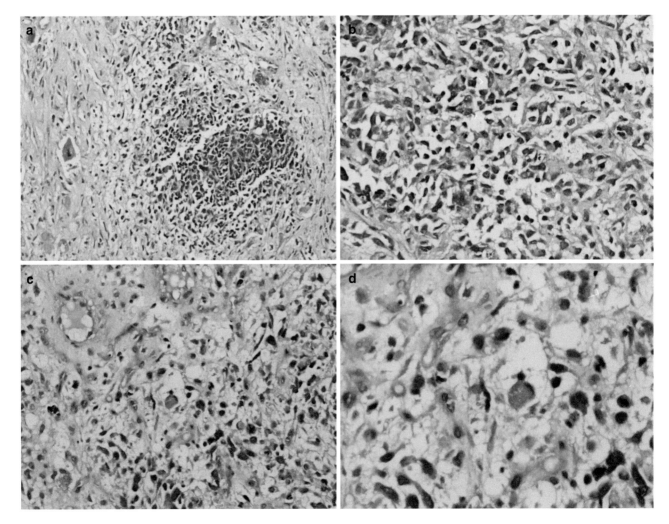

Fig. 3.54 (**a**) Rhabdomyosarcoma: focal collection of tumour cells. (**b**) Rhabdomyosarcoma: oval to spindle tumour cells. (**c**) Rhabdomyosarcoma: discrete tumour cells with round moderately pleomorphic nuclei. (**d**) Rhabdomyosarcoma: rhabdoid differentiation of the cells. Note deep pink cytoplasm and eccentric nuclei

Endometrial Stromal Sarcoma

Image gallery: Fig. 3.55a, b

Endometrial stromal sarcoma of the cervix is very rare. It is usually secondarily involved in the cervix.

The primary tumour in the cervix develops from the endometriotic foci.

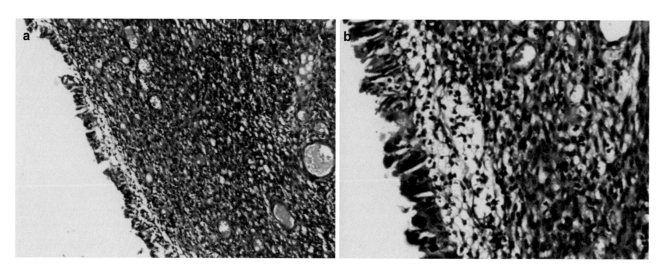

Fig. 3.55 (**a**) Endometrial stromal sarcoma: the diffuse sheets of tumour cells underneath the endocervical lining. (**b**) Endometrial stromal sarcoma: the tumour cells resemble endometrial stromal cells

Mixed Epithelial Mesenchymal Tumour

Adenomyoma

Image gallery: Fig. 3.56a, b
Clinical features

- Rare tumour
- Average age 40 year
- Either asymptomatic or mass protruding from cervical canal
- Polypoid mass

Gross

- Polyp
- Usually circumscribed
- Variable size
- Greyish
- Trabecular appearance on cut section

Histopathology

- Multiple endocervical or endometrial glands
- Usually endocervical glandular component
- The glands are encircled by smooth muscle tissue

Differential diagnosis

- Minimal deviation adenocarcinoma: Not circumscribed, desmoplastic reaction present

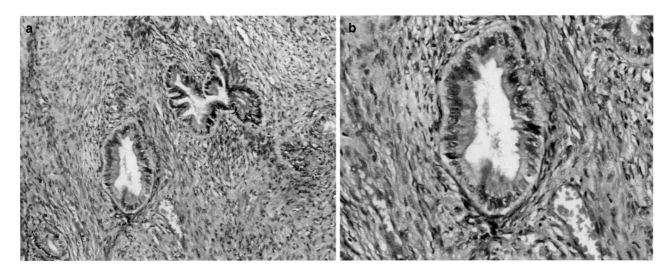

Fig. 3.56 (**a**) Adenomyoma: multiple endocervical glands surrounded by smooth muscle. (**b**) Adenomyoma: the endocervical mucin secreting columnar lining

Adenosarcoma

Image gallery: Fig. 3.57a–e
   Definition: It is a mixed Müllerian tumour that consists of benign epithelial component glands along with sarcoma.
   Epidemiology

- Extremely rare
- Only 2% of adenosarcoma of the female genital tract

   Clinical features

- Mean age 38 year
- Vaginal bleeding
- Polypoid mass in the cervix

   Gross

- Polypoid mass

Histopathology

- Multiple uniformly distributed benign glands
- Mostly endocervical glands
- Stroma is cellular and composed of oval to spindle cells
- Mitosis: At least 2 per 10 high power field is mandatory for the diagnosis of sarcoma

Differential diagnosis

- Adenomyoma: Smooth muscle present
- Atypical endocervical polyp: No stromal overgrowth and mitosis
- Prolapsed leiomyoma of cervix: Smooth muscle cells with no atypia

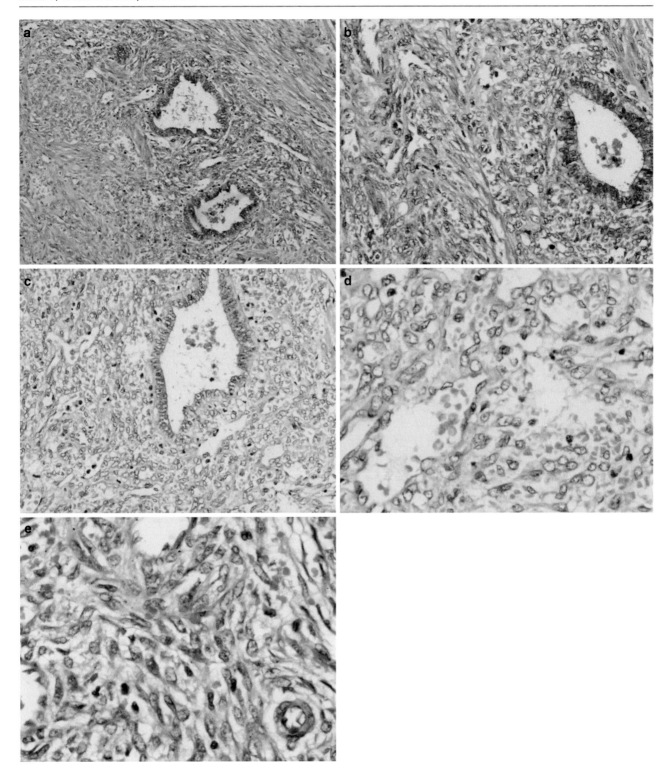

Fig. 3.57 (**a**) Adenosarcoma: multiple uniformly distributed benign glands. (**b**) Adenosarcoma: stroma is cellular and composed of oval to spindle cells. (**c**) Adenosarcoma: the stromal cells are condensed around the benign gland. (**d**) Adenosarcoma: the pleomorphic stromal cells showing high mitotic activity. (**e**) Adenosarcoma: note the moderately pleomorphic oval to spindle cells in the stroma with high mitosis

Carcinosarcoma

Image gallery: Fig. 3.58a–e
  Epidemiology

- Uncommon tumour in cervix
- Only 0.005% of all cervical cancer

  Clinical features

- It is present in post-menopausal patient
- Mean age 60 year
- Vaginal bleeding

  Gross

- Polypoid fungating mass
- Ulcerated surface
- Fleshy
- Hemorrhage and necrosis

Histopathology

- Epithelial part: commonly squamous, occasionally adenocarcinoma or adenoid cystic carcinoma
- Sarcoma part:
  - Homologous: Bundles of oval to spindle cells
  - heterologous sarcoma: Rhabdoid or chondroid material

Differential diagnosis

- Low grade adenosarcoma: Benign glandular element is easily recognizable
- Uterine carcinosarcoma extended to cervix: Large area of tumour is located in uterus.

Prognosis and treatment

- Mainly confined locally so may have better prognosis
- Surgery along with radiation

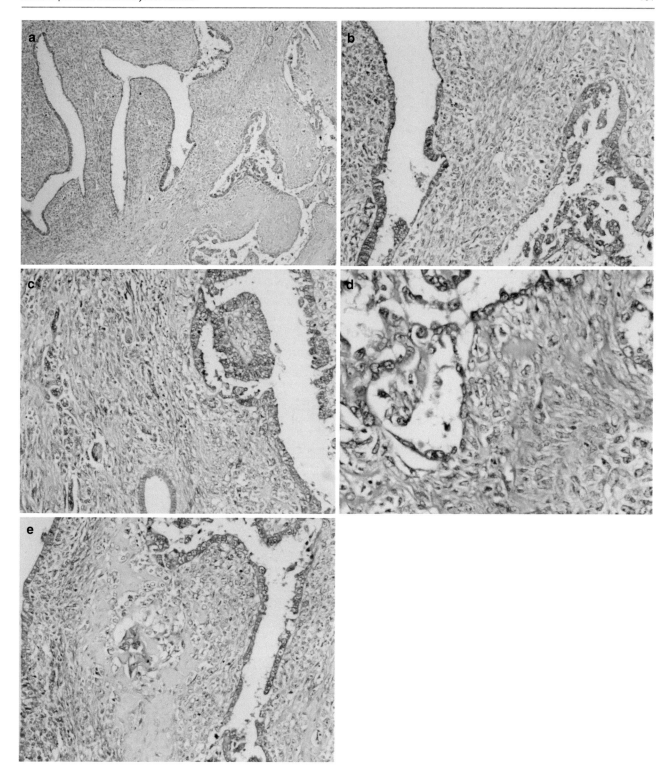

Fig. 3.58 (**a**) Carcinosarcoma: malignant stromal and glandular components. (**b**) Carcinosarcoma: adenocarcinoma elements showing moderately pleomorphic cells of the epithelial lining. The sarcomatous stroma is composed of oval to spindle cells. (**c**) Carcinosarcoma: serous adenocarcinoma and homologous sarcomatous element. (**d**) Carcinosarcoma: higher magnification showing malignant glands and stroma. (**e**) Carcinosarcoma: osteoid elements showing pinkish material and large pleomorphic cells indicating osteosarcoma of the sarcoma part

Miscellaneous

Lymphoma of Cervix

Image gallery: Fig. 3.59a–c
  Incidence

- Primary lymphoma is rare
- Usually secondary to systemic lymphoma

  Clinical feature

- Vaginal bleeding
- Dyspareunia
- Cervical mass

  Types: Diffuse large B cell lymphoma, follicular lymphoma
  Histopathology

- Diffuse sheets, cords, trabeculae
- Immature lymphoid cells

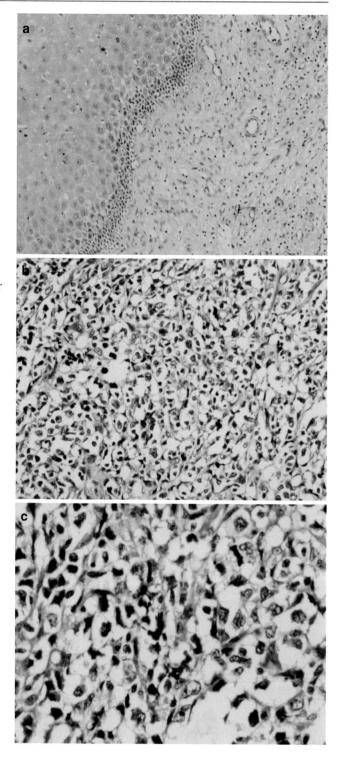

Fig. 3.59 (**a**) Lymphoma of cervix: diffuse loosely arranged cells underneath the squamous epithelium in diffuse large B cell lymphoma secondarily involving the cervix. (**b**) Lymphoma of cervix: the cells are predominantly round to oval with scanty cytoplasm. (**c**) Lymphoma of cervix: higher magnification of the same

Malignant Melanoma

Image gallery: Fig. 3.60a, b
   Incidence: Very rare
   Clinical features

- Adult patient
- Vaginal bleeding

Histopathology

- Diffuse sheets
- Oval to spindle cells with abundant cytoplasm
- Prominent large nucleoli
- Cytoplasmic melanin pigment present
- Junctional activity present

Immunocytochemistry

- Positive for HMB 45 and melan A

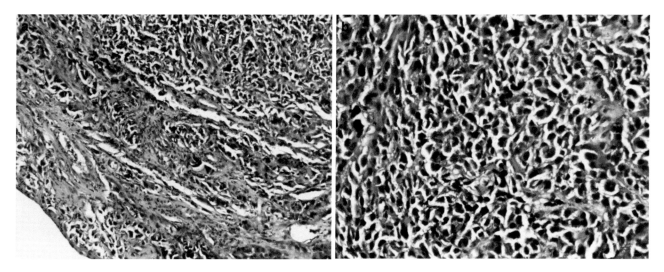

Fig. 3.60 (**a**) Malignant melanoma: the tumour under the squamous epithelium. (**b**) Malignant melanoma: note the sheets of tumour cells with intercellular brownish melanin pigment

Metastasis in Cervix

Isthmus of cervix: Metastatic signet ring carcinoma
Image gallery: Figs. 3.61a, b and 3.62a, b.
Primary sites:

- Commonly it gets metastasis from the other sites of the female genital tract such as uterus, ovary and fallopian tube.

- Rarely breast or gastrointestinal carcinomas metastasize in the cervix.

Histopathology: The histopathological features mainly depend upon the types of primary tumour.

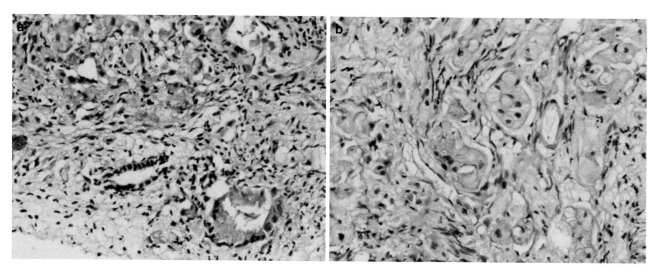

Fig. 3.61 (**a**) Metastatic signet ring carcinoma: the diffuse sheets of tumour cells around the benign endocervical glands. This is a case of metastatic signet ring carcinoma from the stomach. (**b**) Metastatic sig- net ring carcinoma: the individual cells have abundant cytoplasm with eccentric nuclei

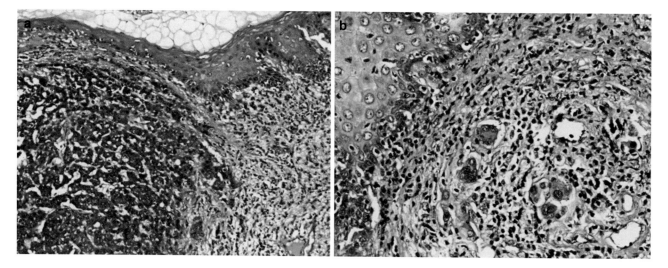

Fig. 3.62 (**a**) Metastatic carcinoma in cervix: the nodular collections of tumour cells underneath the squamous epithelium in a case of metastasis from ovarian serous carcinoma. (**b**) Metastatic carcinoma in cervix: higher magnification showing large pleomorphic tumour cells

Reference

1. Kurman RJ, Carcangiu ML, Herrington S, Young RH. Tumours of the uterine cervix. In: WHO classification of tumours of female genital reproductive organs. 4th ed. Lyon: International Agency for Research on Cancer; 2014.

Suggested Reading

Ahmad AK, Hui P, Litkouhi B, Azodi M, Rutherford T, McCarthy S, Xu ML, Schwartz PE, Ratner E. Institutional review of primary non-hodgkin lymphoma of the female genital tract: a 33-year experience. Int J Gynecol Cancer. 2014;24(7):1250–5.

Alfsen GC, Kristensen GB, Skovlund E, Pettersen EO, Abeler VM. Histologic subtype has minor importance for overall survival in patients with adenocarcinoma of the uterine cervix: a population-based study of prognostic factors in 505 patients with nonsquamous cell carcinomas of the cervix. Cancer. 2001;92(9):2471–83.

Anand M, Deshmukh SD, Gulati HK. Papillary squamotransitional cell carcinoma of the uterine cervix: a histomorphological and immunohistochemical study of nine cases. Indian J Med Paediatr Oncol. 2013;34(2):66–71.

Binesh F, Karimi Zarchi M, Vahedian H, Rajabzadeh Y. Primary malignant lymphoma of the uterine cervix. BMJ Case Rep. 2012;2012.

Chen TD, Chuang HC, Lee LY. Clinicopathologic features of 12 cases with reference to CD117 expression. Int J Gynecol Pathol. 2012;31(1):25–32.

Ditto A, Martinelli F, Carcangiu M, Solima E, de Carrillo KJ, Sanfilippo R, Haeusler E, Raspagliesi F. Embryonal rhabdomyosarcoma of the uterine cervix in adults: a case report and literature review. J Low Genit Tract Dis. 2013;17(4):e12–7.

Doshi B, Shetty S, Safaya A. Leiomyosarcoma of cervix. J Obstet Gynaecol India. 2013;63(3):211–2.

Farley JH, Hickey KW, Carlson JW, Rose GS, Kost ER, Harrison TA. Adenosquamous histology predicts a poor outcome for patients with advanced-stage, but not early-stage, cervical carcinoma. Cancer. 2003;97(9):2196–202.

Fluhmann CF. Focal hyperplasia (tunnel clusters) of the cervix uteri. Obstet Gynecol. 1961;17:206–14.

Gilks CB, Young RH, Aguirre P, DeLellis RA, Scully RE. Adenoma malignum (minimal deviation adenocarcinoma) of the uterine cervix. A clinicopathological and immunohistochemical analysis of 26 cases. Am J Surg Pathol. 1989;13(9):717–29.

Ganesan R, Hirschowitz L, Dawson P, Askew S, Pearmain P, Jones PW, Singh K, Chan KK, Moss EL. Neuroendocrine carcinoma of the cervix: review of a series of cases and correlation with outcome. Int J Surg Pathol. 2016;24(6):490–6.

Greeley C, Schroeder S, Silverberg SG. Microglandular hyperplasia of the cervix: a true "pill" lesion? Int J Gynecol Pathol. 1995;14:50–4.

Hasegawa K, Nagao S, Yasuda M, Millan D, Viswanathan AN, Glasspool RM, Devouassoux-Shisheboran M, Covens A, Lorusso D, Kurzeder C, Kim JW, Gladieff L, Bryce J, Friedlander M, Fujiwara K. Gynecologic Cancer InterGroup (GCIG) consensus review for clear cell carcinoma of the uterine corpus and cervix. Int J Gynecol Cancer. 2014;24(9 Suppl 3):S90–5.

Hasiakos D, Papakonstantinou K, Kondi-Paphiti A, Fotiou S. Low-grade endometrial stromal sarcoma of the endocervix. Report of a case and review of the literature. Eur J Gynaecol Oncol. 2007;28(6):483–6.

Huang PS, Chang WC, Huang SC. Müllerian adenosarcoma: a review of cases and literature. Eur J Gynaecol Oncol. 2014;35(6):617–20.

Kalof AN, Cooper K. Our approach to squamous intraepithelial lesions of the uterine cervix. J Clin Pathol. 2007;60(5):449–55.

Koyfman SA, Abidi A, Ravichandran P, Higgins SA, Azodi M. Adenoid cystic carcinoma of the cervix. Gynecol Oncol. 2005;99(2):477–80.

Lataifeh IM, Al-Hussaini M, Uzan C, Jaradat I, Duvillard P, Morice P. Villoglandular papillary adenocarcinoma of the cervix: a series of 28 cases including two with lymph node metastasis. Int J Gynecol Cancer. 2013;23(5):900–5.

Maniar KP, Nayar R. HPV-related squamous neoplasia of the lower anogenital tract: an update and review of recent guidelines. Adv Anat Pathol. 2014;21(5):341–58.

Martin CM, O'Leary JJ. Histology of cervical intraepithelial neoplasia and the role of biomarkers. Best Pract Res Clin Obstet Gynaecol. 2011;25(5):605–15.

McCluggage WG. New developments in endocervical glandular lesions. Histopathology. 2013;62(1):138–60.

McCluggage WG, Sumathi VP, McBride HA, Patterson A. A panel of immunohistochemical stains, including carcinoembryonic antigen, vimentin, and estrogen receptor, aids the distinction between primary endometrial and endocervical adenocarcinomas. Int J Gynecol Pathol. 2002;21(1):11–5.

Mount S, Evans MF, Wong C, et al. Human papillomavirus induced lesions of the cervix: a review and update on the grading of cervical dysplasia. Pathol Case Rev. 2003;8:145–51.

Mulvany NJ, Monostori SJ. Adenoma malignum of the cervix: a reappraisal. Pathology. 1997;29(1):17–20.

Niu X, Gilbert L. Neuroendocrine carcinoma of the uterine cervix: a single institution case review. Eur J Gynaecol Oncol. 2011;32(4):377–80.

Nucci MR. Symposium part III: tumour-like glandular lesions of the uterine cervix. Int J Gynecol Pathol. 2002;21(4):347–59.

Nucci MR, Clement PB, Young RH. Lobular endocervical glandular hyperplasia, not otherwise specified: a clinicopathologic analysis of thirteen cases of a distinctive pseudoneoplastic lesion and comparison with fourteen cases of adenoma malignum. Am J Surg Pathol. 1999;23:886–91.

Nucci MR, Crum CP. Redefining early cervical neoplasia: recent progress. Adv Anat Pathol. 2007;14:1–10.

Omranipour R, Mahmoodzadeh H, Jalaeefar A, Abdirad A, Parsaei R, Ebrahimi R. Primary malignant melanoma of uterine cervix. J Obstet Gynaecol. 2014;34(1):111.

Ostör AG. Early invasive adenocarcinoma of the uterine cervix. Int J Gynecol Pathol. 2000;19(1):29–38.

Östör AG, Duncan A, Quinn M, Rome R. Adenocarcinoma in situ of the uterine cervix: an experience with 100 cases. Gynecol Oncol. 2000;79:207–10.

Reig Castillejo A, Membrive Conejo I, Foro Arnalot P, Rodríguez de Dios N, Algara López M. Neuroendocrine small cell carcinoma of the uterine cervix. Clin Transl Oncol. 2010;12(7):512–3.

Ronnett BM. Endocervical adenocarcinoma: selected diagnostic challenges. Mod Pathol. 2016;29(Suppl 1):S12–28.

Sharma NK, Sorosky JI, Bender D, Fletcher MS, Sood AK. Malignant mixed mullerian tumour (MMMT) of the cervix. Gynecol Oncol. 2005;97(2):442–5.

Tamimi HK, Ek M, Hesla J, Cain JM, Figge DC, Greer BE. Glassy cell carcinoma of the cervix redefined. Obstet Gynecol. 1988;71(6 Pt 1):837–41.

Togami S, Kasamatsu T, Sasajima Y, Onda T, Ishikawa M, Ikeda S, Kato T, Tsuda H. Serous adenocarcinoma of the uterine cervix: a clinicopathological study of 12 cases and a review of the literature. Gynecol Obstet Investig. 2012;73(1):26–31.

Tseng CJ, Pao CC, Tseng LH, Chang CT, Lai CH, Soong YK, Hsueh S, Jyu-Jen H. Lymphoepithelioma-like carcinoma of the uterine cervix: association with Epstein-Barr virus and human papillomavirus. Cancer. 1997;80(1):91–7.

Zaino RJ. Symposium part I: adenocarcinoma in situ, glandular dysplasia, and early invasive adenocarcinoma of the uterine cervix. Int J Gynecol Pathol. 2002;21(4):314–26.

Zhou C, Gilks CB, Hayes M, Clement PB. Papillary serous carcinoma of the uterine cervix: a clinicopathologic study of 17 cases. Am J Surg Pathol. 1998;22(1):113–20.

Pathology of Endometrium: Benign Lesions, Preneoplastic Lesions and Carcinomas

4

Classification of the tumours of the uterine corpus according to World Health Organization [1] have been highlighted in the Fig. 4.1.

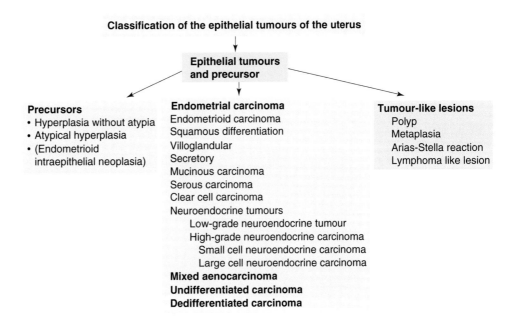

Classification of the epithelial tumours of the uterus

Epithelial tumours and precursor

Precursors
- Hyperplasia without atypia
- Atypical hyperplasia
- (Endometrioid intraepithelial neoplasia)

Endometrial carcinoma
Endometrioid carcinoma
Squamous differentiation
Villoglandular
Secretory
Mucinous carcinoma
Serous carcinoma
Clear cell carcinoma
Neuroendocrine tumours
    Low-grade neuroendocrine tumour
    High-grade neuroendocrine carcinoma
      Small cell neuroendocrine carcinoma
      Large cell neuroendocrine carcinoma
Mixed aenocarcinoma
Undifferentiated carcinoma
Dedifferentiated carcinoma

Tumour-like lesions
Polyp
Metaplasia
Arias-Stella reaction
Lymphoma like lesion

Fig. 4.1 Classification of epithelial tumours of the uterine body by World Health Organization

© Springer Nature Singapore Pte Ltd. 2019
P. Dey, *Color Atlas of Female Genital Tract Pathology*, https://doi.org/10.1007/978-981-13-1029-4_4

Cyclic Endometrium

- There are three stages of physiological cyclic endometrial cycle: proliferative, secretory and menstrual phase.
- Duration of each complete endometrial cycle is 28 days
- Ovulation occurs 14 days before the menstruation

Proliferative Endometrium

Image gallery: Fig. 4.2a, b.
Features

- Small, uniform tubular glands
- Lining of the gland is cuboidal epithelial cells
- Stroma is compact and cellular
- Focal stromal edema may be present in the later part of this stage

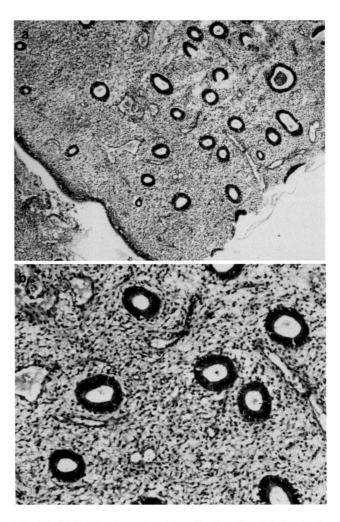

Fig. 4.2 (**a**) Proliferative endometrium: Small, uniform tubular glands. (**b**) Proliferative endometrium: The glands are lined by cuboidal epithelial cells

Secretory Phase

Image gallery: Figs. 4.3a–c, 4.4, 4.5a–f, and 4.6a–c.

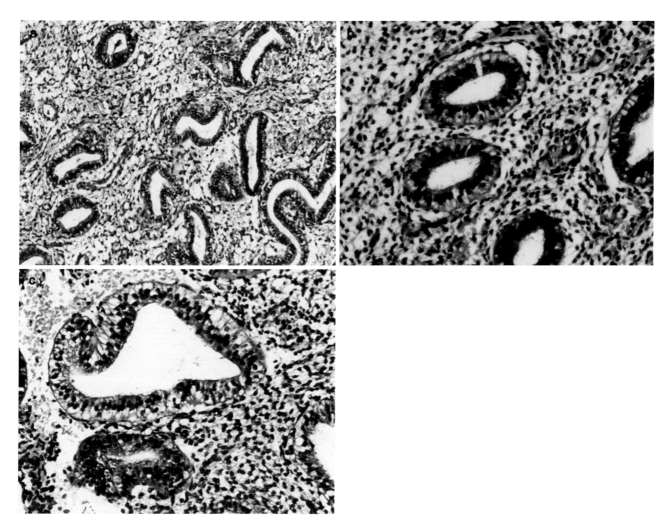

Fig. 4.3 (**a**) Early secretory: All the glands show subnuclear vacuolation. (**b**) Early secretory: Regular subnuclear vacuolation. (**c**) Early secretory: Higher magnification of the same

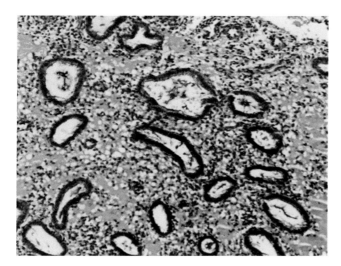

Fig. 4.4 Mid secretory: Secretion within the glands along with marked stromal oedema

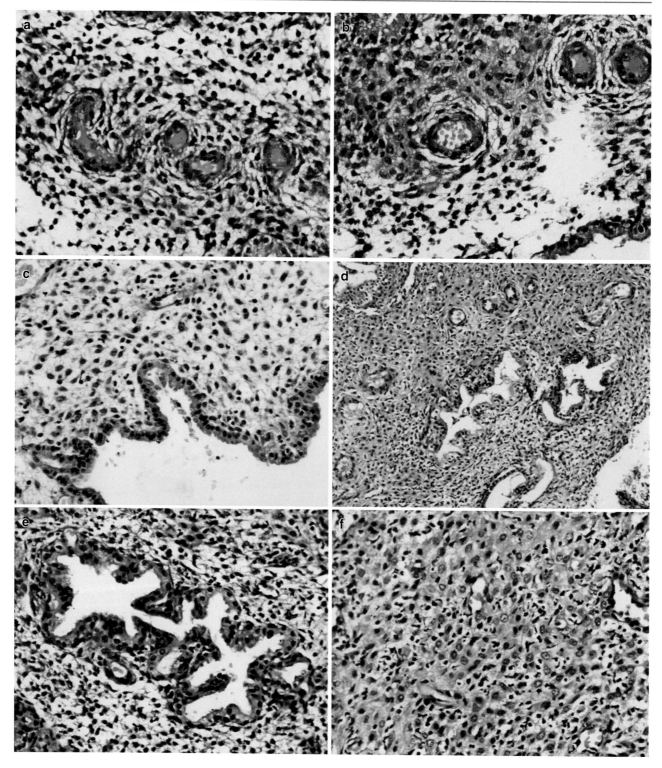

Fig. 4.5 (**a**) Late secretory, 23rd day: Prominent stromal vessels. (**b**) Late secretory, 23rd day: Perivascular decidua formation. (**c**) Late secretory, 24th day: Decidual cells become confluent beneath the surface epithelium. (**d**) Late secretory, 25th day: Secretory glands with confluent decasualized stroma underneath the epithelium. (**e**) Late secretory, 25th day: Corkscrew like secretory glands. (**f**) Late secretory 26th day: Large sheets of decidua

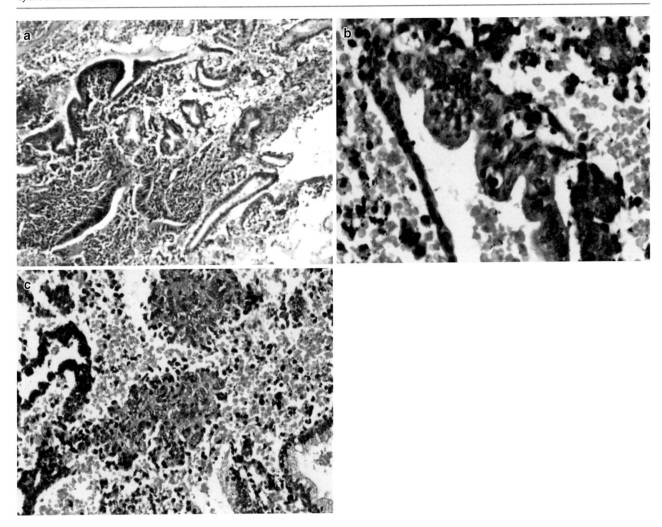

Fig. 4.6 (a) Menstrual endometrium: Broken and fragmented endometrial glands. (b) Menstrual endometrium: Higher magnification showing the piling up of the epithelial cells. (c) Menstrual endometrium: Many broken glands with stromal granulocytes

Early Secretory

Features

- Duration: 16th–19th day of the cycle considering 1st day as the strating day of bleeding.
- 16th day: At first irregular subnuclear vacuolation appears in the gland
- 17th day: The vacuoles become more regular
- 18th day: Both sub and supranuclear vacuoles appear
- 19th day: Secretion appears in the lumen of the gland. Nuclei are all placed in basal position

Mid Secretory

Features

- Duration: 20th–22nd day
- Abundant intraluminal secretion
- Significant stromal edema

Late Secretory

Features

- Duration: 23rd–28th day
- 23rd day: Spiral arterioles become prominent and decidua forms around the small vessels

- 24th day: Decidual cells become confluent and extends in the stroma
- 25th day: Decidua underneath the stroma
- 26th day: Large sheet of decidua
- 27th day: More extensive decidua formation
- 28th day: Fibrin thrombi appears in the small vessels, stromal granulocytes, haemorrhage

Menstrual Endometrium

Features

- Duration: 1st–4th day
- Glands are broken and fragmented
- Discontinuation of the surface epithelium
- Stroma disintegrates and collapses
- Crowding of the stromal cells
- Polymorphs infiltration and necrosis

Precautions During Interpretation of the Endometrial Curetting

Image gallery: Figs. 4.7a, b, 4.8a, b, 4.9a, b, 4.10a, b, and 4.11a, b.

Collapsed glands may simulate hyperplasia

- The glands may collapse and come close together resembling false crowding

Lower uterine segment

- Endometrial curettings may come from the lower uterine segment and provide false impression on dating as they do not properly response to hormone

Secretory hyperplasia

- At times the glands may show exaggerated secretory activity and may false look like hyperplastic

Telescopic gland

- Proliferative glands and even secretory endometrium may give gland in gland appearance. The telescopic gland has no additional significance.

Aberrant focal subnuclear vacuolation

- There may be aberrant subnuclear vacuolation in the glands in different phases of endometrium. This subnuclear vacuolation is only focal.

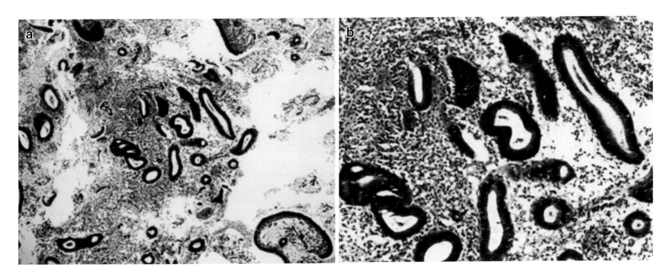

Fig. 4.7 (**a**) The collapsed glands may simulate hyperplasia. (**b**) Due to the collapsing of the stroma the glands have come close and are simulating hyperplastic

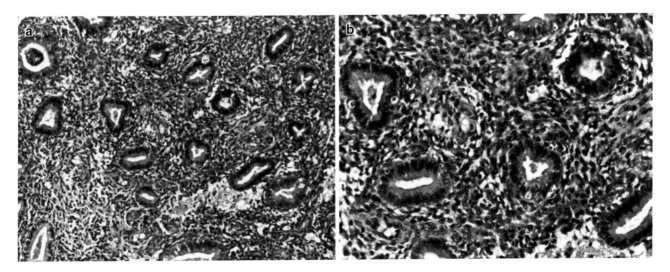

Fig. 4.8 (**a**) Lower uterine segment: The glands of the lower uterine segment may often give wrong impression in dating. (**b**) Lower uterine segment: the endocervical glands in the lower uterine segment may often mislead the pathologists

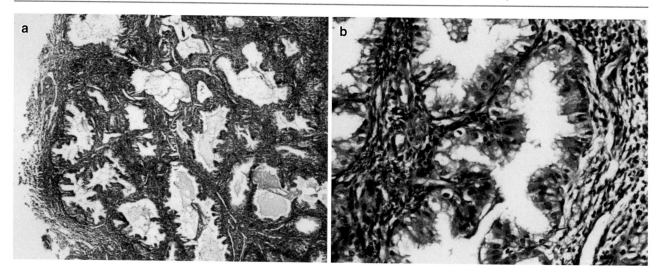

Fig. 4.9 (**a**) Secretory hyperplasia: The glands showing exaggerated secretory activity. (**b**) Secretory hyperplasia: The lining epithelial cells showing pseudostratification

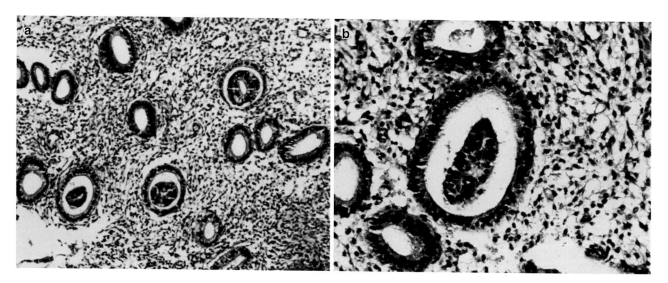

Fig. 4.10 (**a**) Telescopic gland: Proliferative glands showing in gland appearance. (**b**) Telescopic gland: Higher magnification of the same

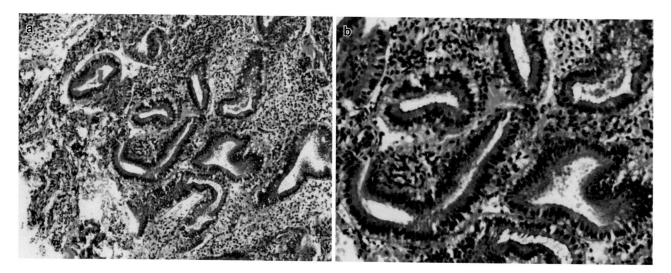

Fig. 4.11 (**a**) Aberrant subnuclear vacuolation in a late secretory endometrium. (**b**) Higher magnification of the same showing subnuclear vacuolation

Post Menopausal Endometrium

Image gallery: Fig. 4.12a, b.
  Features

- Atrophic glands
- Cuboidal to flattened epithelial lining
- Occasionally cystically dilated glands
- Fibrous stroma

Atrophic Polyp

Image gallery: Fig. 4.13.
  Figure 4.13 Atrophic polyp: Atrophic epithelium forms a polypoid projections to make a polyp.
  Features

- At times atrophic endometrium may show polypoid projection
- The atrophic polyp shows cystically dilated glands lined by flattened epithelium

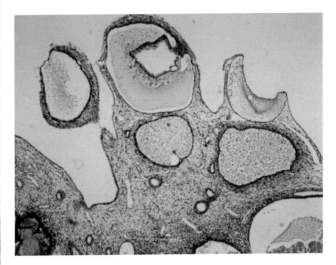

Fig. 4.13 Atrophic polyp: Atrophic epithelium forms a polypoid projections

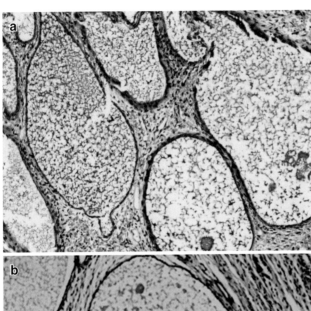

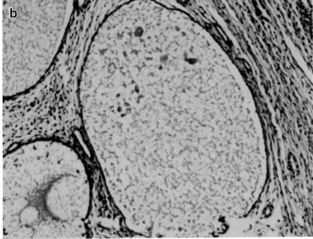

Fig. 4.12 (**a**) Post menopausal endometrium: Large cystically dilated glands. (**b**) Post menopausal endometrium: The lining epithelium of the gland is flattened

Hormone Induced Changes

Progesterone Effect

Atrophic Pattern

Image gallery: Fig. 4.14a, b.
  Features

- Extensive decidual changes
- Glands become small tubular or elongated
- Atrophic looking glands with poor secretory activities

Secretory Pattern

Image gallery: Fig. 4.14c.
  Features

- Abundant pre-decidua
- Secretory glands

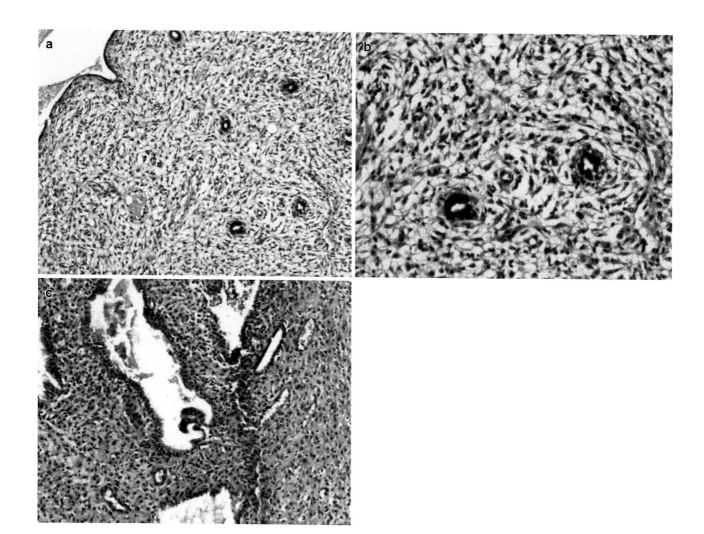

Fig. 4.14 (**a**) Progesterone effect: Small tubular glands with abundant decidua. (**b**) Progesterone effect: Atrophic looking glands in the midst of abundant decidua. (**c**) Progesterone effect: Secretory pattern showing Secretory glands and abundant decidua

Endometritis

Chronic Endometritis

Image gallery: Fig. 4.15a, b.

Causes: Bacterial infections such as Streptococcus, Chlamydia trachomatis, Neisseria gonorrhoeae and various viruses.

Predisposing factors: intrauterine contraceptive device, instrumentation, pregnancy, leiomyoma, endometrial polyp.

Clinical feature

- Reproductive age period
- Intermenstrual bleeding
- Menorrhagia

Histopathology

- Infiltration of lymphocytes and plasma cells
- The presence of plasma cell is a valuable indicator of chronic endometritis
- Commonly underdeveloped atrophic glands
- Poor secretory activity of the gland

Differential diagnosis

- Menstrual endometrium: Occasional plasma cells in the late menstrual period may be noted
- Endometrial polyp: Occasional presence of plasma cells may be misinterpreted as endometritis
- Lymphoproliferative disease: Rarely simulate endometritis. In lymphoproliferative disease the endometrium is diffusely involved.

Prognosis and treatment

- Systemic antibiotic therapy
- Improvement within few days

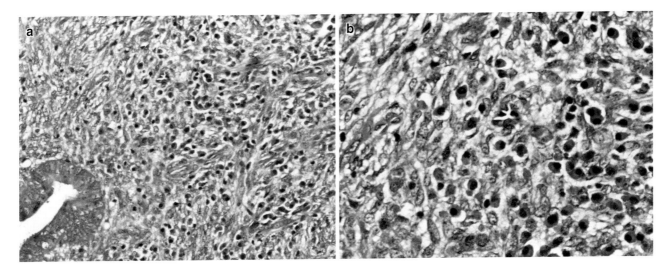

Fig. 4.15 (**a**) Chronic endometritis: Endometrial stroma shows lymphocytes and plasma cell infiltration. (**b**) Chronic endometritis: Higher magnification showing abundant plasma cells

Granulomatous Endometritis

Tuberculosis

Image gallery: Fig. 4.16a–c.
   Causative organism: Mycobacterium tubercle infection.
   Clinical feature

- Infertility is the commonest presentation
- Postmenopausal patient: Menorrhagia

   Histopathology

- Multiple epithelioid cell granulomas
- Multinucleated giant cells

- Necrosis
- Improper development of the endometrial glands

   Ancillary study

- Ziehl Neelsen stain
- Mycobacterial culture or polymerase chain reaction

   Differential diagnosis

- Foreign body granuloma
- Granuloma in endometrioid carcinoma in reaction to keratin
- Rarely sarcoid

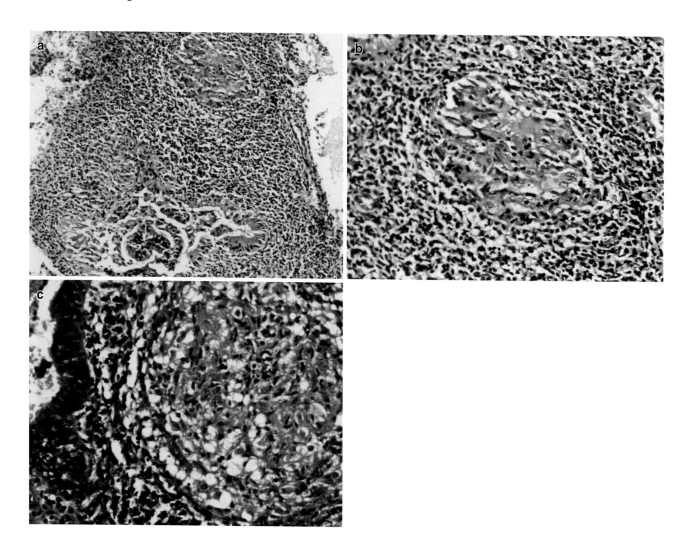

Fig. 4.16 (**a**) Granulomatous endometritis: Multiple epithelioid cell granulomas in the endometrial stroma. (**b**) Granulomatous endometritis: Well circumscribed granulomas along with dense lymphocytes. (**c**) Granulomatous endometritis: Higher magnification of the epithelioid granuloma

Epithelial Tumours and Precursors

Endometrial Hyperplasia without Atypia

Image gallery: Figs. 4.17a, b, 4.18a–c, and 4.19a, b.

Synonym: Simple hyperplasia without atypia, complex hyperplasia without atypia and benign endometrial hyperplasia.

Epidemiology

- Endometrial hyperplasia without atypia occurs more frequently than endometrial carcinoma.

Clinical features

- Majority of the patients are asymptomatic
- Usually detected during the investigation of infertility
- Occasionally the patient may have abnormal uterine bleeding

Risk factors

- Unopposed estrogenic stimulation due to
  - Anovulatory cycle
  - Estrogen intake
  - Polycystic ovarian syndrome
  - Ovarian neoplasm releasing excess estrogen

Histopathology

- Multiple glands with varying size and shape
- Cystically dilated gland

- Outpouching and branching of the glands in case of complex hyperplasia
- Glands are focally crowded
- Tubal or ciliated metaplasia may be seen
- Epithelium may be stratified with mitotic figures

Differential diagnosis (Fig. 4.20)

- Cystic atrophy: Postmenopausal patients, the epithelial lining of the glands show flattened epithelial cells
- Disordered proliferation: Mild excess of glands but no crowding of glands present
- Endometrial polyp: At times difficult to diagnose the endometrial polyp.
  - It is lined by endometrial epithelial cells in all three sides.
  - Normal looking endometrium may be admixed

Prognosis

- Rarely progress to endometrial carcinoma (1–3% only)

Treatment

- Progesterone administration followed by repeated curetting to follow up

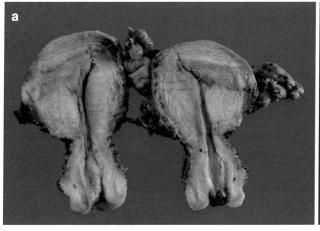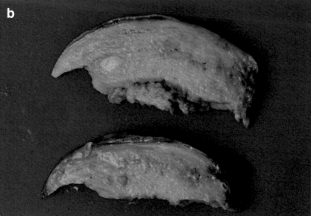

Fig. 4.17 (**a**) Gross picture of endometrial hyperplasia: Endometrium is thickened. (**b**) Gross picture of endometrial hyperplasia: Sections from the wall showing thickened endometrium

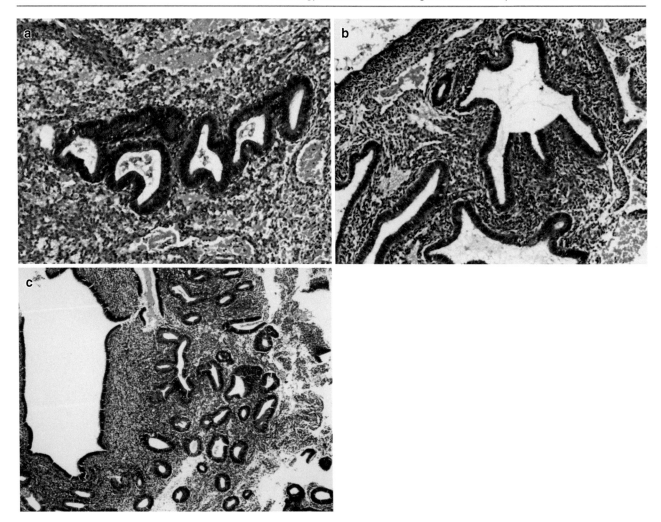

Fig. 4.18 (**a**) Simple hyperplasia: Focally crowded glands. (**b**) Simple hyperplasia: Dilated glands showing simple branching. (**c**) Simple hyperplasia: Variably sized glands

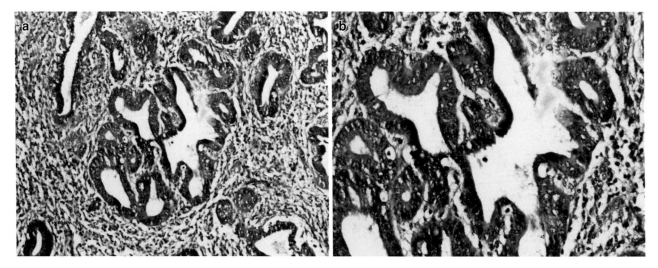

Fig. 4.19 (**a**) Complex hyperplasia without atypia: Closely packed variably sized glands with complex branching. (**b**) Complex hyperplasia without atypia: The glands with little intervening stroma

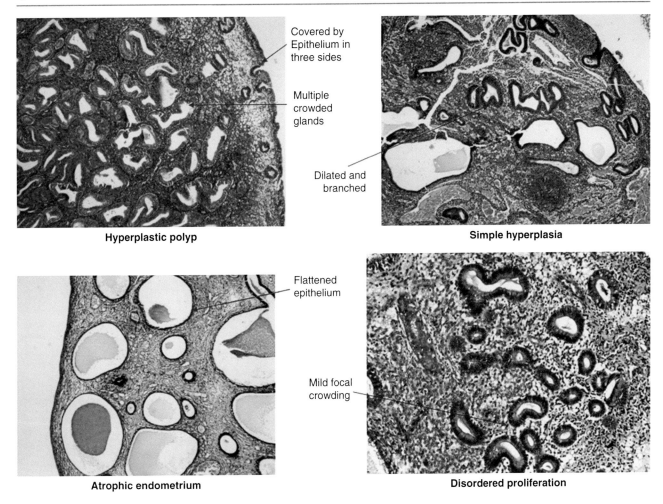

Hyperplastic polyp

Covered by Epithelium in three sides

Multiple crowded glands

Dilated and branched

Simple hyperplasia

Flattened epithelium

Mild focal crowding

Atrophic endometrium

Disordered proliferation

Fig. 4.20 Distinguishing features of simple hyperplasia from other mimickers

Disordered Proliferation

Image gallery: Fig. 4.21a, b.
  Histopathology

- Glands are much more in number than the normal endometrium

- The overall glandular proliferation is less than that of endometrial hyperplasia
- No crowding of the endometrial glands

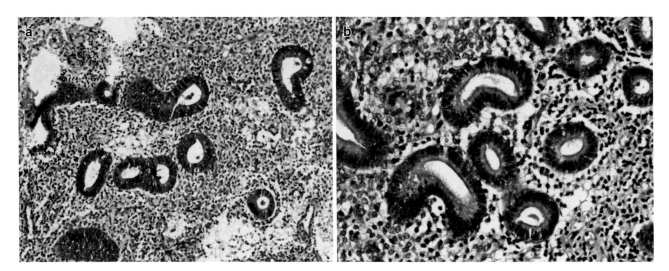

Fig. 4.21 (**a**) Disordered proliferation: Glands are more in number than the normal endometrium, however the overall glandular proliferation is less than that of endometrial hyperplasia. (**b**) Disordered proliferation: Variably sized glands

Atypical Hyperplasia/Endometrial Intraepithelial Neoplasia (EIN)

Image gallery: Fig. 4.22a–c.

Synonym: Endometrial intraepithelial neoplasia, complex hyperplasia with atypia, simple endometrial hyperplasia with atypia.

Epidemiology

- Typically occurs in elderly postmenopausal patients

Risk factors

- Unopposed estrogenic activity: exogenous estrogen administration, tamoxifen therapy, estrogen producing ovarian tumours etc.
- Obesity
- Genetic risk factors: Hereditary non-polyposis colon cancer, Cowden's syndrome

Clinical features

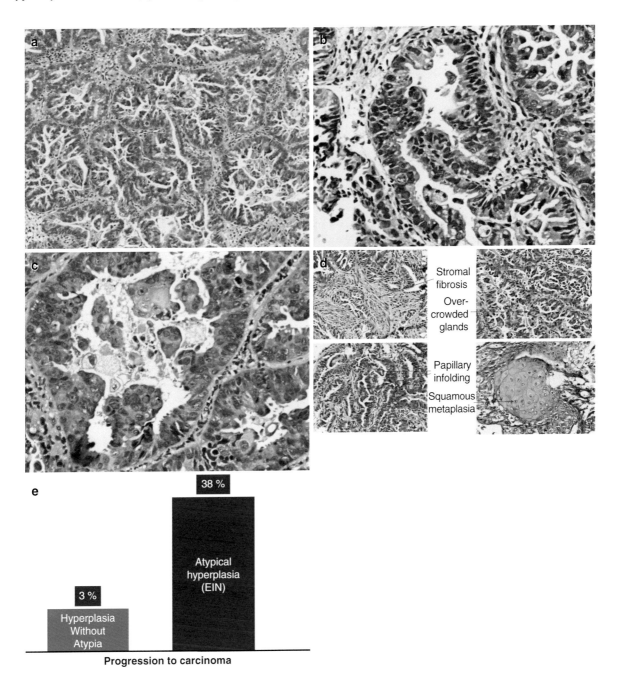

Fig. 4.22 (**a**) Endometrial intraepithelial neoplasia: The glands showing back to back arrangement. (**b**) Endometrial intraepithelial neoplasia: Truly stratified lining epithelium of the glands. (**c**) Endometrial intraepithelial neoplasia: Note the nuclear pleomorphism of the lining epithelium. (**d**) Important features of endometrial adenocarcinoma to distinguish it from atypical hyperplasia on curetting. (**e**) Rate of progression of hyperplasia to carcinoma

- Abnormal vaginal bleeding

Histopathology

- Overcrowded glands with back to back arrangement
- Marked increase of glands versus stromal ratio
- Nuclear atypia of the glandular epithelial cells characterized by:
  - Nuclear enlargement
  - Pleomorphism
  - Loss of orientation of nuclei and the polarity is lost
  - Nuclei become more round
- The lining epithelial cells show true stratification

Essential diagnostic criteria of EIN

- Architectural: Area occupied by the gland is always more than stromal area (gland versus stromal ration is more than 0.5).
- Cytology: The glandular lining epithelial cells show nuclear atypia
- Size: The linear dimension of the lesion should be more than 1 mm.
- Exclusion of mimickers: Various benign conditions that mimic the lesion should be excluded such as endometrial polyp, collapsed endometrial stroma, hyperplasia without atypia, reactive changes due to instrumentation etc.
- Exclusion of cancer: The cancer often shows cribriform arrangement, myometrial invasion, stromal fibrosis etc.

Molecular profile

- Mutation of PTEN, KRAS and beta catenin
- Inactivation of PAX 2
- Microsatellite instability

Prognosis

- Majority of the cases (25–33%) develop adenocarcinoma in follow up
- Risk of development of malignancy is almost 15 folds

Differential diagnosis (see Fig. 4.22d)

- Well differentiated adenocarcinoma: The features indicating carcinoma include stromal fibrosis, glandular overcrowding, papillary structures and squamous metaplasia (Box 4.1).
- Reactive changes in the endometrium: The common causes of reactive changes are infection, instrumentation or pregnancy.
- Endometrial polyp: The variably shaped irregular glands in the polyp may be misinterpreted as EIN.
- Endometrial breakdown: Collapsed endometrial glands and pilling of the lining epithelial cells in menstrual endometrium may be over interpreted as EIN.

- Artifactual displacement of gland: Telescoping of the gland and the displaced glands in lateral direction may mimic EIN
- Simple hyperplasia: EIN should be distinguished from simple hyperplasia (see Box 4.2)

Prognosis (see Fig. 4.22e)

- It is often associated with endometrial carcinoma (30–40% cases).
- If untreated chance of malignant transformation is about 28–45%.

Treatment

- Hysterectomy: Due to higher chance of malignant conversion and associated carcinoma, hysterectomy is preferable in such lesion in post-menopausal patients.
- Combination treatment of progesterone and gonadotrophin releasing hormone: This can be applied in the younger patient who wants to retain the uterus. The patient should be regularly followed up by USG and endometrial curetting.

Box 4.1 Endometrial Carcinoma Versus EIN (Atypical Hyperplasia)

Features favouring carcinoma are:

- Glandular overcrowding without any intervening stroma
- Desmoplastic stromal reaction
- Glandular epithelium forming papillae like structures
- Squamous metaplasia

Box 4.2 Simple Hyperplasia Versus EIN (Atypical Hyperplasia)

Note:

- Is there any glandular overcrowding?
  - If yes, favors EIN
- Gland versus stromal ratio?
  - Much high in EIN
- Complex branching present?
  - Almost always present in EIN
  - Essential features and must be present in EIN: Nuclear enlargement, pleomorphism, prominent nucleoli and loss of polarity of the nuclei.

Endometrial Carcinomas

Epidemiology

- The most common cancer of the female genital tract in developed countries.
- 10 cases per 100,000 women in each year.
- There are 150,000 cases of endometrial cancer diagnosed in year throughout the world.
- High in the Caucasian woman

Risk factors

- Obesity
- Early menarche and late menopause
- Dietary factors: High calorie and protein intake
- Nulliparous and diabetic person
- Estrogen: Continuous estrogenic stimulation
- Ethnic factor: Whites more affected
- Genetic Factors: Mutation of PTEN, PIK3CA, K-RAS and p53. Microsatellite instability due to hypermethylation of hMSH 2, 3, 6, gene.

Type of tumour: Endometrial adenocarcinoma is divided into Type I and Type II. (see Table 4.1).

Table 4.1 Type I versus type II endometrial carcinoma

Features	Type I	Type II
Age	Average age is 50–60 year	Average age is 60–70 year
Estrogenic stimulation	Present	Absent
Relation with atypical hyperplasia	Present	Absent
Grade of tumour	Usually low grade tumour	Usually high grade tumour
Histology type	Endometrioid carcinoma and mucinous carcinoma	Serous and clear cell carcinoma
Myometrial invasion	Minimal	Much deeper
Tumour spread	Lymph node involved	Peritoneal spread more common
Genetic abnormality	Microsatellite instability, PTEN, and K-RAS mutation	p53 mutation

Endometrioid Carcinoma

Image gallery: Figs. 4.23, 4.24, 4.25, 4.26, and 4.27.
     Clinical features

- Mean age 55 year
- Abnormal vaginal bleeding in post-menopausal patient
- Menorrhagia in peri-menopausal patient

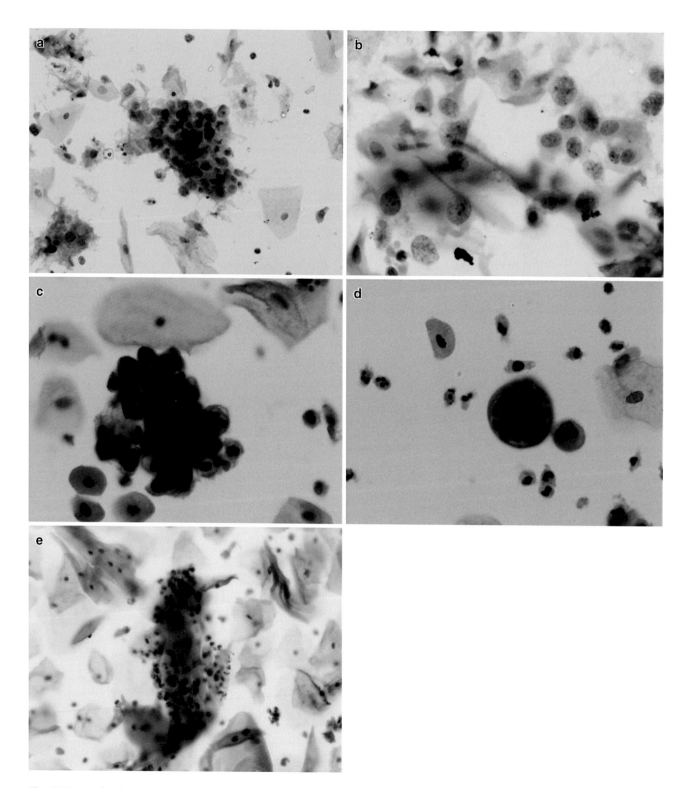

Fig. 4.23 (**a**) Cervical cytology smear of endometrial carcinoma: Cohesive round cells with enlarged nuclei. (**b**) Cervical cytology smear of endometrial carcinoma: The scattered isolated cells with vacuolated cytoplasm. (**c**) Cytology smear: Round cells with scanty cytoplasm hav-ing hyperchromatic nuclei. (**d**) Cervical cytology smear of endometrial carcinoma: Bag of polymorphs. (**e**) Cervical cytology smear of endo-metrial carcinoma: Tumour diathesis

Gross features

- Exophytic growth
- Solid, grey white friable mass
- Hemorrhage and necrosis
- Tumour invades in the deeper myometrium either by pushing margin or by infiltration

Cytology of endometrioid carcinoma

- Cohesive tight clusters and also discrete cells
- Round cells with high nucleocytoplasmic ratio
- Cytoplasmic vacuolation may be present

- Cell may be full of polymorphs giving the look of "bag of poly"
- Thin tumour diathesis

Histopathology of endometrioid carcinoma

- Resembles normal endometrium
- Back to back arrangement of the glands
- Complex branching
- Variable amount of solid area
- Cuboidal cells with moderate nuclear enlargement and pleomorphism
- Prominent nucleoli

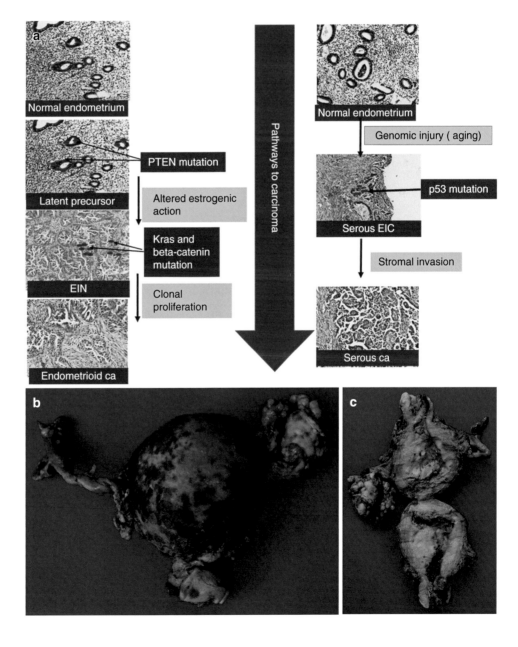

Fig. 4.24 (**a**) Pathogenesis of endometrial carcinoma. (**b**) Endometrial carcinoma: Gross picture showing bulky uterus. (**c**) Endometrial carcinoma: Cut section showing grey white tumour with foci of haemorrhage

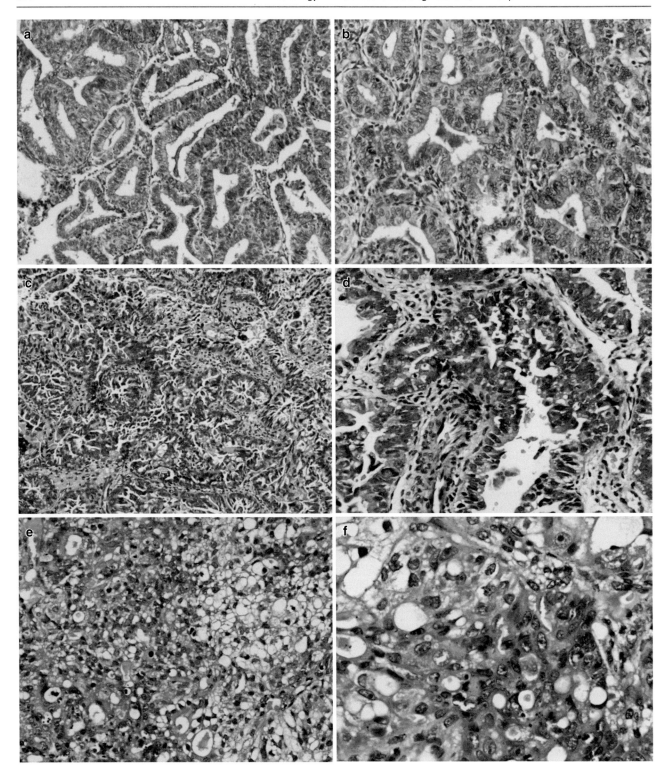

Fig. 4.25 (a) Endometrioid carcinoma: Well differentiated endometrial carcinoma showing predominantly gland component. (b) Endometrioid carcinoma: The back to back arrangement of the glands. The lining epithelial cells of the glands are cuboidal with pleomorphic nuclei having prominent nucleoli. (c) Endometrioid carcinoma: Moderately differentiated endometrial carcinoma showing glands within the solid areas. (d) Endometrioid carcinoma: Moderately differentiated endometrial carcinoma showing multiple glands lined by moderately pleomorphic nuclei.

(e) Endometrioid carcinoma: Poorly differentiated endometrial carcinoma showing occasional glands in a large amount of solid area. (f) Endometrioid carcinoma: Poorly differentiated endometrial carcinoma showing markedly pleomorphic cells in the solid area. (g) Endometrioid carcinoma: Lymphovascular invasion. (h) Endometrioid carcinoma: Pushing margin of the tumour. (i) Endometrioid carcinoma: Pushing margin of the tumour indicated by red line and arrow. (j) Endometrioid carcinoma: infiltrating margin indicated by red arrow

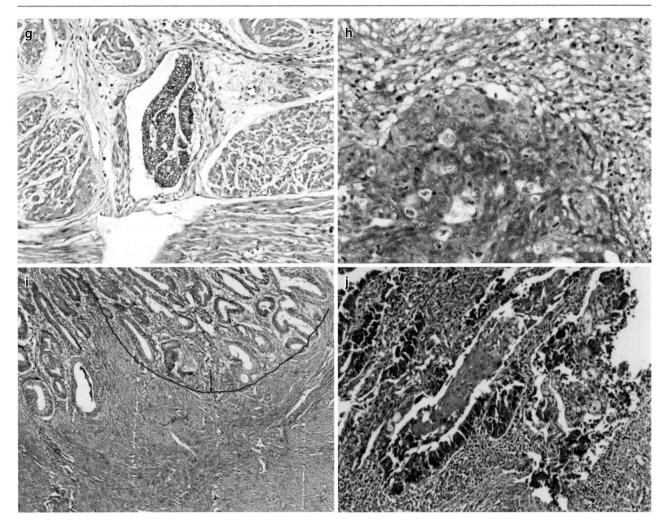

Fig. 4.25 (continued)

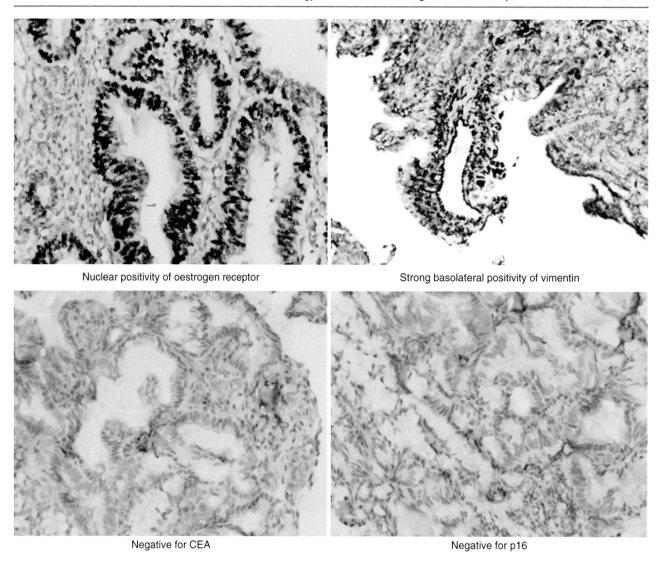

| Nuclear positivity of oestrogen receptor | Strong basolateral positivity of vimentin |
| Negative for CEA | Negative for p16 |

Fig. 4.26 Essential helpful immunostains for the confirmation of endometrial origin

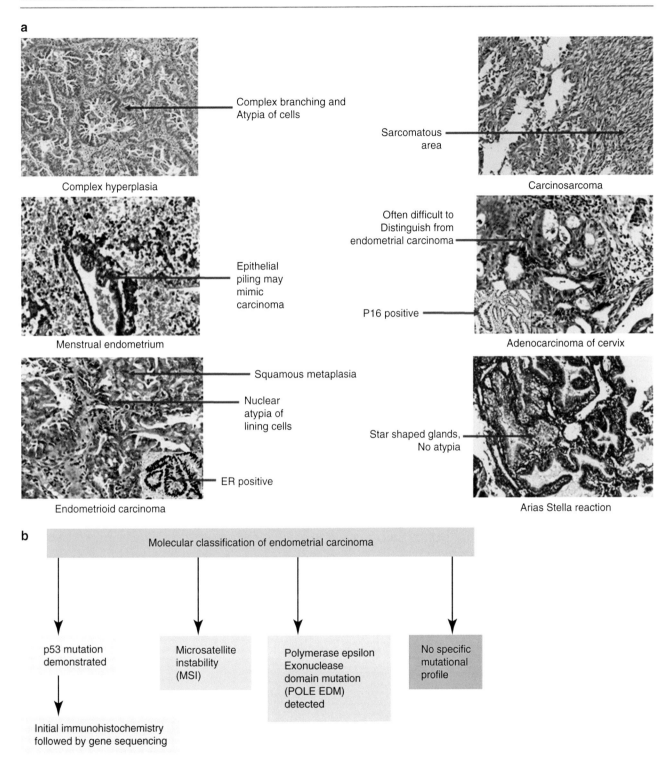

Fig. 4.27 (**a**) Differential diagnosis of endometrial carcinoma. (**b**) Proposed molecular classification of endometrial carcinoma

Grading

Architectural Grade
Excluding squamous or morular component

- Grade 1: Solid area is 5% or less
- Grade 2: Solid area is 6–50%
- Grade 3: Solid area is over 50%

Nuclear grade

- Grade 1: Mildly enlarged and pleomorphic nuclei with prominent nucleoli. Nuclear chromatin is fine.
- Grade 2: In between grade 1 and 2
- Grade 3: Severely pleomorphic nuclei with markedly enlarged prominent nucleoli.

Overall grade: In the presence of significant nuclear atypia, one will be added with the score of the architectural grade. Such as grade 2 architectural grade with significant atypia will be considered as overall grade 3.

Myometrial invasion

- Measurement: The distance between the junction of the endomyometrium and the deeper point of tumour tissue.
- Types of invasion:
  - Pushing: The broad margin of the tumour pushes the myometrial tissue
  - Infiltrating: Multiple cords or islands of tumour tissue invades the deeper myometrium.

Immunohistochemistry (see Fig. 4.26).
Positive for: Pan-cytokeratin, epithelial membrane antigen, Ber EP4, and B72.3, estrogen receptor, vimentin, CK 7.
Negative: p16, and ProExC, CK 20.
Differential diagnosis (Fig. 4.27a).

- Atypical polypoid adenomyomata
  - Atypia is relatively less
  - No desmoplastic reaction
  - No evidence of myometrial invasion
- Menstrual endometrium
  - Simulating factors are: Broken glands of varying sizes, piling of stromal cells, hemorrhage and necrosis.
  - Differentiating points: Presence of late secretory endometrial glands, normal decidual cells, bland looking endometrial glandular epithelial cells
- Arias-Stella reaction
  - Young age
  - History of pregnancy

- The presence of decidual cells
- Lack of papillary pattern
- No desmoplastic reaction
- No mitosis
- Endocervical adenocarcinoma
  - Mass predominantly in the endocervix
  - No squamous morules
  - Glands may show adenocarcinoma in situ
  - Dysplastic squamous epithelial cells may be present
  - Immunocytochemistry: Positive for p16, ProExC, CEA and negative for vimentin, ER/PR
- Malignant mixed Mullerian tumour
  - The stromal spindle cell component is pleomorphic with increased mitosis
  - The epithelial and mesenchymal component are sharply distinguished

Molecular profiling (Fig. 4.27b)

- Mutation of PTEN KRAS, p 53 and PIK 3R1
- Microsatellite instability
- Methylation of MLH 1 gene promoter region

Reporting of endometrial carcinoma: See Box 4.3.

Box 4.3 Reporting Endometrial Adenocarcinoma
- Type of specimen: Total, subtotal or radical hysterectomy
- Weight and measurement of uterus
- Size of the tumour
- Distance of the tumour from the inferior surgical margin
- Depth of invasion in the myometrium
- Involvement of the cervical wall along with depth of the tumour in the cervical wall
- Tumour proper
  - Type of tumour
  - Grade of tumour
  - Microscopic depth of myometrial invasion
  - Lymphovascular involvement: in the tumour stromal interface or deep in the myometrium
- Residual endometrium: Atrophic/hyperplastic/no change
- Cervical involvement: Mucosa or wall, if wall then depth of invasion
- Cervical lymphovascular involvement
- Parametrium involvement
- Lymph node involvement

Endometrioid Carcinoma with Squamous Differentiation

Image gallery: Fig. 4.28a–d.

Incidence: Near about 20% of endometrioid carcinoma shows squamoid differentiation.

Criteria: At least 10% of the area of the carcinoma should show squamoid differentiation.

Diagnostic guideline for the determination of squamous cell

1. The evidence of keratinization in the routine section
2. Presence of cell to cell junction
3. At least any three features:
   - Sheet of cells without any glandular differentiation
   - Presence of eosinophilic cytoplasm
   - Keratin pearl
   - Cells with cytoplasmic eosinophilia

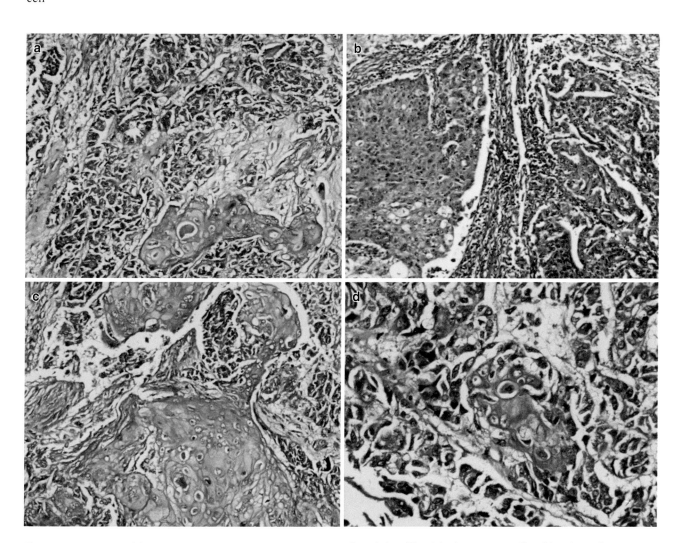

Fig. 4.28 (**a**) Endometrioid carcinoma with squamous differentiation: Adenocarcinoma with foci of squamous cell carcinoma component. (**b**) Endometrioid carcinoma with squamous differentiation: Adenocarcinoma component along with large areas of squamous cell carcinoma component. (**c**) Endometrioid carcinoma with squamous dif- ferentiation: Keratinized squamous cells with polygonal appearance and intracellular keratinization. (**d**) Endometrioid carcinoma with squamous differentiation: Note the nuclear enlargement and pleomorphism of the squamous cell component

Villoglandular Carcinoma

Image gallery: Fig. 4.29a–e.
  Incidence

- About 20–30% of endometrioid carcinoma
- Median age: 61 year

Histopathology

- Multiple slender villi with fibrovascular core
- Lining cells are stratified columnar epithelial cells
- Mild nuclear atypia
- Nuclear axis of the cells are perpendicular to the basement membrane
- Variable mitosis

Differential diagnosis (Fig. 4.29e)

- Serous carcinoma
  - Short and stout papillae
  - Significant nuclear atypia
  - Large prominent macronucleoli
  - Micropapillary structure present
  - Strong p53 and occasionally p16 positive

Key diagnostic points: see Box 4.4.

Box 4.4 Key Diagnostic Points of Villoglandular Carcinoma
- Tall and slender papillae
- Multilayered columnar lining epithelial cells of the papillae
- Tumour cells show mildly pleomorphic nuclei
- Predominantly superficial

Note: The absence of marked nuclear pleomorphism and large prominent nucleoli. Villi are tall and slender.

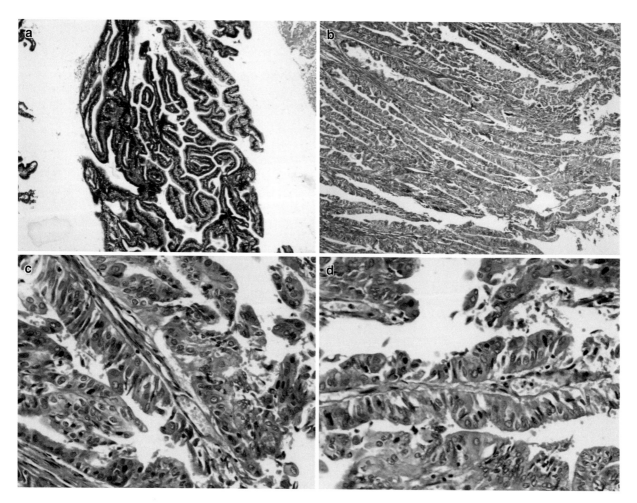

Fig. 4.29 (**a**) Villoglandular carcinoma: Slender villi like structures. (**b**) Villoglandular carcinoma: Long villi with thin vascular core. (**c**) Villoglandular carcinoma: Nuclear axis of the cell is perpendicular to the basement membrane of the villi. (**d**) Villoglandular carcinoma: The villi are lined by cuboidal epithelial cells. (**e**) Differential diagnosis of villoglandular carcinoma of uterus

e

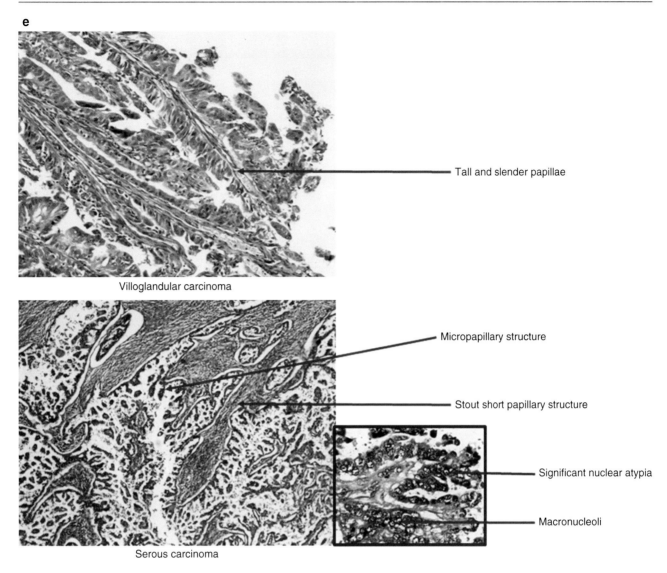

Villoglandular carcinoma

Serous carcinoma

Fig. 4.29 (continued)

Secretory Carcinoma

Image gallery: Fig. 4.30a–d.
   Incidence: Less than 1% of endometrioid carcinoma.
   Histopathology

- Simulates early secretory endometrium however the glands are relatively large and arranged closely with little intervening stroma.

- Glands are lined by tall columnar epithelial cells with distinct subnuclear and supranuclear vacuoles
- Mild to moderate nuclear atypia present
- Usually well differentiated

Differential diagnosis (Fig. 4.30e).

- Secretary endometrium

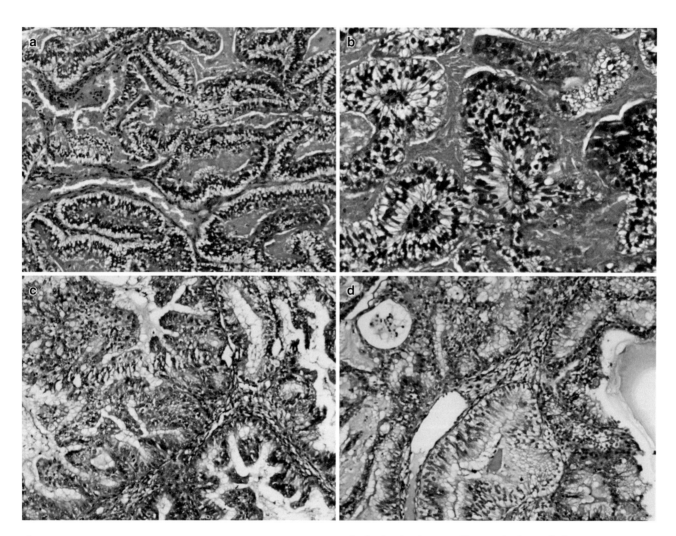

Fig. 4.30 (**a**) Secretory carcinoma: The tumour in lower magnification simulates secretory endometrium. (**b**) Secretory carcinoma: The glands are relatively large with no intervening stroma. Note the nuclear pleomorphism of the lining cells of the glands. (**c**) Secretory carcinoma: The glands showing inner papillary projections. (**d**) Secretory carcinoma: Significant nuclear atypia of the cells. (**e**) Differential diagnosis of secretory carcinoma

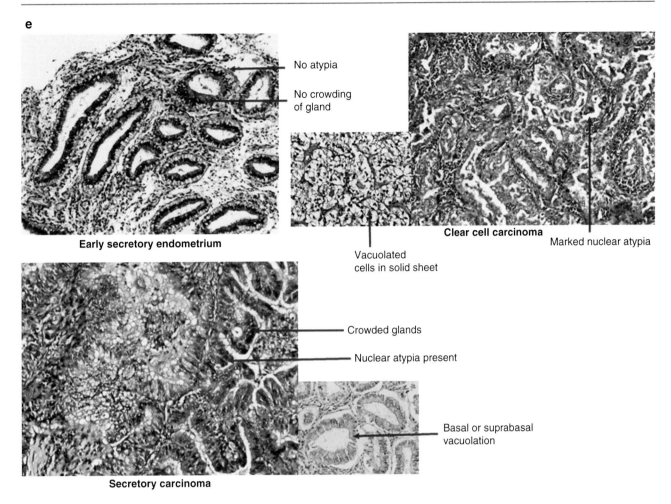

Fig. 4.30 (continued)

– Unlike postmenopausal patient in secretory carcinoma, the secretary endometrium is seen in reproductive age
– Back to back appearance is absent in secretory endometrium
• Clear cell carcinoma
– Nuclear pleomorphism is more
– High nucleo-cytoplasmic ratio
– The cells with cytoplasmic vacuolation are usually in solid sheet
• *Key diagnostic points*: Box 4.5

Box 4.5 Key Diagnostic Points of Secretory Carcinoma
• Overcrowding of glands without any intervening stroma
• Nuclear enlargement and pleomorphism
• Sub and supranuclear cytoplasmic vacuolation
• Typical endometrioid carcinoma may be present in the adjacent areas of the curetting

Note: Usually no sloid area present, predominantly glandular area with mild nuclear pleomorphism. So it is a well differentiated adenocarcinoma.

Mucinous Carcinoma

Image gallery: Fig. 4.31a–e.

Incidence: Approximately 10% of endometrial carcinoma.

Clinical feature

- Age varies from 50 to 80 year
- Post-menopausal bleeding

Criteria

- At least 50% of the malignant cells should show mucinous differentiation
- The mucinous material is PAS positive and diastase resistant

Histopathology

- Multiple glands with no intervening stroma
- Papillary structures
- Glands lined by mucin secreting columnar epithelial cells
- Nuclei are basally placed with mild atypia
- Mucinous material is positive for PAS, Alcian blue and mucicarmine

Differential diagnosis

- *Endocervical mucinous carcinoma*
  - Difficult to differentiate on the basis of morphology alone. However, p16, ER and PR immunostaining are helpful to distinguish the lesion from endocervical mucinous carcinoma

- *Clear cell carcinoma*
  - Tumour cells show predominantly papillary structures
  - Polygonal clear cells rather than columnar
  - Typical hobnail appearance
  - Cell contain glycogen so they are PAS positive and diastase sensitive

- *Key diagnostic points*: Box 4.6

Box 4.6 Key Diagnostic Points of Mucinous Carcinoma
- Confluent glands without any intervening stroma
- Tumour containing mucinous cytoplasm should be more than 50% area. The cells are PAS positive and diastase resistant
- Glandular and also villoglandular pattern present
- Nuclear enlargement and pleomorphism

Note: If mucinous area is less than 50% then it should be labelled as just endometrioid carcinoma.

Prognosis and Treatment

- As most of them are low grade tumour with minimal myometrial invasion so the prognosis of these tumours is better.
- Total abdominal hysterectomy with bilateral salpingo oophorectomy is the treatment of choice.

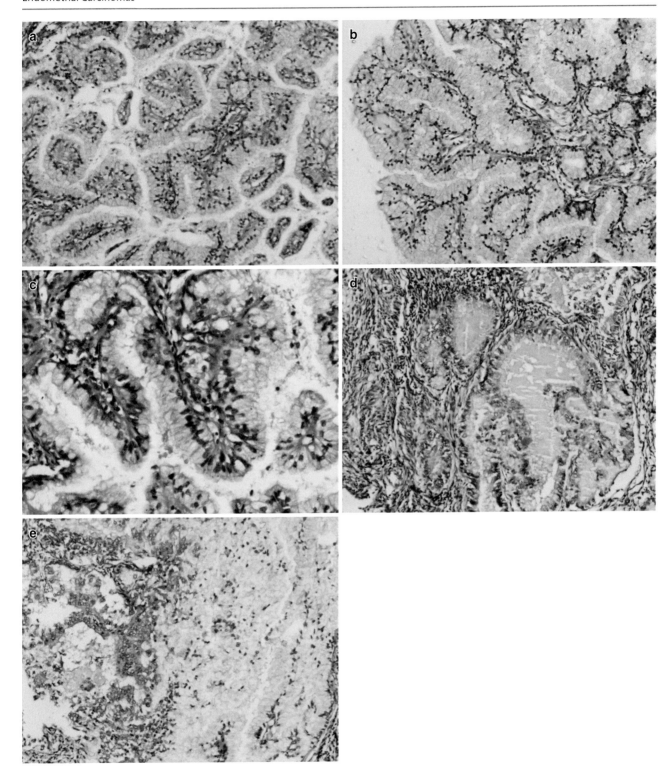

Fig. 4.31 (a) Mucinous carcinoma: Multiple mucinous glands with no intervening stroma. (b) Mucinous carcinoma: Glands lined by mucin secreting columnar epithelial cells. (c) Mucinous carcinoma: Higher magnification of the same. Note abundant mucinous cytoplasm with basally places nuclei. (d) Endometrioid carcinoma with foci of mucinous differentiation: Occasional gland showing mucinous epithelium. (e) Endometrioid carcinoma with foci of mucinous differentiation: Typical mucinous differentiation along with endometrioid carcinoma

Clear Cell Carcinoma

Image gallery: Figs. 4.32 and 4.33a–e.
  Epidemiology

- It represents about 2–5% of endometrial carcinoma
- Mainly occurs in postmenopausal patients
- Mean age: 65 years

Genetic profiling

- Mutation of p 53 and PTEN in 40% cases
- Mutation of PIK3CA

Clinical features

- Post-menopausal bleeding
- No relation with diethylstilbestrol exposure

Gross features

- Enlarged bulky uterus
- Soft and fleshy growth
- Polypoid at times

Histopathology

- Papillary, solid and tubular pattern
- Tubular pattern:
  - Multiple gland like structure
  - Prominent hobnail appearance: Nuclei that bulge out from the cells
  - Eosinophilic material in lumen
  - Lining cells are polygonal with abundant clear cytoplasm
- Papillary pattern
  - Multiple small papillae
  - Core of papillae is edematous and hyalinized
  - Single layer of lining cells
  - Nuclei are markedly pleomorphic having prominent nucleoli
  - No exfoliation of papillae or cellular tufting
- Solid pattern
  - Solid sheet of cells
  - Cells with abundant clear cytoplasm with central nuclei
- Eosinophilic hyaline globules are present in 3/4th cases: PAS positive and diastase sensitive

Immunohistochemistry

- Rarely p53 positive
- ER/PR negative
- Positive for CK 7, Leu M1, vimentin
- Ki67 less than 25% tumour cells are positive
- HNF Iβ positivity is unique and helps to differentiates the clear cell carcinoma from serous carcinoma

Differential diagnosis (see Fig. 4.33f)

- Secretory carcinoma:
  - Low nucleocytoplasmic ratio
  - Mild pleomorphism
  - Cells are in glandular arrangement and cytoplasmic vacuolation is basal and suprabasal in position
- Serous carcinoma (see Table 4.2):

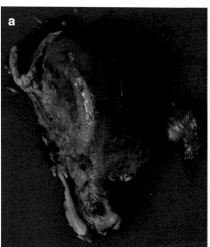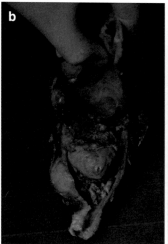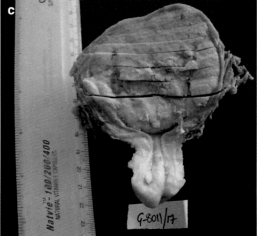

Fig. 4.32 (**a**) Clear cell carcinoma of uterus: Bulky uterus. (**b**) Clear cell carcinoma of uterus: Cut section showing fleshy growth occupying the whole uterine cavity. (**c**) Clear cell carcinoma of uterus: Cut section showing sloid firm growth occupying the entire uterine cavity

- Papillae are relative larger
- Presence of micropapillae
- Pseudostratification is present
- Round cells with moderate nuclear pleomorphism
- No hyaline globule seen
- HNF Iβ negative
- Strong and diffuse p53 positivity
- High Ki 67 positive cells

- Mucinous carcinoma:
  - Predominant glandular arrangement
  - No hobnail appearance
  - The cells are columnar
  - PAS positive and diastase resistant cytoplasmic content
- Yolk sac tumour
  - Very rare in uterus and occurs in young patient

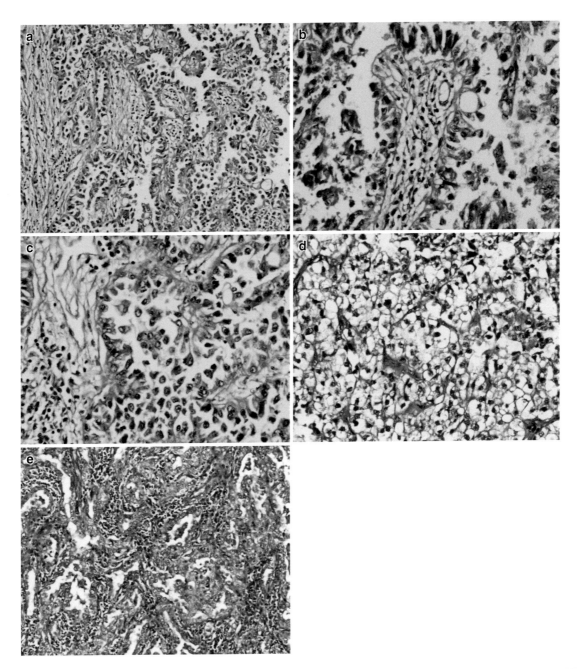

Fig. 4.33 (**a**) Clear cell carcinoma: Multiple papillary structures. (**b**) Clear cell carcinoma: Papillae with fibrovascular core. (**c**) Clear cell carcinoma: Prominent hobnail appearance is seen. Note the pinkish hyaline globules also. (**d**) Clear cell carcinoma: Solid sheet of cells with clear cytoplasm and centrally placed pleomorphic nuclei. (**e**) Clear cell carcinoma: Solid sheet and gland like pattern. (**f**) Differential diagnosis of clear cell carcinoma of uterus

f

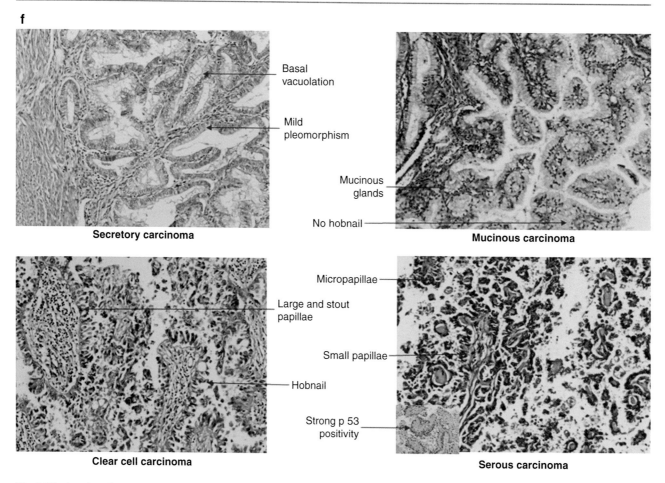

Secretory carcinoma

Mucinous carcinoma

Clear cell carcinoma

Serous carcinoma

Fig. 4.32 (continued)

Table 4.2 Clear cell versus serous carcinoma

Features	Clear cell carcinoma	Serous carcinoma
Papillae	• Relative small • Micropapillae absent	• Stout, thick and branched along with many • Micropapillae present
Solid area	• Usually present	• Absent
Cell cytoplasm	Well defined margin with abundant clear cytoplasm	Occasionally clear cytoplasm
Nuclear pleomorphism	Moderate	Marked
Hyaline globules	Present	Absent
Immunohistochemistry	• Positive for HNF Iβ • Low Ki 67 index	• Positive for p 53, p16 • Very high Ki 67 index

- Characteristic Schiller-Duval bodies present
- High alpha-fetoprotein level in serum

Key diagnostic points: See Box 4.7

Prognosis and management

- High grade tumour
- Variable 5 year survival rate is variable 21 to 75%
- Overall majority reported 5 year survival in stage 1 case as 44%
- Adjuvant chemotherapy is recommended along with total abdominal hysterectomy with bilateral salpingo oophorectomy.

Box 4.7 Key Diagnostic Points of Clear Cell Carcinoma
- Papillary, solid and tubular arrangement
- Hyalinized stroma
- Cell with abundant clear cytoplasm having central enlarged nuclei
- Clear cells are PAS positive and diastase sensitive (due to the cytoplasmic glycogen)
- Hobnail appearance: Nuclei bulging out from the cell
- Hyaline bodies: PAS positive and diastase resistant
- Negative for ER. PR, p53, CK 20 and WT 1
- Characteristically positive for HNF-1β

Endometrial Intraepithelial Carcinoma

Image gallery: Fig. 4.34a–c.

Definition: Serous intraepithelial carcinoma is the precursor of invasive serous carcinoma.

Epidemiology

- Typically occurs in atrophic endometrium
- It may be present in a small focal area of endometrial polyp
- Often associated with underlying serous carcinoma
- No relation with estrogenic hyperactivity

Histopathology

- The endometrial surface lining and the superficial endometrial glands are lined by malignant cells
- The nuclei of the epithelial cells show moderate enlargement, pleomorphism and high nucleocytoplasmic ratio
- High mitotic activity
- Hobnail appearance may be seen

Immunohistochemistry: Strong and diffuse p53 positivity.

Differential diagnosis:

- Eosinophilic metaplasia or tubal metaplasia
  - Less pleomorphic nuclei
  - Low Ki 67 index and P 53 negative

Diagnostic key points: See Box 4.8.

Box 4.8 Diagnostic Key Points of Endometrial Intraepithelial Carcinoma
- Only endometrial surface lining or superficial endometrial glands showing marked nuclear atypia and high mitosis
- Hobnail appearance
- Absence of confluent gland pattern
- Absence of stromal desmoplasia
- Greatest dimension is less than 1 mm
- Strong p 53 expression, high Ki 67 index

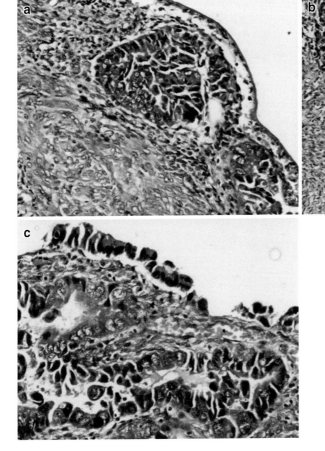

Fig. 4.34 (**a**) Endometrial intraepithelial carcinoma: Only the surface endometrial glands are involved. (**b**) Endometrial intraepithelial carcinoma: The nuclei of the surface epithelial cells show moderate enlargement, pleomorphism and high nucleocytoplasmic ratio. (**c**) Endometrial intraepithelial carcinoma: The glands on the surface of endometrium showing marked nuclear atypia

Serous Carcinoma

Image gallery: Figs. 4.35, 4.36a–I, and 4.37.
  Epidemiology

- It consists of 5–10% of endometrial carcinoma
- Typical prototype of type 2 endometrial carcinoma
- Unrelated with estrogenic hyperactivity
- Patients are not obese
- Common in nulliparous women

  Genetic features

- p53 mutation: 90% cases
- PIK3C mutation: 40% cases
- FBXW7 mutation: 20% cases

  Clinical features

- Post-menopausal patients in late sixty
- Commonly complaints of vaginal bleeding
- Uterus usually enlarged, however occasionally the tumour may be microscopic and no uterine enlargement is evident

  Gross features

- Uterus may be small in size due to old age
- Exophytic growth fills up the uterine cavity
- Occasionally the tumour is seen within the endometrial polyp

  Histopathology

- Predominantly papillary pattern and occasionally glandular and solid areas
- Tumour cells
    - The lining cells are large, cuboidal to polygonal with abundant eosinophilic cytoplasm
    - Nuclei show high N/C ration with moderate to marked pleomorphism.
    - Large macro nucleoli

- Multinucleated giant cells
- High mitotic activity
- Deeper myometrial invasion and lymphovascular permeation are frequent
- Marked hobnail appearance
- Psammoma bodies
- Papillary and glandular pattern
    - Short, stout and often branching papillae
    - Frequent sloughing of papillae gives rise to many small islands of cells that float freely
    - There may be multiple glands
- Slit like spaces
    - In lower magnification the tumour looks like slit like spaces formed by glands.
    - The slit like glands are lined by tumour cells
- Poorly differentiated solid component
    - The tumour cells are in diffuse solid sheets
    - Occasional papillae
    - Large cells with abundant cytoplasm
    - Nuclei show severe pleomorphism
- Microcystic pattern
    - Multiple small cystic spaces
    - Cyst wall is lined by tumour cells

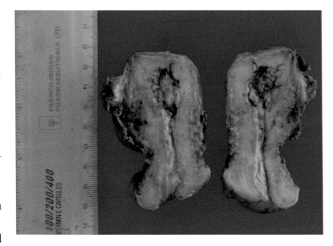

Fig. 4.35 Gross picture of uterine serous carcinoma showing a polypoid projecting growth in the endometrial cavity

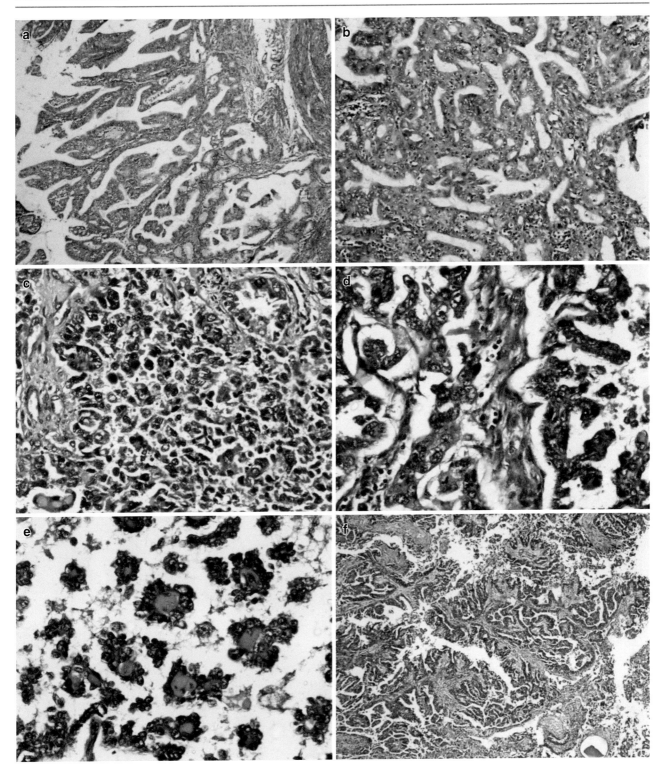

Fig. 4.36 (**a**) Serous carcinoma: Predominantly papillary pattern. (**b**) Serous carcinoma: The glandular pattern. (**c**) Serous carcinoma: Solid sheets of cells having moderately pleomorphic nuclei with large prominent nucleoli. (**d**) Serous carcinoma: Multiple short papillae. (**e**) Serous carcinoma: Micropapillae present. (**f**) Serous carcinoma: Tumour with many slit like spaces. (**g**) Serous carcinoma: Marked nuclear atypia in the glandular lining cells. (**h**) Serous carcinoma: Tufts of cell showing nuclear pleomorphism. (**i**) Serous carcinoma: Nuclei of the lining cells show moderate pleomorphism

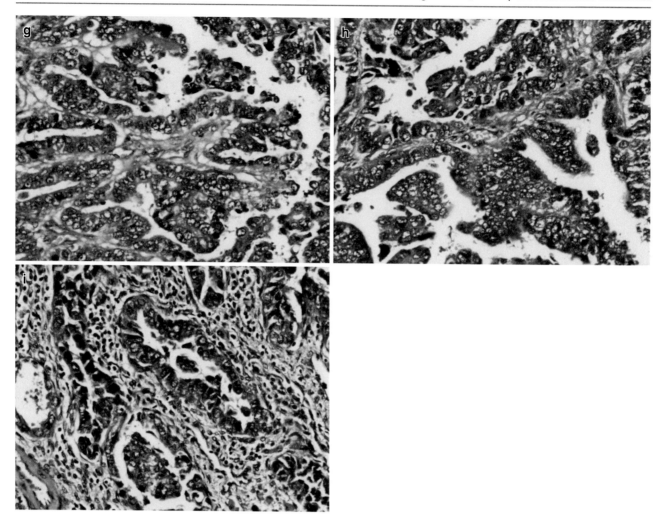

Fig. 4.36 (continued)

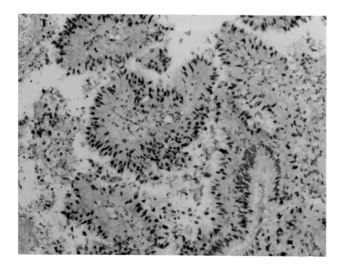

Fig. 4.37 Serous carcinoma: Strong nuclear p53 positive cells

Immunohistochemistry

Positive:

- Strong and diffuse positivity of p53, p16, CK, EMA, IMP 3
- IMP 3 positivity is important to differentiate the serous carcinoma from high grade endometrial carcinoma

- *Key diagnostic points*: Box 4.9

Box 4.9 Key Diagnostic Points of Serous Carcinoma
- Papillae, gland and solid areas
- Mainly short, stout and branched papillae
- Small sloughed papillary tuft
- Hobnail appearance
- Marked nuclear pleomorphism, multinucleation and even giant cells in a tumour with papillary pattern should be considered as serous carcinoma
- Immunohistochemistry pattern: Strong diffuse p 53 positivity, high Ki 67 index and negative ER/PR
- Diffuse and strong p16 positivity

Note:

- This is a prototype of Type II endometrial carcinoma. Always distinguish it from (a) villoglandular carcinoma, (b) Grade III endometrioid carcinoma
- In morphologically difficult situation: Put a panel of p53, ER/PR, Ki 67

Differential diagnosis

- Clear cell carcinoma: discussed before
- Endometrioid carcinoma (see Table 4.3):
  - Significant areas are solid (>50%)
  - High nuclear grade
  - Nuclear polarity preserved
  - Positive for p16, ER/PR
- Villoglandular carcinoma: discussed before

Prognosis

- Frequent lymphovascular emboli and deep myometrial invasion
- Metastasis in pelvic region is common
- Overall 5 year survival is 36% to 57%
- Poor prognostic factors include higher age group, lymphovascular invasion and deeper myometrial invasion (>50%)

Table 4.3 Serous versus grade III endometrioid carcinoma

Features	Serous carcinoma	Grade III endometrioid carcinoma
Solid area	Both papillary and solid areas	Predominant solid areas
Papillae	Short and stout and often tips are detached forming sloughed out micropapillae	Thick
Nuclear pleomorphism	Marked and even the glands and papillae show significant pleomorphism	Only solid areas show marked pleomorphism
Hobnail appearance	Frequently present	Absent
Immunohistochemistry	• Positive for p53, p16 • High Ki 67 index • Negative for ER/PR	• Often positive for p53, ER/PR • Low Ki 67 index

Mixed Carcinomas

Image gallery: Figs. 4.38 and 4.39a–c.

Definition: The mixed carcinomas consist of both type I and type II carcinoma together and one of the component should be more than 5% of the tumour mass.

Histopathology

- Endometrioid and serous component: The commonest combination
- Endometrioid and clear cell component

Prognosis

- It depends on the admixture of the highest grade component of the tumour. The presence of serous carcinoma has bad prognosis

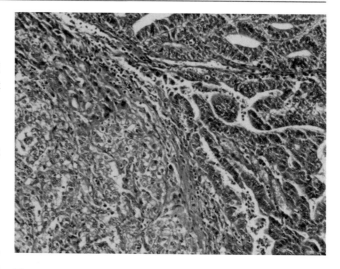

Fig. 4.38 Mixed clear cell and endometrioid carcinoma: Both clear cell carcinoma (left side) and endometrioid carcinoma (right side) are coexisting

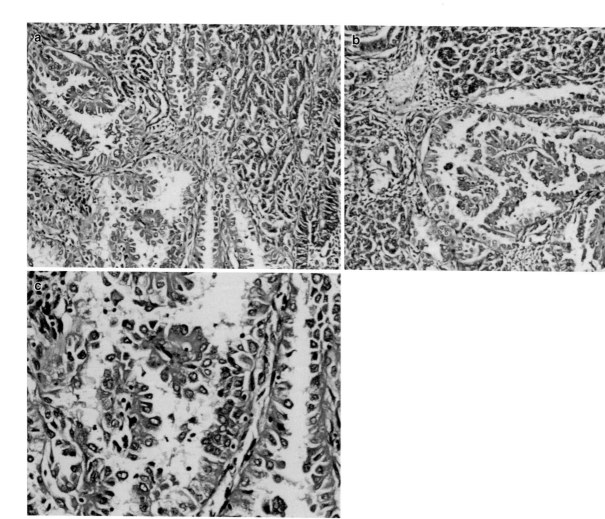

Fig. 4.39 (**a**) Mixed serous and endometrioid carcinoma: Note the hobnail pattern of serous carcinoma (left part) and gland pattern of endometrioid carcinoma. (**b**) Mixed serous and endometrioid carcinoma: Glandular component of endometrioid carcinoma along with papillary architecture of serous carcinoma showing multiple papillae and hobnailing appearance. (**c**) Mixed serous and endometrioid carcinoma: Higher magnification of the serous component showing the papillae lined by moderately pleomorphic cells with large prominent nucleoli

Tumour like Lesions of Uterus

Arias–Stella Reaction

Image gallery: Fig. 4.40a–c.
  Association

- Mostly associated with intrauterine or ectopic pregnancy
- Rarely seen due to progestin administration

  Clinical features: No symptoms.
  Histopathology

- Tortuous and star shaped glands

- Lining epithelial cells of the glands are large with clear vacuolated cytoplasm
- Enlarged nuclei with mild hyperchromasia and pleomorphism
- Hobnail appearance
- Epithelial tufting
- Decidua

  Differential diagnosis

- Clear cell carcinoma
    - Nucleo-cytoplasmic ratio is altered
    - Unlike Arias-Stella reaction, here the normal glandular architecture is not maintained

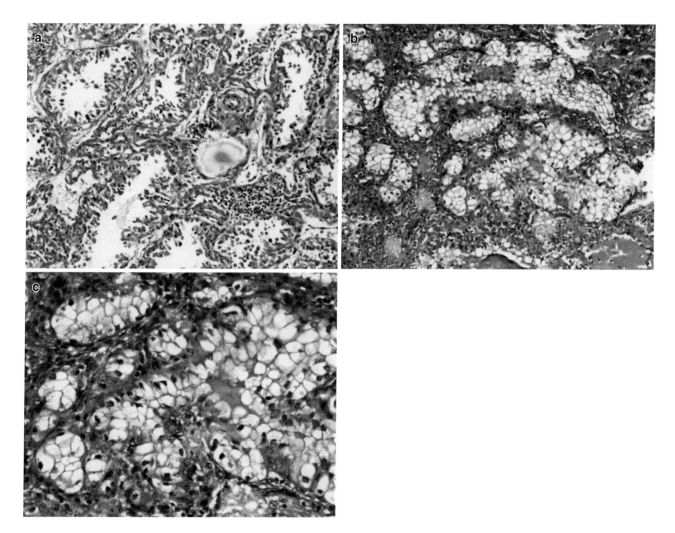

Fig. 4.40 (**a**) Arias-Stella reaction: Multiple star shaped glands. (**b**) Arias-Stella reaction: Many irregular glands with papillary infolding. The glands are lined by cells with abundant clear cytoplasm. (**c**) Arias-Stella reaction: Higher magnification showing glands with clear vacuolated cytoplasm and basally placed monomorphic nuclei

Endometrial Polyp

Image gallery: Figs. 4.41 and 4.42a–g.
  Epidemiology:

- Common, near about 25% patients
- Often associated with hormone replacement therapy
- It occurs around 40 years of age
- Both pre and post-menopausal patients are affected
- About 5% polyps are associated with carcinoma

Histogenesis

- Monoclonal proliferation of endometrial stromal cells
- Reactive polyclonal proliferation of the glands

Clinical features

- Small polyps are asymptomatic
- Larger polyp presents with abnormal uterine bleeding

Gross features

- Polypoid structure
- Single to multiple
- Sessile or pedunculated
- Soft and fleshy with smooth surface

Diagnostic criteria

- Tissue covered with surface epithelium in three sides
- Abnormal in architecture of the glands: Dilated, out-pouching and crowded
- Glands in the polyp look different than the normal adjacent endometrial gland
- Thick walled blood vessels in stroma
- Fibrotic and hyalinized stroma

Histopathological patterns of polyp

- Hyperplastic polyp
  - Variable sized irregular shaped glands
  - Focally crowded glands
  - Fibrotic stroma
  - Lining epithelium may show metaplastic changes
- Functional polyp
  - Proliferative or secretory glands
  - Abnormally oriented glands
  - Thick walled blood vessels
- Atrophic polyp
  - Cystically dilated glands
  - Flattened to small cuboidal cells

Differential diagnosis

- Lower uterine segment
  - No thick walled blood vessels
  - No irregularity of the glandular architecture
- Adenosarcoma
  - Atypia and increased mitosis of stromal cells
  - Stromal condensation around glands
- Atypical polypoid adenomyoma
  - Fibromyomatous stroma
  - Atypia in the glandular epithelium

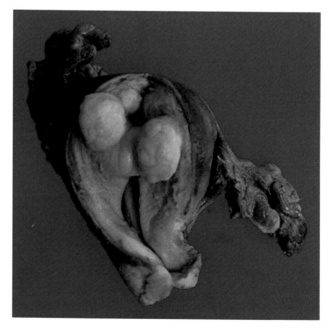

Fig. 4.41 Gross picture of benign endometrial polyp showing multiple grey white polyp

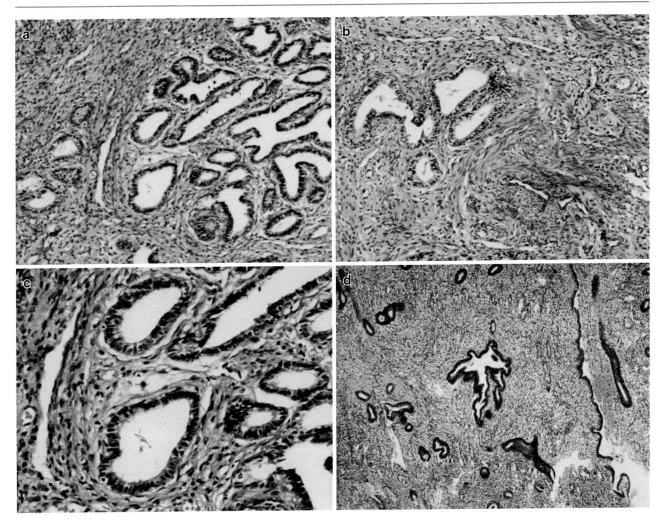

Fig. 4.42 (**a**) Hyperplastic polyp: Overcrowded variable sized irregular shaped glands. (**b**) Hyperplastic polyp: The glands are surrounded by smooth muscle. (**c**) Hyperplastic polyp: The glands are lined by cuboidal cells. (**d**) Endometrial functional polyp: Abnormally oriented proliferative gland embedded in the endometrial stroma. (**e**) Endometrial functional polyp: Abnormal branching of the glands. (**f**) Atrophic polyp: Many cystically dilated glands lined by flattened to cuboidal cells. (**g**) Atrophic polyp: The flattened to cuboidal lining cells of the glands in higher magnification

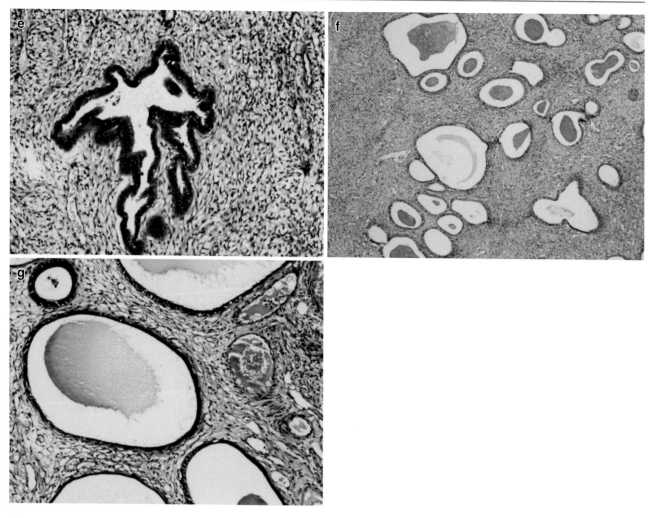

Fig. 4.42 (continued)

Metaplasia

Image gallery: Fig. 4.43.

Definition: Metaplasia indicates the replacement of one type of cells into other type of mature cells that are not normally present in that organ.

In true sense many types of endometrial metaplasia are not true metaplasia and those changes are better defined as "altered differentiation" rather than metaplastic changes.

Histogenesis

- From the sub columnar reserve cells
- Direct transition of the endometrial cells to squamous cells or ciliated cells

- The stimulation of the transition comes due to chronic irritation or abnormal hormonal stimulation

Significance

- Morules: High risk of malignancy
- Squamous metaplasia: Occasional risk of malignancy
- Ciliary, tubal and mucinous metaplasia are often related with malignancy
- Papillary syncytial metaplasia: Never related with malignancy
- Clear cell metaplasia has no relation with malignancy

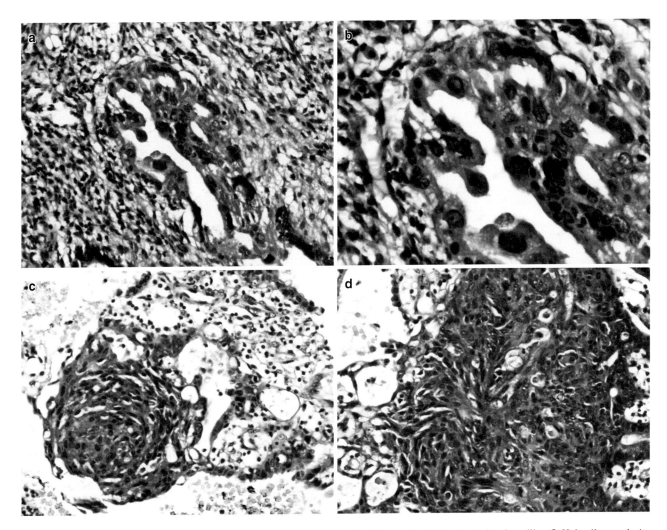

Fig. 4.43 (**a**) Squamous metaplasia: The cells with polyhedral in shape having dense eosinophilic cytoplasm. (**b**) Squamous metaplasia: Higher magnification of the same highlighting the cytoplasmic character. (**c**) Squamous morule: The round to oval cells arranged concentrically like a granuloma. (**d**) Squamous morule: Higher magnification showing polyhedral to elongated cells. (**e**) Tubal metaplasia: The lining cells of the endometrial glands showing cilia. (**f**) Hobnail metaplasia: The hobnail appearance in the endometrial glands. (**g**) Clear cell metaplasia: Marked clear cell changes in the glandular lining epithelium. (**h**) Papillary syncytial metaplasia: Focal piling up of the endometrial lining epithelium giving syncytial appearance. The cell showing eosinophilic cytoplasm

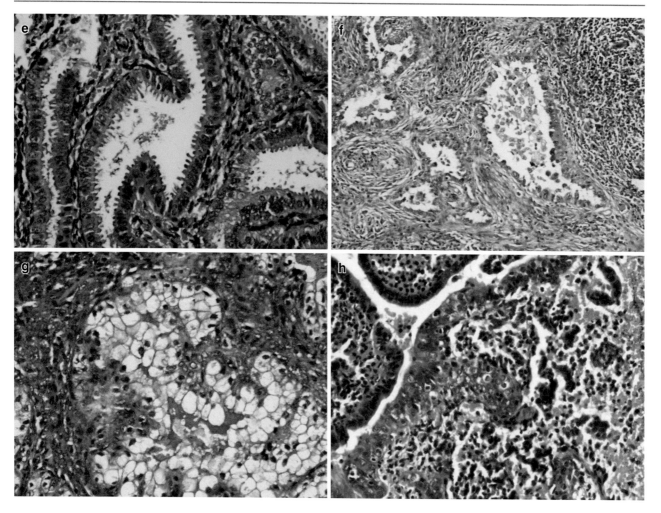

Fig. 4.43 (continued)

Different Types of Metaplasia

Squamous metaplasia

- Polyhedral cells with well-defined margin
- Dense eosinophilic cytoplasm
- Intercellular bridge

Squamous morules

- In morular metaplasia the cells are round to oval and arranged concentrically like a granuloma
- Morules are present in between the glands
- Occasionally central necrosis is present

Ciliated and tubal metaplasia

- Association: Endometrial hyperplasia, endometritis, endometrial polyps and adenocarcinoma
- The epithelial cells of the glands and surface lining of the uterus are replaced by ciliated columnar epithelial cells.

Eosinophilic metaplasia

- Association: Endometrial polyp and endometritis
- Cuboidal cells with abundant eosinophilic cytoplasm resembling oncocytic appearance
- Electron microscope: Abundant mitochondria in the cytoplasm

Hobnail metaplasia

- Association: endometrial polyp, clear cell carcinoma
- Round cells with eosinophilic cytoplasm
- Nuclei protruding out from the cytoplasm at the luminal side

Clear cell metaplasia

- Association: Pregnancy and progesterone therapy
- Cells have abundant clear cytoplasm

Mucinous metaplasia

- Association: Endometriosis, tamoxifen induced polyp, glands in adenofibroma
- The tall columnar cells with abundant mucinous cytoplasm
- Rarely goblet cells and neuroendocrine cells are noted
- Simple mucinous metaplasia: The glands are architecturally normal
- Complex mucinous metaplasia: The gland show complex branching and crowding.

Papillary syncytial metaplasia

- Association: Mainly seen during menstrual breakdown of the endometrial cells
- Tufts of epithelial cells with eosinophilic cytoplasm
- Nuclear pleomorphism and occasional mitotic activity
- Fibrovascular core present

Reference

1. Kurman RJ, Carcangiu ML, Herrington S, Young RH. WHO classification of tumours of female genital reproductive organs. 4th ed. Lyon: International Agency for Research on Cancer; 2014.

Suggested Reading

Ambros RA, Malfetano JH. Villoglandular adenocarcinoma of the endometrium. Am J Surg Pathol. 2000;24(1):155–6.

Baak JP, Mutter GL, Robboy S, van Diest PJ, Uyterlinde AM, Orbo A, Palazzo J, Fiane B, Løvslett K, Burger C, Voorhorst F, Verheijen RH. The molecular genetics and morphometry-based endometrial intraepithelial neoplasia classification system predicts disease progression in endometrial hyperplasia more accurately than the 1994 World Health Organization classification system. Cancer. 2005;103(11):2304–12.

Bhola V, Hafeez MA, Shukla CB. Tuberculous endometritis. J Indian Med Assoc. 1984;82(5):149–51.

del Carmen MG, Birrer M, Schorge JO. Uterine papillary serous cancer: a review of the literature. Gynecol Oncol. 2012;127:651–61.

Gadducci A, Cosio S, Spirito N, Cionini L. Clear cell carcinoma of the endometrium: a biological and clinical enigma. Anticancer Res. 2010;30(4):1327–34.

Gatius S, Matias-Guiu X. Practical issues in the diagnosis of serous carcinoma of the endometrium. Mod Pathol. 2016;29(Suppl 1):S45–58.

Hentati D, Belghith B, Kochbati L, Driss M, Maalej M. Tunis Med. 2010;88(4):230–3.

Jalloul RJ, Elshaikh MA, Ali-Fehmi R, Haley MM, Yoon J, Mahan M, Munkarah AR. Mucinous adenocarcinoma of the endometrium: case series and review of the literature. Int J Gynecol Cancer. 2012;22(5):812–8.

Kaspar HG, Crum CP. The utility of immunohistochemistry in the differential diagnosis of gynecologic disorders. Arch Pathol Lab Med. 2015;139(1):39–54.

Kendall BS, Ronnett BM, Isacson C, Cho KR, Hedrick L, Diener-West M, Kurman RJ. Reproducibility of the diagnosis of endometrial hyperplasia, atypical hyperplasia, and well-differentiated carcinoma. Am J Surg Pathol. 1998;22(8):1012–9.

Kurman RJ, Kaminski PF, Norris HJ. The behaviour of endometrial hyperplasia. Along-term study of "untreated" hyperplasia in 170 patients. Cancer. 1985;56:403–12.

Kurman RJ, Norris HJ. Evaluation of criteria for distinguishing atypical endometrial hyperplasia from well–differentiated carcinoma. Cancer. 1982;49:2547–57.

Malpica A. How to approach the many faces of endometrioid carcinoma. Mod Pathol. 2016;29(Suppl 1):S29–44.

Melhem MF, Tobon H. Mucinous adenocarcinoma of the endometrium: a clinico-pathological review of 18 cases. Int J Gynecol Pathol. 1987;6:347–55.

Michels TC. Chronic endometritis. Am Fam Physician. 1995;52(1):217–22.

Mittal K, Salem A, Lo A. Diagnostic criteria for distinguishing endometrial adenocarcinoma from complex atypical endometrial hyperplasia. Hum Pathol. 2014;45(1):98–103.

Mondal SK. Histopathologic analysis of female genital tuberculosis: a fifteen-year retrospective study of 110 cases in eastern India. Turk Patoloji Derg. 2013;29(1):41–5.

Ng AB, Reagan JW, Storaasli JP, Wentz WB. Mixed adenosquamous carcinoma of the endometrium. Am J Clin Pathol. 1973;59:765–81.

Nicolae A, Preda O, Nogales FF. Endometrial metaplasias and reactive changes: a spectrum of altered differentiation. J Clin Pathol. 2011;64(2):97–106.

O'Connor KA, Holman DJ, Wood JW. Menstrual cycle variability and the perimenopause. Am J Hum Biol. 2001;13(4):465–78.

Owings RA, Quick CM. Endometrial intraepithelial neoplasia. Arch Pathol Lab Med. 2014;138(4):484–91.

Rose PG. Endometrial carcinoma. N Engl J Med. 1996;335(9):640–9. Review. Erratum in: N Engl J Med 1997 May 1;336(18):1335.

Stelloo E, Nout RA, Osse EM, Jurgenliemk-Schulz IJ, Jobsen JJ, Lutgens LC, et al. Improved risk assessment by integrating molecular and clinicopathological factors in early-stage endometrial cancer – combined analysis of PORTEC cohorts. Clin Cancer Res. 2016;22:4215–24.

Talhouk A, McAlpine JN. New classification of endometrial cancers: the development and potential applications of genomic-based classification in research and clinical care. Gynecol Oncol Res Pract. 2016;3:14.

Tobon H, Watkins GJ. Secretory adenocarcinoma of the endometrium. Int J Gynecol Pathol. 1985;4:328–35.

Treloar AE, Boynton RE, Behn BG, Brown BW. Variation of the human menstrual cycle through reproductive life. Int J Fertil. 1967;12(1 Pt 2):77–126.

Zaino RJ, Kurman RJ. Squamous differentiation in carcinoma of the endometrium: a critical appraisal of adenoacanthoma and adenosquamous carcinoma. Semin Diagn Pathol. 1988;5(2):154–71.

Pathology of Mesenchymal and Other Miscellaneous Tumours of Uterine Corpus

5

Classification of uterine mesenchymal and other tumours (excluding epithelial tumours) according to World Health Organization [1] is highlighted in the Fig. 5.1.

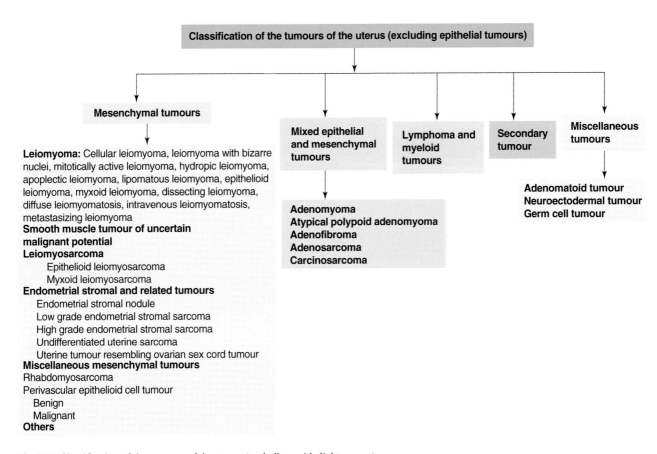

Fig. 5.1 Classification of the tumours of the uterus (excluding epithelial tumours)

© Springer Nature Singapore Pte Ltd. 2019
P. Dey, *Color Atlas of Female Genital Tract Pathology*, https://doi.org/10.1007/978-981-13-1029-4_5

Mesenchymal Tumours of Uterus

Leiomyoma

Image gallery: Figs. 5.2, 5.3, 5.4, 5.5, 5.6, 5.7, 5.8, 5.9, and 5.10.

Epidemiology

- Commonest uterine neoplasm
- Approximately 20% females are affected
- It is present in 70% hysterectomy specimen
- Higher rate of occurrence in black women

Clinical features

- Asymptomatic: 25% patients
- Menorrhagia, pain abdomen, and pressure symptoms
- Submucosal leiomyoma: Abortion, infertility, malformed fetus

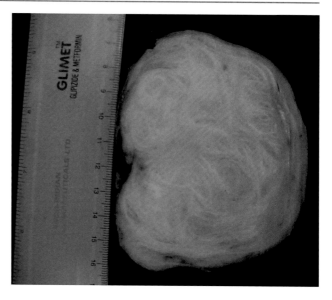

Fig. 5.2 Gross of leiomyoma: Solid grey white and whorled appearance

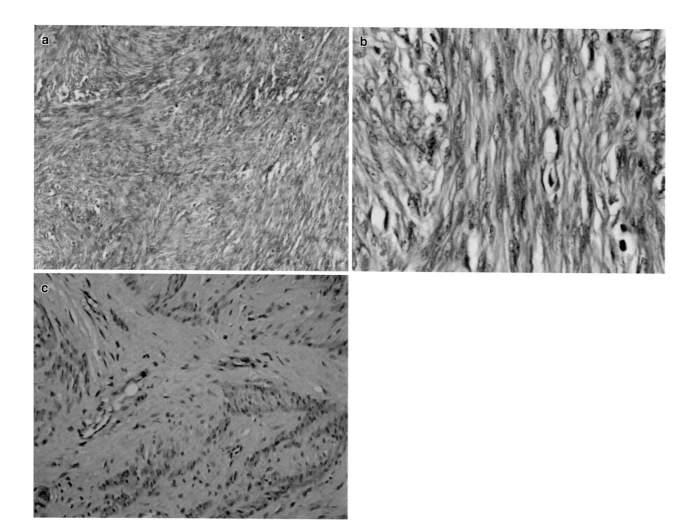

Fig. 5.3 (**a**) Leiomyoma: Small and large fascicles of smooth muscle. (**b**) Leiomyoma: The cells are elongated with blunt ended nuclei. (**c**) Leiomyoma: Marked hyaline changes

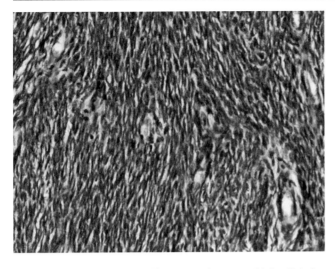

Fig. 5.4 Cellular leiomyoma: The tumour shows very high cellularity. This has no additional significance

- Large leiomyoma: Pressure symptoms such as constipation, urinary problems
- Subserosal leiomyoma: Torsion, infection and fever
- Abdominal pain due to bleeding within leiomyoma

Gross features

- Well encapsulated with sharp demarcated margin
- White to pinkish in colour
- Firm to rubbery in consistency
- Cut surface: Grey white with whorled appearance

Histopathology

- Interlacing bundles of cells
- Elongated cells

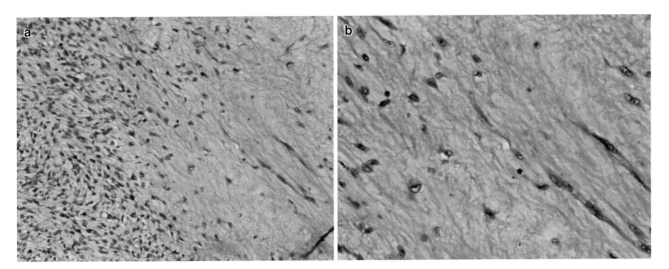

Fig. 5.5 (**a**) Myxoid leiomyoma: Large amount of myxoid stromal material along with oval to elongated cells. (**b**) Myxoid leiomyoma: Scanty elongated spindle cells in the myxoid material

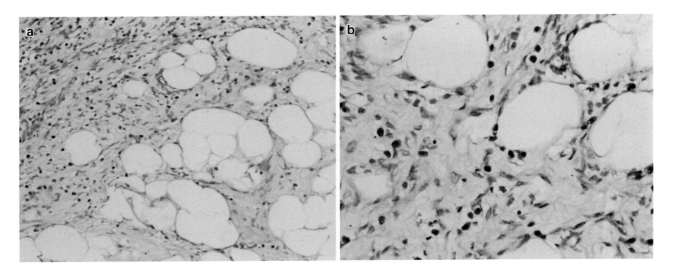

Fig. 5.6 (**a**) Lipoleiomyoma: Large areas of mature fat along with leiomyomatous component. (**b**) Lipoleiomyoma: Higher magnification of the same showing mature fat and spindle cells

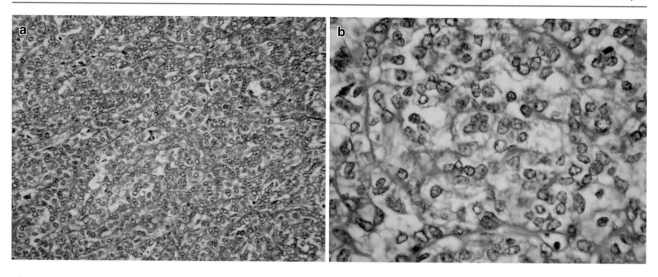

Fig. 5.7 (**a**) Epithelioid leiomyoma: Diffuse sheets of cells. (**b**) Epithelioid leiomyoma: Polygonal cells with abundant eosinophilic cytoplasm, central nuclei having small nucleoli

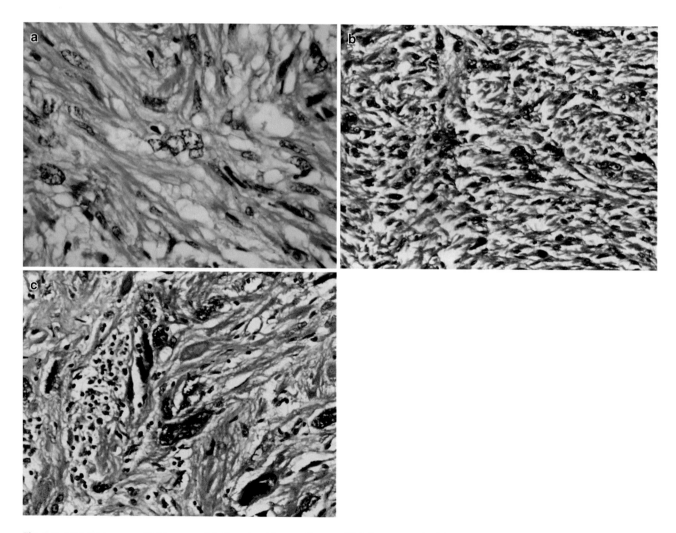

Fig. 5.8 (**a**) Leiomyoma with bizarre nuclei: Occasional large cells seen. (**b**) Leiomyoma with bizarre nuclei: Many large pleomorphic cells present. (**c**) Leiomyoma with bizarre nuclei: Bizarre pleomorphic nuclei with irregular margin

- Spindle shaped nuclei with blunt ends giving cigar shaped appearance
- Fine chromatin with tiny nucleoli
- Hyalinization, oedema, cystic degeneration may be present

- Many vascular channels may be present
- Foci of haemopoietin elements containing lymphocytes, histiocytes and mast cells may be seen

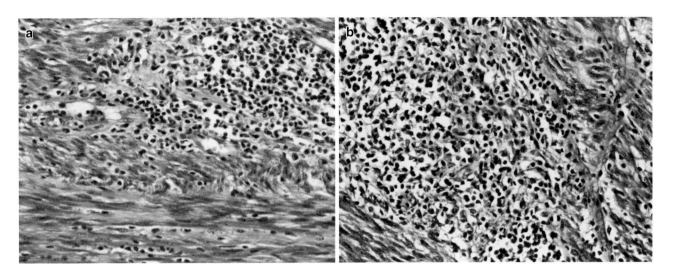

Fig. 5.9 (**a**) Leiomyoma: Aggregations of lymphoid cells within the leiomyoma. (**b**) Leiomyoma: Predominantly mature lymphocytes are infiltrated

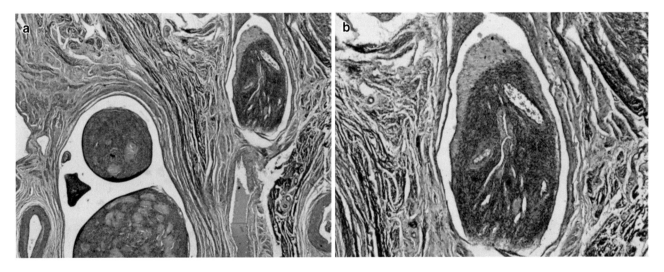

Fig. 5.10 (**a**) Intravenous leiomyoma: Small clusters of smooth muscle cells covered with endothelial cells of the blood vessels. (**b**) Intravenous leiomyoma: Higher magnification shows leiomyoma within the blood vessel

Types of Leiomyoma

Cellular leiomyoma

- Abundant cellularity
- Nuclear crowding and nuclear overlapping
- No necrosis or mitosis
- No additional significance
- Differential diagnosis: (a) Endometrial stromal sarcoma, b) Leiomyosarcoma

Myxoid leiomyoma

- Large amount of myxoid stromal material: Pale basophilic colour in haematoxylin and eosin stain
- Low cellularity
- Spindle shaped smooth muscle cells
- No increase in mitosis (less than 2 per 10 high power field) or pleomorphism
- Differential diagnosis: myxoid liposarcoma

Lipoleiomyoma

- Mixed tumour: Bothe mature fat cells and smooth muscle cells are intimately admixed

Epithelioid leiomyoma

- It contains more than 50% round to polygonal cells
- Small ribbon like arrangement of the cells
- Abundant matrix material is present in between the cells
- The cells look like epithelial cells: Polygonal cells with abundant eosinophilic cytoplasm, central nuclei having small nucleoli
- Characterized by HMGA-2 overexpression
- Differential diagnosis: a) Metastatic lobular carcinoma of breast: due to the arrangement of single rows of cells

Leiomyoma with bizarre nuclei

- Scattered large atypical cells present
- Large cell with single to multiple large pleomorphic nuclei
- Irregular nuclear outline
- Clumped chromatin
- Occasional Intranuclear inclusion
- Mitosis: Usually 0 to 5 per 10 high power field

Leiomyoma with lymphoid infiltrate

- Focal or diffuse lymphocytic infiltrate
- Mature lymphocytes and plasma cells
- Usually seen in case of gonadotrophin releasing hormone agonist therapy

Intravenous leiomyoma

- No predisposing factors
- Presence of multiple leiomyoma in the uterus
- Smooth muscle cells covered with endothelial cells of the blood vessels
- Occasionally the intravenous leiomyoma may be present in the inferior vena cava or even in heart

Dissecting leiomyoma

- Rare growth pattern
- Smooth muscle cells are arranged in swirling fashion and dissects the myometrium
- It simulates cotyledons of placenta
- High vascularity and oedema

Immunohistochemistry

Positive for caldesmon, desmin, smooth muscle actin, and histone deacetylase 8
- Variable positivity for CD 10
- Negative for EMA, CK

Cytogenetic profile

- Monoclonal in origin
- Translocation t (12:14) (q15-q23-24) in nearly 40% cases
- MED 12 mutation in occasional cases

Differential diagnosis

- Leiomyosarcoma: Many variants of leiomyoma may be confused with leiomyosarcoma such as
  - Cellular leiomyoma: No nuclear atypia, increased mitosis and necrosis
  - Leiomyoma with bizarre nuclei: Lack of necrosis and mitosis
  - Myxoid leiomyoma: Mitosis is usually less than 2 per 10 HPF
  - Mitotically active leiomyoma: Absence of necrosis and nuclear atypia
  - Epithelioid leiomyoma: Mitosis is usually less than 5 per 10 HPF
- Endometrial stromal sarcoma
  - Round to oval cells
  - Sheet like arrangement
  - Prominent vascular pattern
  - CD 10 positivity and negative caldesmon

Prognosis

- Benign course
- Intravenous leiomyoma may recur
- Most cases of epithelioid and myxoid leiomyoma also follow a benign course

Smooth Muscle Tumours of Uncertain Malignant Potential

Definition: This tumour does not completely fulfil the criteria of leiomyosarcoma and also cannot be put into the group of leiomyoma.

Diagnostic criteria (see Table 5.1)

- Coagulative necrosis is present, however there is no nuclear atypia and mitosis is less than 10 per 10 high power field.
- Coagulative necrosis is absent, moderate to severe nuclear atypia is present along with 5–9 mitosis per 10 high power field.
- Coagulative necrosis is absent, no nuclear atypia, however, mitosis is more than 15 per 10 high power field.

Prognosis

- There is variable rate of recurrence that ranges from 0 to 26% cases
- Immunohistochemistry of p16 and p 53 to classify this lesion has been attempted but these stains are not useful.

Table 5.1 Diagnostic criteria of Smooth muscle tumours of uncertain malignant potential, mitotically active leiomyoma and leiomyoma with bizarre nuclei

Coagulative necrosis	Significant nuclear atypia	Mitosis rate per 10 HPF	Diagnosis
Present	Absent	Less than 10	STUMP
Absent	Present	5–9	STUMP
Absent	Absent	More than 15	STUMP
Absent	Absent	5–15	Mitotically active leiomyoma
Absent	Present	Less than 5	Leiomyoma with bizarre nuclei

STUMP Smooth muscle tumours of uncertain malignant potential, *HPF* High power field

Leiomyosarcoma

Image gallery: Figs. 5.11 and 5.12.
Epidemiology

- It represents 1–2% of all uterine cancer
- About 40% of all uterine sarcomas
- Leiomyoma: leiomyosarcoma = 800:1 ratio

Genetic profile

- Loss of heterozygosity of 10q and 13q
- Gain of 17p, Xp, 1q
- Loss of 2p, 16q
- Frequent numerical chromosomal aberration
- Overexpression of c-MYC gene
- p16 is also associated with the tumorigenesis

Clinical features

- Predominantly occurs after 50 years
- Mean age is 55 year
- Vaginal bleeding
- Pelvic mass and pain abdomen
- Rapid enlargement of uterus in a post-menopausal patient
- Hypercalcemia may be present

Gross features

- Usually large single mass
- Mean size is 10 cm
- Poorly circumscribed mass
- Cut section: Soft and fleshy with haemorrhage and necrosis

Histopathology

- Short and long fascicles of spindle cells
- Elongated spindle cells with eosinophilic cytoplasm
- Spindle shaped nuclei with blunt ends resemble cigar
- Nuclear atypia: Moderate to severe

- Mitosis: Usually more than 10 per 10 HPF
- Coagulative necrosis present
- Vascular invasion is often present

Diagnostic criteria
Any two of the following features

- Mitosis: More than 10 per 10 HPF
- Nuclear atypia: Moderate to severe
- Coagulative necrosis: present

Immunohistochemistry of leiomyosarcoma

- Positive for desmin, caldesmon, smooth muscle actin and HDAC-8
- Occasionally positive for CD 10, CK and EMA
- Diffusely positive p16
- High Ki 67 index
- Thirty percent cases are also positive for ER/PR

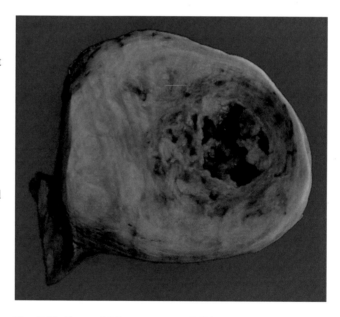

Fig. 5.11 Gross of leiomyosarcoma: Solid grey white tumour with large areas of haemorrhage and necrosis

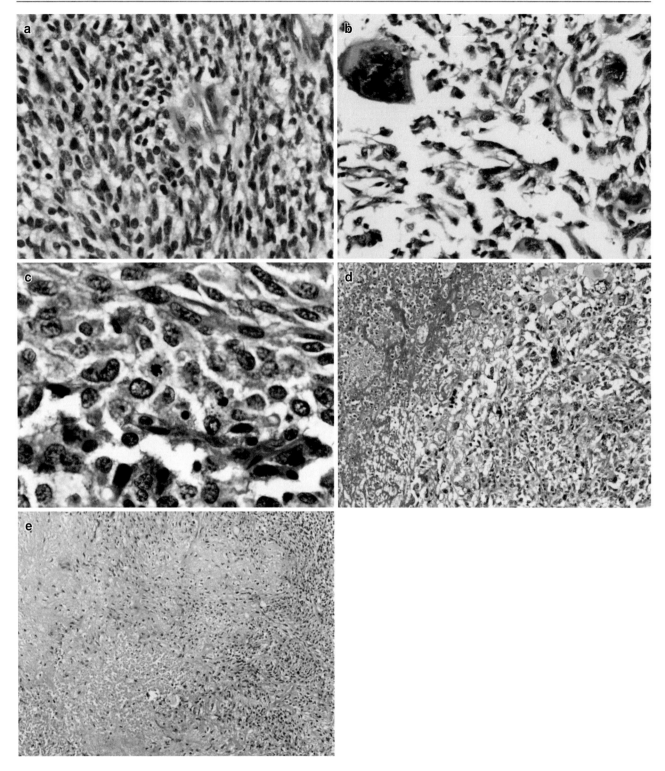

Fig. 5.12 (**a**) Leiomyosarcoma: Moderately pleomorphic oval to spindle cells. (**b**) Leiomyosarcoma: Large mononuclear and multinuclear giant cells. (**c**) Leiomyosarcoma: Many mitotic figures are seen. (**d**) Leiomyosarcoma: Viable tumour cells (right) and coagulative necrosis. (**e**) Leiomyosarcoma: Vast areas of coagulative necrosis

Diagnostic key points of leiomyosarcoma: See Box 5.1.

Box 5.1 Diagnostic Key Points of Leiomyosarcoma
- Oval to spindle cells in fascicles
- Any two of these features below:
    - Coagulative necrosis
    - Significant nuclear atypia
    - Mitotic count: more than 10 per 10 high power field
- Immunohistochemistry: Usually not needed, however tumour cells are positive for SMA, desmin, caldesmon and HDAC 8

Table 5.2 Distinguishing features of leiomyosarcoma and leiomyoma

Features	Leiomyosarcoma	Leiomyoma
Cellularity	Hypercellular	Usually not much cellular
Nuclear pleomorphism	Significant	Usually no nuclear pleomorphism
Mitotic activity	Most of the time elevated and more than 10 per 10 HPF	Variable. Most of the time it is low.
Tumour margin	Infiltrating margin	Well circumscribed and sharp
Necrosis	Coagulative necrosis	Hyaline necrosis

Differential diagnosis:

- Leiomyoma: Leiomyoma particularly cellular leiomyoma or leiomyoma with bizarre nuclei should be distinguished from leiomyosarcoma (Table 5.2).

Myxoid Leiomyosarcoma

Image gallery: Fig. 5.13a–c.
  Histopathology

- Abundant myxoid material: pale blue in haematoxylin and eosin stain
- Hypocellular
- Spindle shaped cells in thin fascicles
- Cells often show mild to moderate atypia
- Coagulative necrosis may be present
- Mitotic activity is more than 2 per 10 HPF
- Low mitotic activity may be present due to relatively low cellularity. However, moderate nuclear atypia should always raise doubt of malignancy

Diagnostic key points of myxoid leiomyosarcoma: See Box 5.2.

> **Box 5.2 Diagnostic Key Points of Myxoid Leiomyosarcoma**
>
> *Diagnostic criteria*: Any one feature below
>
> – Mitotic activity: more than 2 per 10 HPF
> – Moderate nuclear atypia
> – Coagulative necrosis
>
> - Infiltration of the tumour cells in the neighbouring adjacent myometrium
> - Immunohistochemistry: Usually not needed, however tumour cells are positive for SMA, desmin, caldesmon and HDAC 8

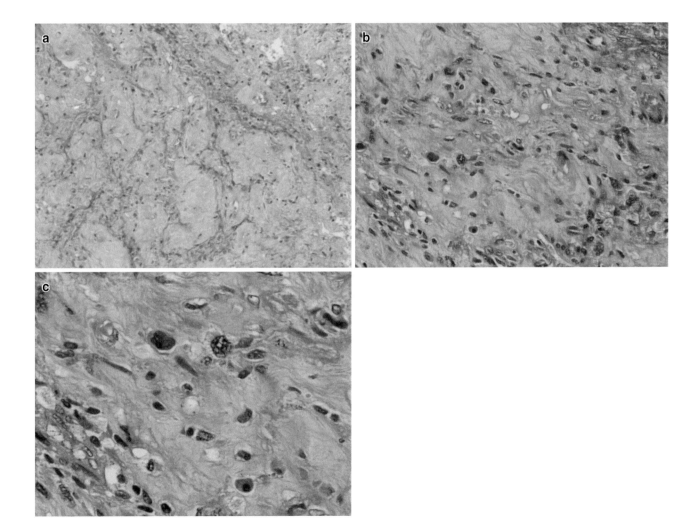

Fig. 5.13 (**a**) Myxoid leiomyosarcoma: Abundant pale blue myxoid material. (**b**) Myxoid leiomyosarcoma: Scattered cells with round mildly pleomorphic nuclei. (**c**) Myxoid leiomyosarcoma: Higher magnification showing the pleomorphic cells in abundant myxoid material

Epithelioid Leiomyosarcoma

Image gallery: Fig. 5.14a–c.
  Histopathology

- Cell arrangement: Sheet, cord and nests
- More than 50% cells are epithelial looking
- Oval to polyhedral cells with abundant cytoplasm
- Centrally placed mildly pleomorphic round nuclei
- Mitosis: More than 5 per 10 HPF
- Coagulative necrosis present

Diagnostic criteria: See Box 5.3.

> **Box 5.3 Diagnostic Key Points of Epithelioid Leiomyosarcoma**
> - Sheet, cord and nests
> - Oval to polyhedral cells with abundant cytoplasm
>
> *Diagnostic criteria of malignancy*:
>
> - More than 5 Mitosis per 10 HPF
> - Coagulative necrosis
> - Nuclear atypia

Prognosis of leiomyosarcoma

- Poor prognosis: overall 5 year survival is only 25%
- Tumour stage is the most important prognostic factor
- Other prognostic factors include:
  - Size: Less than 5 cm diameter tumour has better prognosis
  - Age: Premenopausal patient has good prognosis
  - Mitotic index: High mitotic activity or high ki 67 index is possibly related with bad prognosis.

Clinical management of leiomyosarcoma

- Total abdominal hysterectomy and bilateral salpingo-oophorectomy
- There is little role of adjuvant chemotherapy and radiotherapy on the survival of the patient.

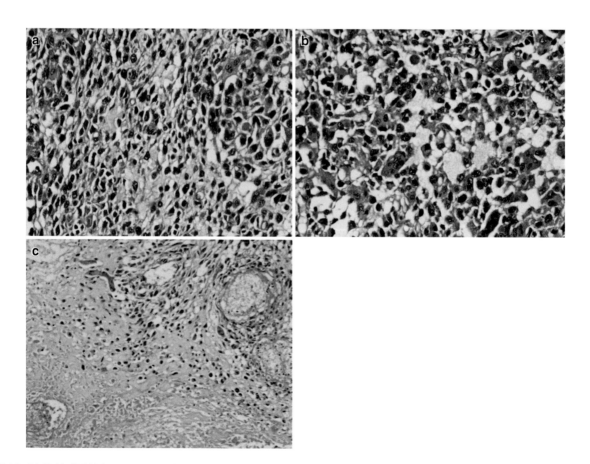

Fig. 5.14 (**a**) Epithelioid leiomyosarcoma: Sheets of tumour cells giving an epithelial look. (**b**) Epithelioid leiomyosarcoma: Oval to polyhedral cells with abundant cytoplasm having centrally placed pleomorphic nuclei. (**c**) Epithelioid leiomyosarcoma: Coagulative necrosis

Endometrial Stromal Tumour

Endometrial Stromal Nodule

Image gallery: Figs. 5.15 and 5.16.

Epidemiology

- Relatively rare tumour
- Endometrial stromal nodule represents 0.2% of all uterine malignancies

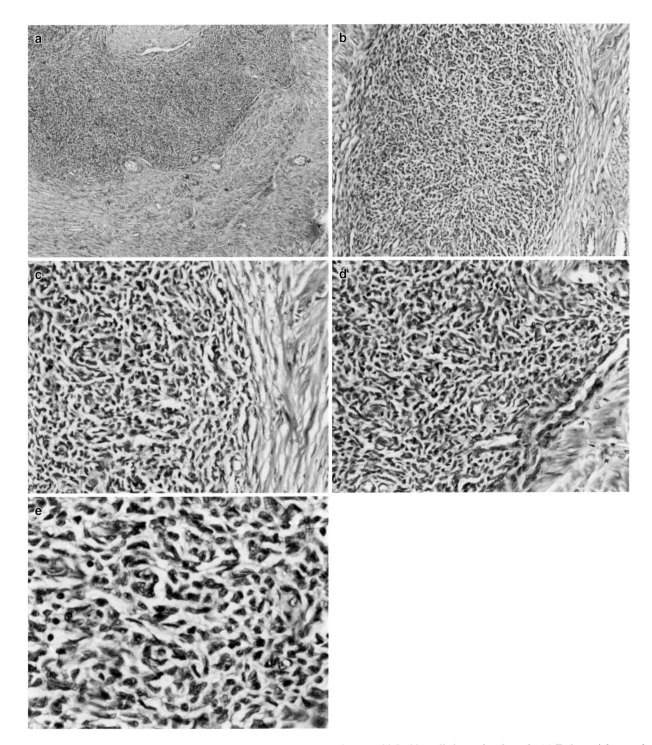

Fig. 5.15 (**a**) Endometrial stromal nodule: Well circumscribed lesion. (**b**) Endometrial stromal nodule: Sharply demarcated margin of the nodule. (**c**) Endometrial stromal nodule: Diffusely small round blue cells with scanty cytoplasm. (**d**) Endometrial stromal nodule: Tumour shows multiple thin walled vascular channels. (**e**) Endometrial stromal nodule: Higher magnification showing individual cell morphology. The cells are small and round with scanty cytoplasm. The nuclei are mildly pleomorphic. Mitosis is almost absent to nil

- It occurs more frequently in fifth and sixth decade
- Mean age 47 year

Histogenesis

- Endometrial stromal cells

Genetic profile

- Translocation t (7:17) (p21: q15): fusion of JAZF1- SUZ12
- Translocation t (6;10) (p21:q22): fusion of EPC 1-PHF1
- Translocation t(6;7)(p21;p15): fusion of PHF1-JAZF1

Clinical features

- Abnormal vaginal bleeding
- Pain abdomen
- Pelvic mass

Gross features

- Location: submucosal
- Polypoid, well circumscribed mass
- Yellowish to tan colour
- Cut section: solid, yellow, necrosis may be present

Histopathology

- Well circumscribed mass
- Highly cellular
- Diffusely small round blue cells with scanty cytoplasm
- Round to oval monomorphic nuclei
- Vascular and shows multiple thin walled vascular channels.
- Tumour cells arranged as whorls around small vascular channels
- Mitosis: variable, usually less than 5 per 10 HPF
- Sex cord like tubules may be seen
- Reticulin network encircles single or group of tumour cells

Immunohistochemistry

- Positive for CD 10 and also WT 1
- Negative for caldesmon, desmin, and SMA

Diagnostic criteria: see Box 5.4.

Box 5.4 Diagnostic Key Points of Endometrial Stromal Nodule
Diagnostic criteria:

- Well circumscribed solitary nodule
- Surface is smooth
- No nuclear pleomorphism
- Mitosis: Less than 5 per 10 HPF
- CD 10 positive and negative for caldesmon and desmin

Differential diagnosis

- Low grade endometrial stromal sarcoma
  - Very difficult to impossible in curetting and the report should be "Endometrial stromal tumour" only
  - Stromal nodule with smooth muscle differentiation may simulate invasion
- Cellular leiomyoma: (Table 5.3 and Fig. 5.16). There are overlapping clinical and gross features of cellular leiomyoma and endometrial stromal nodule. Smooth muscle cells may show CD 10 positivity and therefore it is recommended to use a panel of immunohistochemistry markers including CD 10, desmin, caldesmon.

Prognosis and treatment

- Benign course and does not recur after complete removal
- Hysterectomy is the treatment of choice

Table 5.3 Key distinguishing points of cellular leiomyoma versus endometrial stromal nodule

Features	Endometrial stromal nodule	Cellular leiomyoma
Fascicles	No such arrangement	Focal fascicular appearance and the fascicle merge with the adjacent myometrium
Intra-tumour blood vessels	Thin vascular channels	Thick walled blood vessels
Cleft like spaces	Absent	Present
Immunohistochemistry Panel: CD 10, desmin, caldesmon	CD 10 positive And negative for desmin and caldesmon	Usually CD 10 negative and positive for desmin and caldesmon

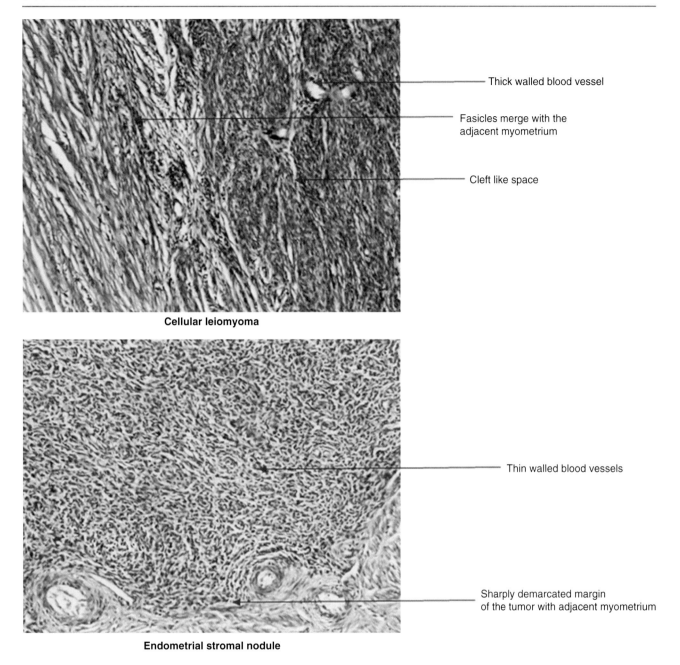

Thick walled blood vessel

Fasicles merge with the adjacent myometrium

Cleft like space

Cellular leiomyoma

Thin walled blood vessels

Sharply demarcated margin of the tumor with adjacent myometrium

Endometrial stromal nodule

Fig. 5.16 Distinguishing morphological features of cellular leiomyoma versus endometrial stromal nodule

Endometrial Stromal Sarcoma Low Grade

Image gallery: Figs. 5.17, 5.18, 5.19, and 5.20.
   Abbreviation: Endometrial stromal sarcoma: ESS.
   Epidemiology

- It consists of 0.2–1% of all cases of uterine malignancies
- Overall ESS represents 15% of uterine mesenchymal tumours

Molecular genetics

- The most common translocation is: Translocation t (7:17) (p21: q15): Fusion of JAZF1- SUZ12
- The second most common: Translocation t(6;7) (p21;p15):Fusion of PHF1-JAZF1

The other translocations include

- Translocation t (6;10) (p21:q22): Fusion of EPC 1-PHF1
- Translocation t(1:6) (p34:q21): Fusion of MEAF6-PHF1

Clinical features

- Average age: 50 years
- Chief complaints: Abnormal uterine bleeding and abdominal pain

Gross features

- Polypoid mass in the uterine cavity
- Nodule in the myometrium

- Diffuse infiltrating lesion in the myometrium
- Combination of above three features
- At times the tumour may look like well circumscribed and may give false impression of benign stromal nodule
- Cut section: Soft and fleshy with areas of haemorrhage and necrosis

Histopathology

- Highly cellular and resembles stromal cells in lower magnification
- Diffuse sheets of cells with tongue like projections in the myometrium
- Round cells with scanty cytoplasm having mild nuclear pleomorphism
- Multiple small vascular channels are present homogenously
- Mitosis: Less than 5 per 10 HPF
- Hyaline plaques, haemorrhage and necrosis may be present
- Lymphovascular invasion
- Metaplasia: Rhabdoid and fatty
- Smooth muscle differentiation may occur:
  - Classical smooth muscle differentiation
  - Nodules of smooth muscle with hyalinised area in the centre
  - Irregular clusters of smooth muscle cells
- Sex cord like differentiation: Cords of cells, trabeculae and rarely tubules
- Focal well-formed endometrial glands may be present indicating divergent differentiation

Reticulin stain:

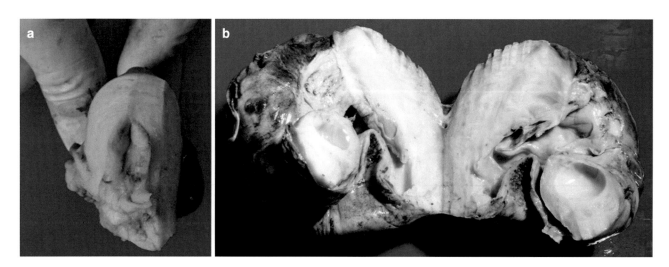

Fig. 5.17 (**a**) Gross photograph of endometrial stromal sarcoma: Grey white tumour in the endometrial cavity. (**b**) Gross photograph of endometrial stromal sarcoma. The solid greyish tumour has replaced whole of the uterine cavity

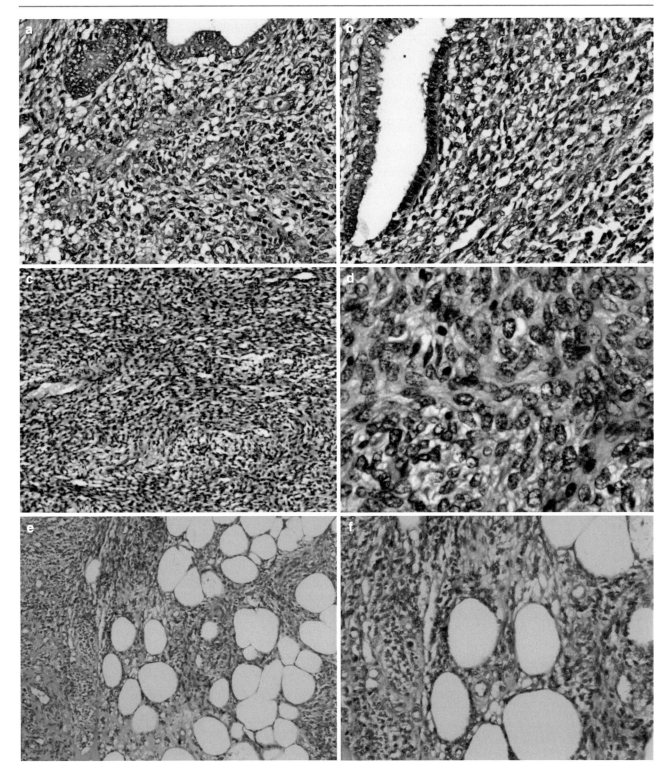

Fig. 5.18 (a) Endometrial stromal sarcoma low grade: Diffuse sheets of cells giving the appearance of endometrial stroma. (b) Endometrial stromal sarcoma low grade: The tumour encircling the normal endometrial gland. (c) Endometrial stromal sarcoma low grade: Tumour cells around multiple vascular channels. (d) Endometrial stromal sarcoma low grade: Individual cells are round to oval with scanty cytoplasm. Mitosis is low. (e) Endometrial stromal sarcoma low grade: Fat infiltration in the tumour. (f) Endometrial stromal sarcoma low grade: Higher magnification of the previous microphotograph. (g) Endometrial stromal sarcoma low grade: Hyaline plaque in the tumour. (h) Endometrial stromal sarcoma low grade: Multiple eosinophilic hyaline plaque. (i) Endometrial stromal sarcoma low grade: Hyaline plaque with oval to spindle cells. (j) Endometrial stromal sarcoma low grade: Myxoid variants showing abundant myxoid changes. (k) Endometrial stromal sarcoma low grade: Myxoid variants showing myxoid changes with slender spindle shaped cells

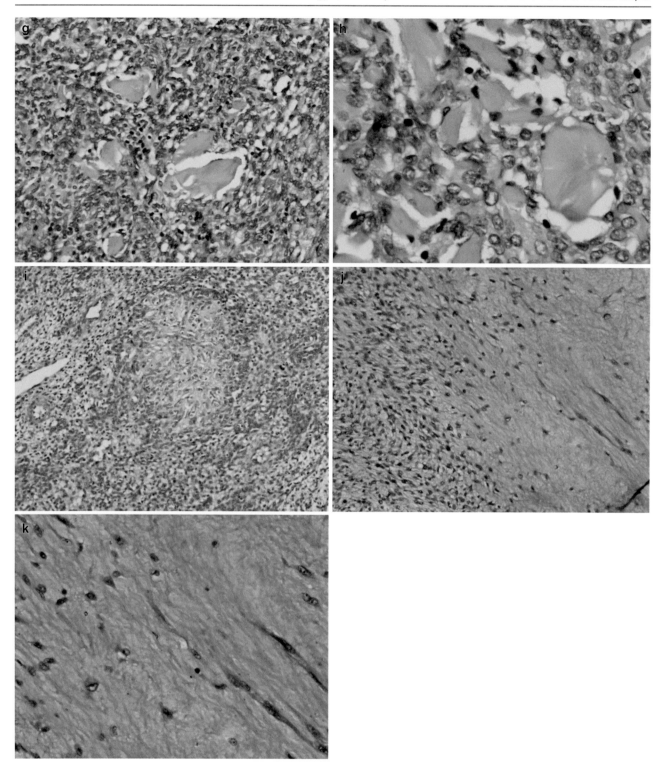

Fig. 5.18 (continued)

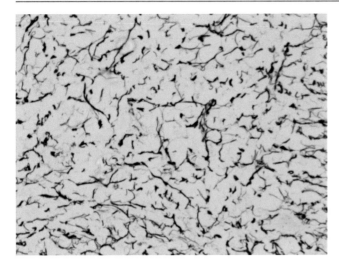

Fig. 5.19 Endometrial stromal sarcoma low grade: Reticulin fibres around the small group of tumour cells resembling 'weave basket" appearance

- Densely connected network of reticulin fibres around the small group of tumour cells that may resemble 'weave basket" appearance.

Immunohistochemistry (see Table 5.4)

- Strongly positive: CD 10
- Also positive: WT1, ER/PR
- Occasionally positive: Desmin and SMA
- Negative: Caldesmon and HDAC-8
- Sex cord differentiated area: Positive for calretinin and inhibin

Diagnostic key points: See Box 5.5.

Box 5.5 Diagnostic Key Points of Low Grade Endometrial Stromal Sarcoma

- Diffuse sheets of small round cells resembling endometrial stromal cells of proliferative endometrium
- Tongue like projections of tumour within the myometrium
- Minimal nuclear pleomorphism
- Mitotic count less than 5 per 10 HPF
- Homogenous distributed prominent vascular structures Immunohistochemistry:
  - Strongly positive for CD 10 and frequently positive for ER/PR
  - Usually negative for SMA, desmin and caldesmon
- Translocation t(7:17) (p21: q15): fusion of JAZF1- SUZ12

Note: A panel of antibody should be used to distinguish cellular leiomyoma from endometrial stromal sarcoma (low grade) as uterine smooth muscle may express CD 10. The panel should include CD 10, Caldesmon, histone deacetylase 8, SMA, desmin.

Differential diagnosis

- Endometrial stromal nodule(see Box 5.6)
  - Well circumscribed
  - No evidence of infiltration or lymphovascular invasion
  - Low mitosis (less than 2 per 10 HPF)
- Undifferentiated uterine sarcoma

Box 5.6 Features Favouring Low Grade Endometrial Stromal Sarcoma over Endometrial Stromal Nodule

- Extensive infiltration in the myometrium
- Vascular invasion
- Multiple nodular growth
- In difficult situation apply the rule of three:
  - More than 3 finger like projections of the tumour
  - More than 3 mm invasion

  - Destructive pushing margin
  - Irregular thick walled blood vessels
  - Marked nuclear pleomorphism
  - High mitosis: More than 10 per 10 HPF
  - CD 10 patchy positive
- Cellular leiomyoma
  - Spindle cells arranged in fascicles
  - Thick walled blood vessels
  - Multiple slit like spaces
  - Positive for smooth muscle markers: Caldesmon and HDAC-8
- Perivascular epithelioid cells

Prognosis

- Slowly growing neoplasm
- Staging of the tumour is the most important prognostic factor
- Five year survival rate of FIGO stage I is 90%
- Median survival: 11 year

Treatment

- Treatment of choice is total abdominal hysterectomy with bilateral salpingo oophorectomy
- In advanced stage: Hormone therapy particularly progestin administration

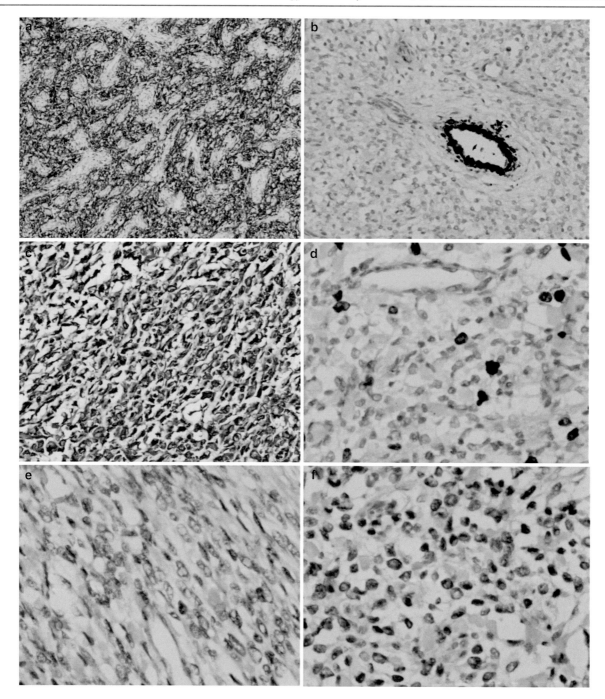

Fig. 5.20 (**a**) Endometrial stromal sarcoma low grade: Tumour is strongly positive for CD 10. (**b**) Endometrial stromal sarcoma low grade: Tumour is negative for caldesmon. (**c**) Endometrial stromal sarcoma, low grade: Strong vimentin positivity. (**d**) Endometrial stromal sarcoma, low grade: Low positive Ki 67. (**e**) Endometrial stromal sarcoma, low grade: Tumour is positive for oestrogen receptor. (**f**) Endometrial stromal sarcoma, low grade: Tumour is positive for progesterone receptor

Table 5.4 Immunohistochemistry of endometrial stromal sarcoma, low grade versus leiomyoma

Diagnosis	CD 10	Caldesmon	IIDAC-8	SMA	desmin
Endometrial stromal sarcoma low grade	+	−	−	−	−
Leiomyoma	−[a]	+	+	+	+

[a]Occasionally smooth muscle tumour may express CD 10

High Grade Endometrial Stromal Sarcoma

Image gallery: Figs. 5.21 and 5.22.
  Epidemiology

- Rare tumour and exact incidence is not known

  Molecular genetics

- Characteristic translocation of t (10:17) (q22;p13) resulting YWHAE-FAM22 gene rearrangement.

  Clinical features

- Wide age range: 25–65 year
- Mean age: 50 years
- Chief complaints: Abnormal uterine bleeding

Gross features: Same as low grade ESS.
Histopathology

- Hypercellular
- The cells simulate endometrial stromal cells
- Confluent diffuse sheet of cells
- Infiltrative and usually shows lymphovascular invasion
- Round cells, scanty cytoplasm
- Moderately pleomorphic nuclei
- Necrosis present
- Mitosis: More than 10 per 10HPF
- Often admixed with low grade ESS

  Immunohistochemistry

- Diffuse and strong positivity of cyclin D1
- Positive: C-Kit
- Negative for CD 10. ER/PR, and DOG1

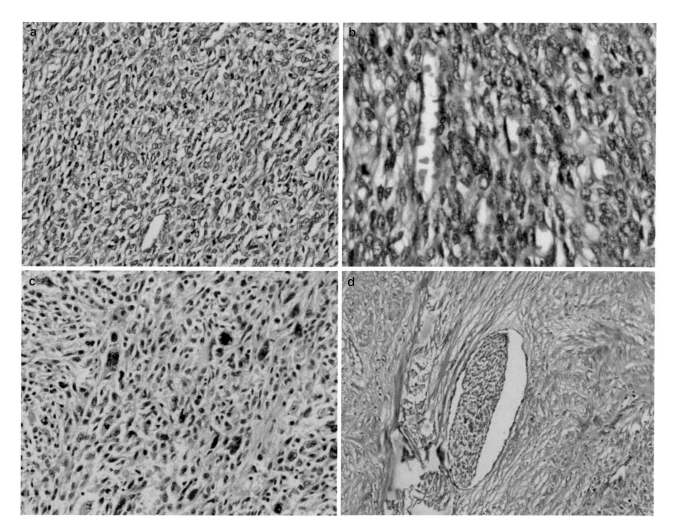

Fig. 5.21 (**a**) Endometrial stromal sarcoma, high grade: Diffuse sheets of tumour cells with many vascular channels. (**b**) Endometrial stromal sarcoma, high grade: Round to oval cells with scanty cytoplasm. Frequent mitotic activity is present. (**c**) Endometrial stromal sarcoma, high grade: Moderately pleomorphic cells with high mitosis. (**d**) Endometrial stromal sarcoma, high grade: Lymphovascular invasion present

Key diagnostic criteria

> **Box 5.7 Key Diagnostic Criteria of High Grade Endometrial Stromal Sarcoma**
> - Moderate nuclear pleomorphism
> - Infiltrative growth with frequent lymphovascular invasion
> - More than 10 mitosis per 10 HPF
> - Characteristic translocation of t(10:17) (q22;p13) causing YWHAE-FAM22 gene rearrangement
> - Strongly positive for cyclin D1
>
> Note: Mitotic count should not be used as a main point to distinguish these two entities.

Differential diagnosis:

- *Low grade endometrial stromal sarcoma*: It is always necessary to distinguish these two entities as high grade one behaves aggressively and does not respond to hormone therapy. See Table 5.5

- *Epithelioid leiomyosarcoma*: The tumour cells are positive for desmin, caldesmon, ER/PR and negative for cyclin D1. Whereas, high grade endometrial stromal sarcoma are strongly positive for cyclin D1 and negative for desmin, caldesmon, and ER/PR.

Prognosis

- Intermediate prognosis between low grade ESS and undifferentiated uterine sarcoma
- High grade ESS recurs in less than 1 year period

Treatment

- Total abdominal hysterectomy with bilateral salpingo-oophorectomy along with pelvic and peritoneal debulking
- Adjuvant chemotherapy

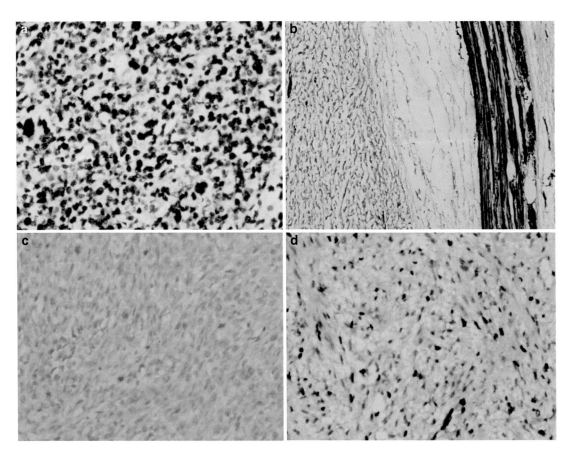

Fig. 5.22 (a) Endometrial stromal sarcoma, high grade: Very high Ki 67 index. Almost 100% cells are showing Ki 67 positivity. (b) Endometrial stromal sarcoma, high grade: Caldesmon is negative in the tumour cells and positive in the peripheral smooth muscle. (c) Endometrial stromal sarcoma, high grade: ER negativity in high grade ESS. (d) Endometrial stromal sarcoma, high grade: Strongly positive for Cyclin D 1

Table 5.5 Distinguishing features of low and high grade endometrial stromal sarcoma

Features	Low grade endometrial stromal sarcoma	High grade endometrial stromal sarcoma
Myometrial invasion	Tongue like projections	Destructive myometrial invasion
Arrangement	Diffuse sheet	Nested or cord like pattern
Cell morphology	Small cells with round nuclei, scanty cytoplasm	Round cells with moderate amount of eosinophilic cytoplasm, moderately pleomorphic nuclei with prominent nucleoli. Nuclei 5 times bigger than normal lymphocytes
Mitosis	Usually less than 10 per 10 HPF	Usually more than 10 per 10 HPF
Coagulative necrosis	Less frequent	Often present
Immunohistochemistry	Characteristically positive for CD 10, ER/PR and focally weak positive for cyclin D1	Negative for CD 10, ER/PR and strongly positive for cyclin D1
Molecular genetics	Translocation t (7:17) (p21: q15): Fusion of JAZF1- SUZ12	Translocation of t (10:17) (q22; p13) resulting YWHAE-FAM22 gene rearrangement.

Undifferentiated Uterine Sarcoma

Image gallery: Fig. 5.23a–c.
  Epidemiology

- It comprises of only 6% of uterine sarcoma
- Postmenopausal patients are commonly affected
- Mean age: 55–60 years

Clinical features

- Chief complaints: abnormal vaginal bleeding, pain abdomen and pelvic mass

Gross features

- Polypoid submucosal mass
- Intramural mass
- Soft and fleshy tumour
- Cut section: soft to firm in feel, yellowish

Histopathology

- Destructive pushing growth in the myometrium
- Arrangement: diffuse sheet or storiform pattern
- Irregular distribution of variable sized blood vessels
- Cell are round to oval with moderate to marked nuclear pleomorphism
- Single or multinucleated bizarre giant cells may be seen
- Mitosis: usually 10 to 20 per 10 HPF

Immunohistochemistry

- Positive: Patchy positivity of CD 10 and ER/PR; cyclin D1 may be diffusely positive
- Negative: Desmin, SMA, caldesmon and EMA

Diagnostic key points: See Box 5.8.

Box 5.8 Points to Remember for the Diagnosis of Undifferentiated Uterine Sarcoma

- It is a disease of exclusion of other tumour
- Extensive tumour sampling is required for the diagnosis
- Tumours cells are severely pleomorphic with destructive myometrial invasion
- Mitotic activity is usually very high
- CD 10 positivity of the tumour cells exclude high grade ESS

Differential diagnosis

- *Low grade ESS*
  - Infiltrative rather than destructive growth pattern
  - Small and regular distribution of the vessels
  - Mild nuclear pleomorphism
  - Low mitosis (usually less than 5 per 10 HPF)
- *Leiomyosarcoma*
  - Spindle cells in short and long fascicles
  - Positive for smooth muscle markers: Desmin, SMA, caldesmon
- *Carcinosarcoma*:
  - Malignant glands present

Prognosis and treatment

- Highly aggressive tumour
- Prognosis depends on the initial stage at the time of presentation
- Patients of stage I disease usually die within 2 year of diagnosis
- Total abdominal hysterectomy with bilateral salpingo-oophorectomy along with radiation and chemotherapy are the treatment of choice

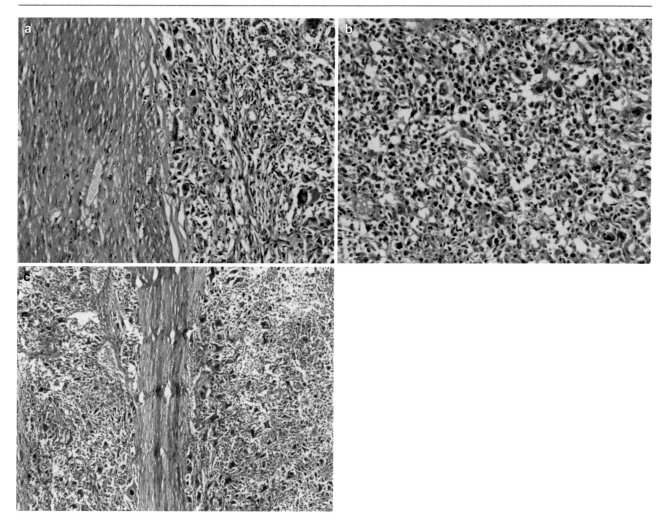

Fig. 5.23 (**a**) Undifferentiated uterine sarcoma: Tumour pushing the normal smooth muscle of uterus. (**b**) Undifferentiated uterine sarcoma: The tumour cells are highly pleomorphic with many mononuclear and multinuclear giant cells. (**c**) Undifferentiated uterine sarcoma: The tumour is infiltrating deep in the uterus with foci of preserved smooth muscle. Note the oval to spindle cells with large bizarre nuclei

Uterine Tumour Resembling Ovarian Sex Cord Tumour

Image gallery: Fig. 5.24a–c.

Definition: These are the endometrial stromal tumours that resemble the ovarian sex cord tumour.

Incidence: Rare tumour.

Clinical features

- Uterine bleeding
- Enlargement of uterus
- The patients may be totally asymptomatic

Gross features

- Intramural, submucosal or may be located towards the endometrial cavity
- Usually well circumscribed
- Mean size 5–6 cm
- Cut surface: yellowish to tan

Histopathology

- Well circumscribed tumour
- The cells are arranged as tubules, cords, and nests.

- Often the cells are in anastomosing trabeculae
- Individuals cells are low columnar with bland nuclei having scanty to abundant eosinophilic cytoplasm
- No mitotic activity

Immunohistochemistry

- Positive for cytokeratin, and smooth muscle markers such as actin and desmin
- The tumour cells are also positive for calretinin, inhibin, CD 99, Melan A, WT1, and CD 56

Molecular profile

- Do not show JAZF1-SUZ12 fusion

Differential diagnosis

- Endometrioid carcinoma
- Endometrial stromal tumors
- Perivascular epithelioid cell tumor
- Epithelioid leiomyomas

Prognosis

- The tumour shows benign behaviour and rarely recurs

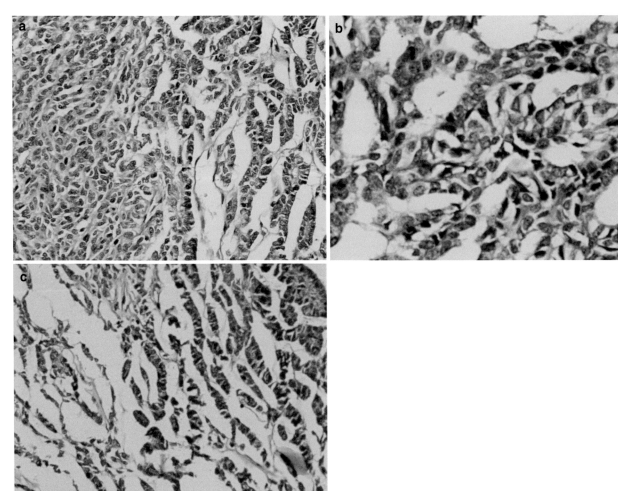

Fig. 5.24 (**a**) Uterine tumour resembling ovarian sex cord tumour: Tubular pattern of the tumour cells. (**b**) Uterine tumour resembling ovarian sex cord tumour: Low columnar cells forming the tubules. (**c**) Uterine tumour resembling ovarian sex cord tumour: Trabecular appearance of the tumour cells

Mixed Epithelial Mesenchymal Tumour

Adenomyoma

Image gallery: Fig. 5.25a, b

Definition: Adenomyoma is characterized by the tumour like masses with the presence of endometrial glands and stroma along with surrounding myometrial tissue.

Epidemiology

- Usually seen in the body of the uterus
- Relatively rare
- Noted in 25–65 years of age

Clinical features

- Incidental
- Abnormal uterine bleeding
- May simulate endometrial polyp

Gross features

- Location: predominantly submucosal, however may be intramural or subserosal
- Size: About 1–15 cm
- Well circumscribed polypoid mass
- Grey-white in cut surface

Histopathology

- Proliferative looking endometrial glands embedded within the endometrial stroma
- Smooth muscle cells arranged as fascicles encompass the endometrial glands and stroma
- Scanty mitotic activity

Differential diagnosis

- Endometrial polyp with smooth muscle metaplasia
  - Here the glands are superficial and smooth muscle is present in the centre, whereas in the adenomyoma the smooth muscle completely surrounds the endometrial gland and stroma
- Entrapped endometrial glands within leiomyoma
  - The glands are present in the periphery of smooth muscle
- Atypical polypoid adenomyoma
  - The glands show focal crowding
  - Cytological atypia of the glandular lining cells

Prognosis

- Benign tumour and does not recur after removal

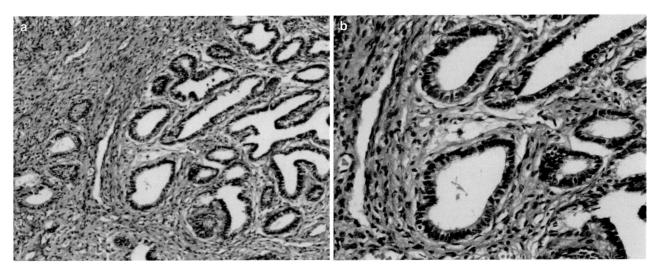

Fig. 5.25 (**a**) Adenomyoma: Endometrial glands embedded within the endometrial stroma. (**b**) Adenomyoma: The glands are surrounded by smooth muscle. The lining of the gland is cuboidal

Atypical Polypoid Adenomyoma

Image gallery: Fig. 5.26a, b.

Definition: Atypical polypoid adenomyoma is characterized by complex proliferation of endometrial glands with cytological atypia in a fibromuscular stroma.

Epidemiology

- Rare tumour
- Mean age: 40 years
- Rarely present in post-menopausal patient

Clinical features

- Abnormal vaginal bleeding
- Polypoid mass coming out from the external os

Gross features

- Solitary polypoid mass
- Sessile or with stalk
- Well-circumscribed
- Size: About 2–5 cm
- Soft to rubbery in consistency
- Cut section: Solid grey-white

Histopathology

- Architecturally complex endometrial glands
- Crowded glands with variable size
- Glandular lining epithelium shows mild to moderate nuclear atypia
- Squamous morules with central necrosis may be present
- Small fascicles of smooth muscle cells with admixed myofibroblast

- Mitotic activity of the stromal cells may be more than 2 per 10 HPF

Immunohistochemistry

- The smooth muscle component is positive for desmin and caldesmon
- The glands are positive for CK, ER/PR

Molecular profile

- MLH-1 promoter hypermethylation
- Microsatellite instability

Diagnostic key points: See Box 5.9.

Box 5.9 Diagnostic Key Points of Atypical Polypoid Adenomyoma
- Complex branching of endometrial glands
- Nuclear atypia of the glandular lining cells
- Squamous morules is almost always present
- The glands are encircled by smooth muscle cells arranged in short fascicles

---

Differential diagnosis

- Well differentiated adenocarcinoma
    - Nuclear atypia is more
    - Stromal desmoplasia present
        - Carcinosarcoma
        Severe nuclear atypia in the glandular epithelium
        Stromal cells show moderate atypia and high mitosis
        Higher age group

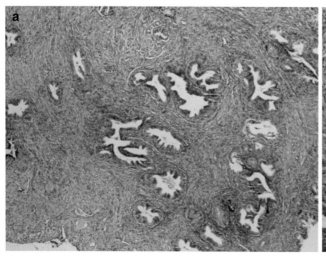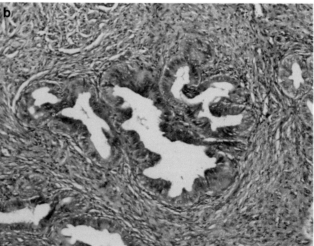

Fig. 5.26 (**a**) Atypical polypoid adenomyoma: Multiple variable sized irregular glands with complex branching encircled by smooth muscle. (**b**) Atypical polypoid adenomyoma: The glandular epithelial cells showing nuclear atypia

– Benign endometrial polyp
   No nuclear atypia in the glandular epithelial cells
   Predominantly fibrous stroma

Prognosis and treatment

• Benign lesion
• Recurrence is common (45%) if not removed thoroughly
• Risk of malignancy is 8%
• The patients who has completed the family: Hysterectomy is the treatment of choice
• The patients who wants to retain the uterus: Removal of the polyp by curetting with subsequent repeated follow up.

Carcinosarcoma

Image gallery: Figs. 5.27, 5.28 and 5.29.

Definition: The tumour consists of both carcinoma and malignant mesenchymal components.

Abbreviation: Uterine Carcinosarcoma (UCS)

Synonym: Malignant mixed Müllerian tumour

Epidemiology

• UCS represents approximately 5% of uterine malignancies
• More frequent in African American women
• Higher risk of UCS in tamoxifen therapy
• Mean age: 65 years

Histogenesis

• Epithelial in origin with mesenchymal metaplasia
• Both epithelial and mesenchymal components are monoclonal in origin
• Similar genetic changes are demonstrated in both the two components

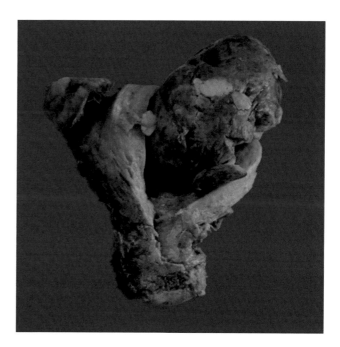

Fig. 5.27 Gross of carcinosarcoma: Large soft fleshy grey white growth arising from the upper part of the body of uterus. Note the areas of haemorrhage

Clinical features

- Postmenopausal bleeding
- Pelvic pain
- Mass coming out from vagina

Gross features

- Polypoid mass within the uterine cavity
- Bulky and soft
- Cut section fleshy with areas of haemorrhage and necrosis

Histopathology

- Homogenously admixed carcinomatous and malignant mesenchymal component
- Carcinoma component:
  - High grade endometrioid carcinoma
  - Serous or clear cell carcinoma
- Sarcomatous component
  - Homologous: leiomyosarcoma, endometrial stromal sarcoma, undifferentiated sarcoma
  - Heterologous: Rhabdomyosarcoma, chondrosarcoma, liposarcoma, osteosarcoma

Immunohistochemistry

- Carcinoma component:
  - Positive: CK, EMA
- Sarcomatous component
  - Positive: Vimentin
  - Homologous component: Positive for CD 34, CD 10
  - Heterologous component:
    Rhabdomyosarcoma positive for desmin, myoglobin, myogenin
    Chondrosarcoma positive for S 100 protein

Diagnostic key points: See Box 5.10.

Box 5.10 Diagnostic Key Points of Carcinosarcoma
- The presence of both carcinoma elements and sarcoma elements
- Carcinoma components may be endometrioid, serous or clear cell type
- Sarcoma components may be non-specific sarcoma, rhabdomyosarcoma or chondrosarcoma
- Immunohistochemistry: Carcinoma component is positive for CK, EMA and sarcoma component is positive for vimentin, SMA, CD 10 etc.

Differential diagnosis

- Sarcomatoid endometrioid carcinoma
  - Gradual transition of carcinoma to spindle cells area
  - Spindle cell component is negative for vimentin
- Endometrioid carcinoma with heterologous elements
  - The heterologous element is benign in nature
- Low-grade Müllerian adenosarcoma with predominant sarcomatous area
  - No malignant epithelial component
- Undifferentiated endometrial carcinoma
  - No spindle cell component

Prognosis

- Poor prognosis
- Overall 5 year survival rate: 35%
- Median survival 2 year
- Prognostic factors
  - Stage of the tumour
  - Advanced age: above 70 year age
  - Lymphovascular invasion
  - Myometrial invasion
  - Non endometrioid carcinoma: clear or serous carcinoma

Treatment

- Total abdominal hysterectomy with bilateral salpingo-oophorectomy along with omentectomy
- Adjuvant chemotherapy (cisplatin) in distant metastasis

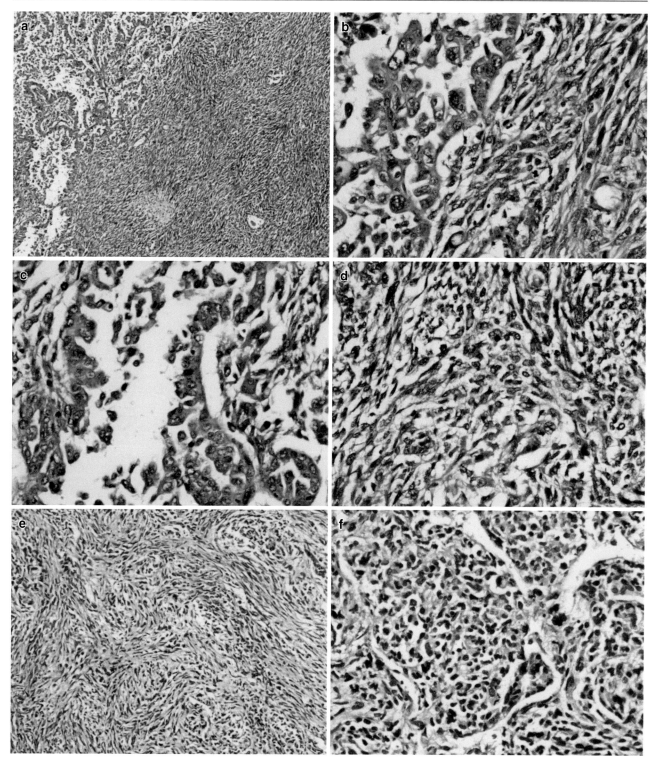

Fig. 5.28 (**a**) Carcinosarcoma: Both adenocarcinoma (left) and sarcoma components are present. Note the serous carcinoma part here. (**b**) Carcinosarcoma: Serous carcinoma (adenocarcinoma) and nonspecific sarcoma area. (**c**) Carcinosarcoma: Hobnail appearance of the serous carcinoma. (**d**) Carcinosarcoma: The sarcoma component is composed of oval to spindle cells with moderate nuclear atypia. The sarcoma component is homologous. (**e**) Carcinosarcoma: Interwoven fascicles of spindle cells in the homologous component of the sarcoma. (**f**) Carcinosarcoma: The cells are pleomorphic showing frequent mitotic activity in the homologous component of the sarcoma. (**g**) Carcinosarcoma: Bony component in the sarcoma area. (**h**) Carcinosarcoma: The heterologous component of the sarcoma showing rhabdomyosarcoma area. (**i**) Carcinosarcoma: The heterologous component of the sarcoma showing osteosarcoma area. Note the adenocarcinoma area in the right side. (**j**) Carcinosarcoma: Osteosarcoma component as heterologous sarcoma part

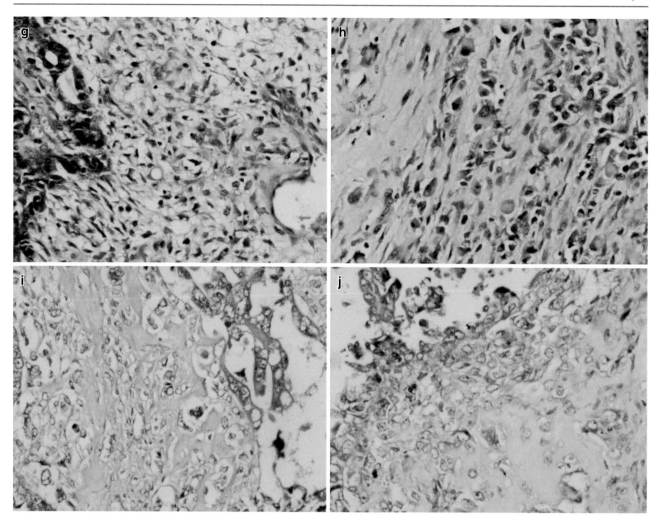

Fig. 5.28   (continued)

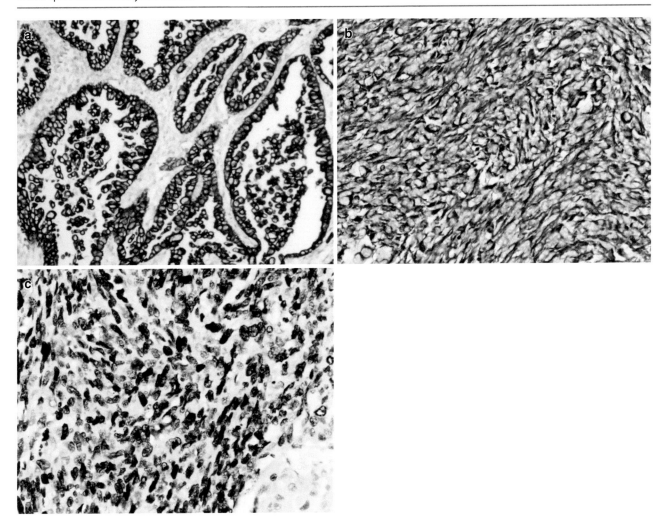

Fig. 5.29 (**a**) Carcinosarcoma: Strong cytokeratin positivity in the adenocarcinoma component. (**b**) Carcinosarcoma: The sarcoma component showing vimentin positivity. (**c**) Carcinosarcoma: Strong nuclear positivity of p 53 immunostaining

Miscellaneous Tumour

Adenomatoid Tumour

Image gallery: Fig. 5.30a, b.

Definition: This is a tumour that develops from mesothelial cells.

Histogenesis

- Mesothelial in origin

Clinical features

- Incidentally detected in hysterectomy specimen
- Mean age: 45 year
- Asymptomatic

Gross features

- Location: subserosal
- Number: Solitary
- Size: Microscopic to several cm
- Cut section: Grey white

Histopathology

- Anastomosing channels of pseudo vascular structures or gland like spaces
- Lining epithelial cells are cuboidal to flat
- Cell with scanty cytoplasm
- Monomorphic bland nuclei
- Smooth muscle proliferation around the pseudovascular channels

Immunohistochemistry

- Lining epithelial cells are positive: WT 1, calretinin, D2-40, CK 7, CK 18 CAM 5.2

Prognosis

- Benign in nature

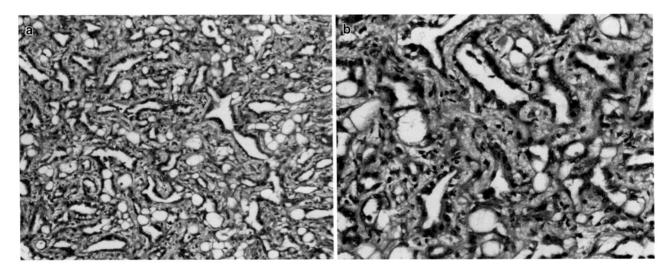

Fig. 5.30 (**a**) Adenomatoid tumour: Multiple anastomosing channels of pseudo vascular structures or gland like spaces. (**b**) Adenomatoid tumour: The channels are lined by cuboidal to flat epithelial cells

Neuroendocrine Tumour

Image gallery: Fig. 5.31a, b.

Definition: Neuroendocrine tumours of uterus are malignant neoplasm with neuroendocrine differentiation.

Incidence: It represents about 1% of endometrial carcinoma.

Clinical features

- Mean age 60 years
- Vaginal bleeding

Gross features

- Enlarged uterus
- Polypoid fleshy mass in uterine cavity

Histopathology

- Tumour cells are arranged in nests, cords, diffuse sheet
- Occasional rosette like structure
- Small cell neuroendocrine carcinoma: small ovoid cells with scanty cytoplasm and nuclear moulding

- Large cell neuroendocrine carcinoma: The cells are larger in size with vesicular nuclei having prominent nucleoli.

Immunohistochemistry

- Positive: CD 56, chromogranin, synaptophysin, CK

Molecular profile

- Characteristic translocation of t (11:22) (q24;q12) causing EWS/FL-1 fusion gene

Diagnostic criteria

- The presence of neuroendocrine pattern
- Expression of CD 56/chromogranin

Prognosis

- Overall poor

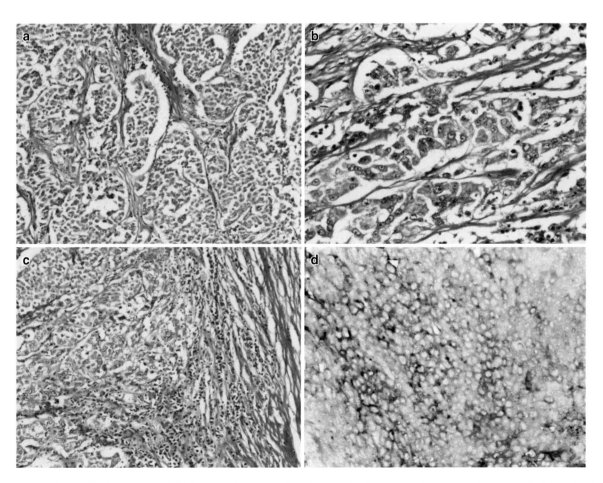

Fig. 5.31 (**a**) Neuroendocrine tumour: Multiple nests of tumour cells separated by thin fibrous tissue. (**b**) Neuroendocrine tumour: The cells are larger in size with vesicular nuclei having prominent nucleoli. (**c**) Neuroendocrine tumour: The nests of tumour cells infiltrating in the myometrium. (**d**) Neuroendocrine tumour: Tumour cells show synaptophysin positivity

Lymphoid and Myeloid Tumours

Lymphoma

Image gallery: Figs. 5.32a–e and 5.33a, b.
  Incidence

- Rare

  Clinical features

- Variable age range 20–60 year
- Abnormal vaginal bleeding
- Pain abdomen
- Pelvic mass

  Gross features

- Ill circumscribed soft and grey white mass

  Histopathology

- Morphology depends on the subtype of lymphoma
- Usually dissociated round cells infiltrate into the myometrium

- Common: Diffuse large B cell lymphoma
- Less common subtypes: Follicular lymphoma, Burkitt's lymphoma

  Immunohistochemistry

- Positive for CD 45
- B cell markers: CD 19, 20
- T cell marker: CD 3

  Differential diagnosis

- Leiomyoma with lymphocytic infiltrate
  - Well circumscribed
  - Monomorphic cells
- Pseudolymphoma
  - The lymphoid cells are mainly present near the endometrial surface

  Prognosis

- Lymphoma restricted to uterus has good prognosis
- Disseminated advanced lymphoma has bad prognosis

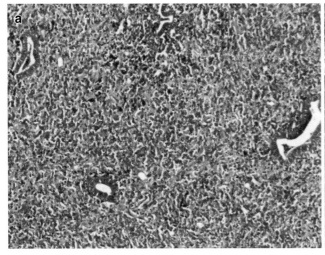
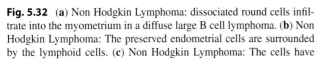
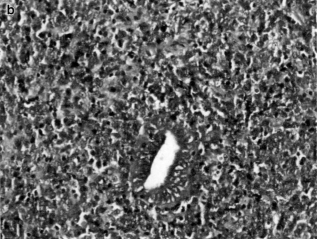

Fig. 5.32 (**a**) Non Hodgkin Lymphoma: dissociated round cells infiltrate into the myometrium in a diffuse large B cell lymphoma. (**b**) Non Hodgkin Lymphoma: The preserved endometrial cells are surrounded by the lymphoid cells. (**c**) Non Hodgkin Lymphoma: The cells have scanty cytoplasm and large nuclei. (**d**) Non Hodgkin Lymphoma: Tumour cells showing strong cytoplasmic CD 45 positivity. (**e**) Non Hodgkin Lymphoma: CD 20 positivity of the lymphoid cells indicating the B cell origin

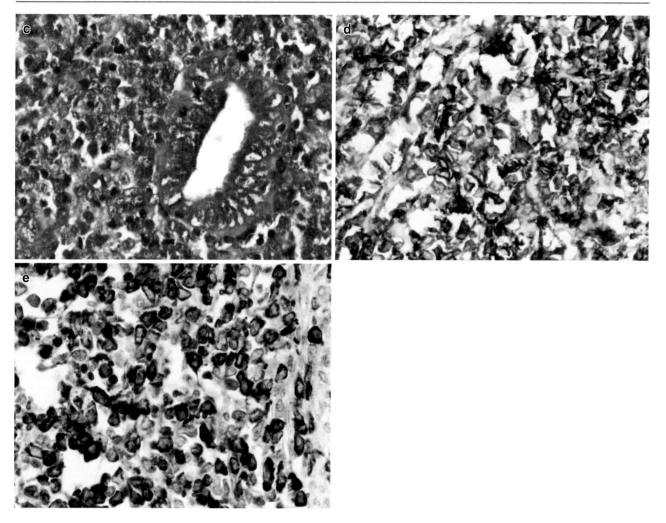

Fig. 5.32 (continued)

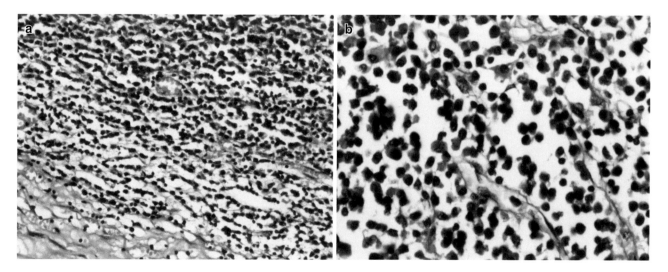

Fig. 5.33 (**a**) Plasmacytoma: Diffuse infiltration of round monomorphic cells. (**b**) Plasmacytoma: Higher magnification showing the plasma cells

Metastasis

Image gallery: Fig. 5.34a, b.
  Clinical feature

- Abnormal vaginal bleeding
- Asymptomatic

  Primary sites

- Female genital tract
    - Common than extra genital tract
    - Fallopian tube, ovary and cervix are the sources
- Extra Female genital tract
    - Rarely from breast, colon and stomach

Histopathology
The diagnostic signals of metastasis are:

- Diffuse involvement of the uterus with preserved endometrial glands
- No evidence of any pre neoplastic endometrial glandular lesion
- Out of proportion involvement of the different parts of the uterus
- Unusual histopathological features that does not fit with conventional endometrial carcinoma

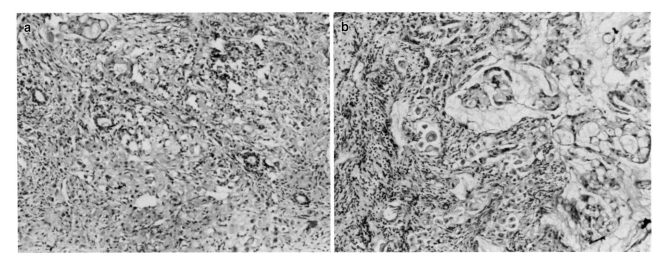

Fig. 5.34 (**a**) Metastatic signet ring carcinoma from stomach: The scattered tumour cells around the benign endometrial glands. (**b**) Metastatic signet ring carcinoma from stomach: The tumour cells are floating in the pool of mucin. Note the signet ring morphology of the cells

Reference

1. Kurman RJ, Carcangiu ML, Herrington S, Young RH. WHO classification of tumours of female genital reproductive organs. 4th ed. Lyon: International Agency for Research on Cancer; 2014.

Suggested Reading

Agrawal A, Ofili G, Allan TL, Mann BS. Malignant lymphoma of uterus: a case report with a review of the literature. Aust N Z J Obstet Gynaecol. 2000;40(3):358–60.

Ali RH, Rouzbahman M. Endometrial stromal tumours revisited: an update based on the 2014 WHO classification. J Clin Pathol. 2015;68(5):325–32.

Arend R, Doneza JA, Wright JD. Uterine carcinosarcoma. Curr Opin Oncol. 2011;23(5):531–6.

Bell SW, Kempson RL, Hendrickson MR. Problematic uterine smooth muscle neoplasms. A clinicopathologic study of 213 cases. Am J Surg Pathol. 1994;18:535–58.

Conklin CM, Longacre TA. Endometrial stromal tumours: the new WHO classification. Adv Anat Pathol. 2014;21(6):383–93.

El-Nashar SA, Mariani A. Uterine carcinosarcoma. Clin Obstet Gynecol. 2011;54(2):292–304.

Fukunaga M, Endo Y, Ushigome S, Ishikawa E. Atypical polypoid adenomyomas of the uterus. Histopathology. 1995;27(1):35–42.

Giuntoli RL, Metzinger DS, et al. Retrospective review of 208 patients with leiomyosarcoma of the uterus: prognostic indicators, surgical management, and adjuvant therapy. Gynecol Oncol. 2003;89(3):460–9.

Irving JA, Carinelli S, Prat J. Uterine tumors resembling ovarian sex cord tumors are polyphenotypic neoplasms with true sex cord differentiation. Mod Pathol. 2006;19:17–24.

Jiang QY, Wang L, Wu RJ. A multiple perspectives on atypical polypoid adenomyoma of uterus. Gynecol Endocrinol. 2013;29(7):623–5.

King ME, Dickersin GR, Scully RE. Myxoid leiomyosarcoma of the uterus: a report of six cases. Am J Surg Pathol. 1982;6:589–98.

Kurman RJ, Norris HJ. Mesenchymal tumours of the uterus. VI. Epithelioid smooth muscle tumours including leiomyoblastoma and clear cell leiomyoma: a clinical and pathological analysis of 26 cases. Cancer. 1976;37:1853–65.

Mandato VD, Palermo R, Falbo A, Capodanno I, Capodanno F, Gelli MC, Aguzzoli L, Abrate M, La Sala GB. Primary diffuse large B-cell lymphoma of the uterus: case report and review. Anticancer Res. 2014;34(8):4377–90.

McCluggage WG. Uterine tumors resembling ovarian sex-cord tumors: immunohistochemical evidence for true sex cord differentiation. Histopathology. 1999;34:374–5.

McCluggage WG. Malignant biphasic uterine tumours: carcinosarcomas or metaplastic carcinomas? J Clin Pathol. 2002;55:321–5.

Nogales FF, Isaac MA, Hardisson D, et al. Adenomatoid tumours of the uterus: an analysis of 60 cases. Int J Gynecol Pathol. 2002;21:34–40.

Nucci MR. Practical issues related to uterine pathology: endometrial stromal tumours. Mod Pathol. 2016;29(Suppl 1):S92–103.

Prayson RA, Hart WR. Pathologic considerations of uterine smooth muscle tumours. Obstet Gynecol Clin N Am. 1995;22(4):637–57.

Pradhan D, Mohanty SK. Uterine tumors resembling ovarian sex cord tumors. Arch Pathol Lab Med. 2013;137(12):1832–6.

Rauh-Hain JA, del Carmen MG. Endometrial stromal sarcoma: a systematic review. Obstet Gynecol. 2013;122(3):676–83.

Schmidt D. Neuroendocrine tumours of the uterus. Verh Dtsch Ges Pathol. 1997;81:260–5.

Singh R. Review literature on uterine carcinosarcoma. J Cancer Res Ther. 2014;10(3):461–8.

Tavassoli FA, Norris HJ. Mesenchymal tumours of the uterus. VII. A clinicopathological study of 60 endometrial stromal nodules. Histopathology. 1981;5:1–10.

Toledo G, Oliva E. Smooth muscle tumours of the uterus: a practical approach. Arch Pathol Lab Med. 2008;132(4):595–605.

Tropé CG, Abeler VM, Kristensen GB. Diagnosis and treatment of sarcoma of the uterus. A review. Acta Oncol. 2012;51(6):694–705.

Ueda G, Yamasaki M. Neuroendocrine carcinoma of the uterus. Curr Top Pathol. 1992;85:309–35.

Primordial Follicle

Image gallery: Fig. 6.1.
    Histopathology

- Primary oocytes
- It is enclosed by a single layer of granulosa cells

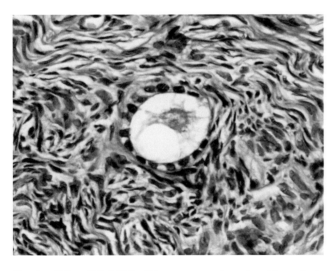

Fig. 6.1 Primordial follicle: Primary oocytes is enclosed by a single layer of granulosa cells

Primary Follicle

Image gallery: Fig. 6.2.
    Histopathology

- The oocyte increases in size
- The granulosa cells surrounding the oocyte become cuboidal to flattened
- In course of time the single layer of the granulosa cells become multi-layered
- Thick zona pellucida of the outer coat of the oocyte appears

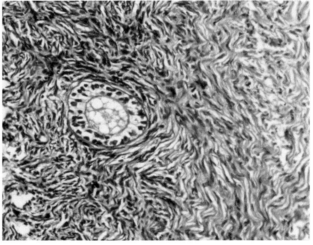

Fig. 6.2 Primary follicle: The granulosa cells surrounding the oocyte are cuboidal. Thick zona pellucida around the ovum appears

© Springer Nature Singapore Pte Ltd. 2019
P. Dey, *Color Atlas of Female Genital Tract Pathology*, https://doi.org/10.1007/978-981-13-1029-4_6

Secondary Follicle

Image gallery: Fig. 6.3a, b.
   Histopathology

- The granulosa cells proliferate

- Theca interna: Spindle shaped theca interna cells appear around the outer layer of the granulosa cells
- Theca externa: Thick fibrous layer of the theca externa appears around the outer aspect of theca interna cells.
- Antrum: The cavity filled with fluid grows within the granulosa cells

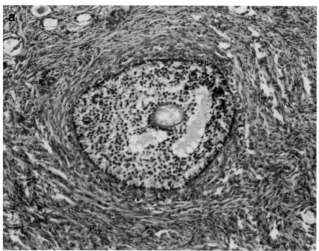 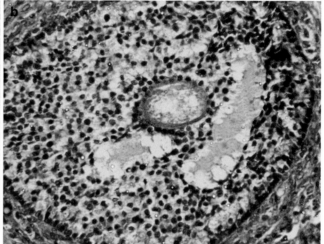

Fig. 6.3 (**a**) Secondary follicle: The granulosa cells around the oocytes. Note the thick fibrous layer of the theca externa around the outer aspect of theca interna cells. (**b**) Secondary follicle: The higher magnification showing the oocytes, granulosa cells and small cystic spaces within the follicle

Tertiary Follicle

Image gallery: Fig. 6.4a–c.
  Histopathology

- Fluid is collected within the antrum and the size of the follicle increase

- Now oocyte along with the ring of granulosa cells detaches and floats within the antral cavity.
- Primary oocyte now complete its first meiotic division.
- A polar body and secondary oocyte develop
- The secondary oocyte divides up to the metaphase of the second meiotic division.
- It waits for fertilization

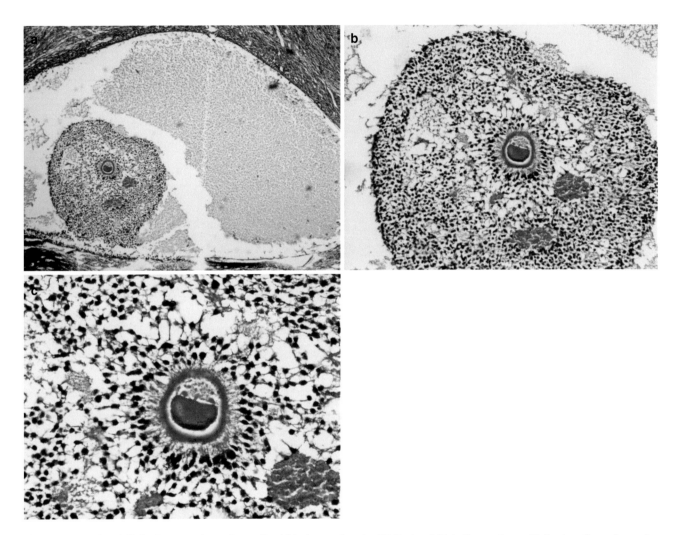

Fig. 6.4 (**a**) Tertiary follicle: Oocyte and granulosa cells within the antral cavity. (**b**) Tertiary follicle Oocyte along with the ring of granulosa cells. (**c**): Tertiary follicle: Note the central oocyte with thick zona pellucida and ring of granulosa cells

Corpus Luteum

Image gallery: Fig. 6.5a–c.

Origin: It is developed from the Graafian follicle after ovulation.

Gross appearance: Yellow colour, cystic.

Histopathology

- Corpus luteal cells: Polygonal cells with abundant eosinophilic cytoplasm and central round monomorphic nuclei
- Theca cells are also present

Functions

- Granulosa cells: Progesterone secretion
- Theca cells: Oestrogen

Fate

- No fertilization: Complete regression
- Fertilization: Corpus luteum persists and enlarges

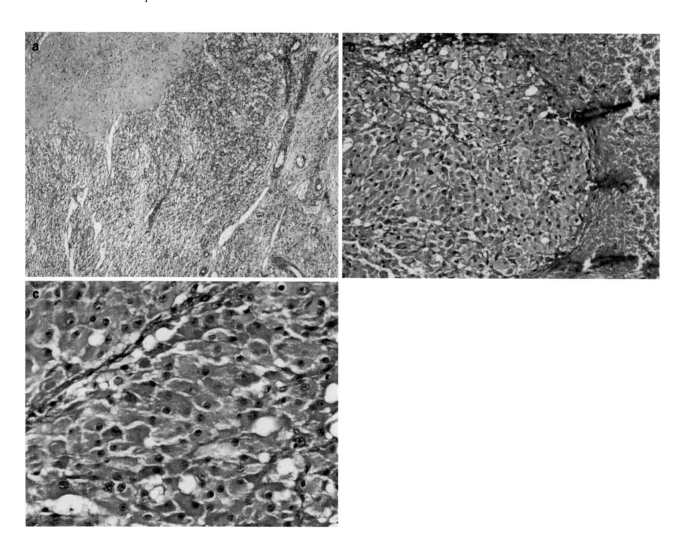

Fig. 6.5 (**a**) Corpus luteum: Haemorrhage surrounded by corpus luteal cells. (**b**) Corpus luteum: The Polygonal cells with abundant eosinophilic cytoplasm and central round monomorphic nuclei. (**c**) Corpus luteum: Higher magnification of the previous one

Corpus Albecans

Image: Fig. 6.6.
  Origin: It develops from the regressed corpus luteum.
  Histology: Scar like deep pink acellular material.

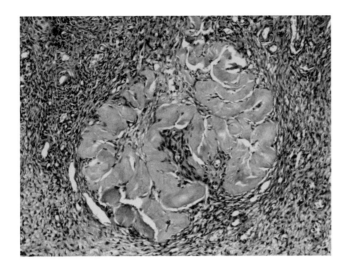

Fig. 6.6 Corpus albecans: Well circumscribed deep pink acellular material

Cysts in Ovary

Follicular Cyst

Image gallery: Fig. 6.7a–c.
  Definition: This is the functional cyst that develops from the Graafian follicle and more than 3 cm in diameter.
  Incidence

- Frequently present in the women of reproductive age period
- Transient and may disappear after sometime
- Rarely seen in postmenopausal patient

Clinical features

- Incidental finding
- Occasionally amenorrhea and irregular menstrual bleeding
- Uncommonly sudden pain abdomen due to rupture of the follicular cyst resulting in hemoperitoneum

Gross features

- Variable in size: ranges from 3–10 cm
- Solitary
- Regular margin
- Contains thin fluid

Histopathology

- Cyst lining: Multiple layers of granulosa cells and outer theca interna cells
- Granulosa cells: Moderate amount of cytoplasm, central round nuclei
- Poor reticulin stain in theca interna cells

Immunohistochemistry

- Positive: Calretinin and inhibin are positive in granulosa cells and theca interna cells

Differential diagnosis

- Cystic granulosa cell tumour
    - Large in size
    - Disorganized proliferation of granulosa cells
    - Presence of Call Exner bodies
- Surface epithelial cyst such as serous cyst adenoma
    - Single layer of cuboidal to ciliated columnar cells
    - Negative for inhibin
- Endometriotic cyst
    - Endometrial glands and stroma present
    - Haemorrhage

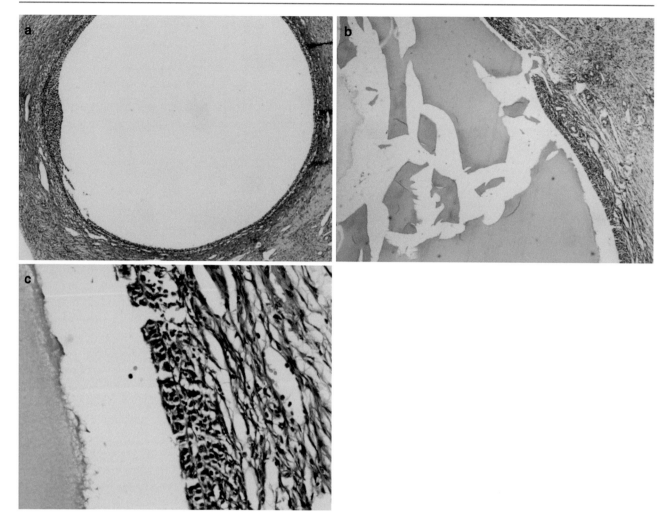

Fig. 6.7 (**a**) Follicular cyst: The cyst lined by granulosa cells. (**b**) Follicular cyst: Two to three layers granulosa cells form the lining of the cyst. (**c**) Follicular cyst: Higher magnification of the previous one

Corpus Luteal Cyst

Image gallery: Fig. 6.8a, b.

Definition: This is the cystic corpus luteum measuring more than 3 cm diameter.

Incidence

- It commonly occurs during the reproductive age period
- Present in corpus luteum of pregnancy, or in menstruation

Clinical features

- Usually asymptomatic and incidentally detected
- Occasionally complaints of amenorrhea and abnormal vaginal bleeding
- Sudden abdominal pain may occur due to rupture of the cyst

Gross features

- Size of the cyst varies from 3 cm to several cm
- Wall of the cyst is thick, convoluted and yellowish colour
- Cut section: Orange yellow in colour
- Contents: Serous fluid or old blood

Histopathology

- Composed of luteinized granulosa and theca interna cells
- Cells show abundant eosinophilic cytoplasm and central monomorphic nuclei

Behaviour

- Spontaneously regress within couple of months

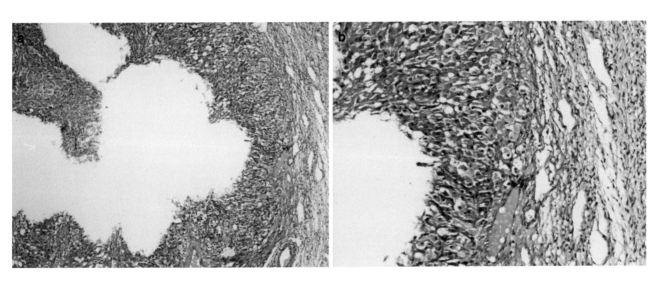

Fig. 6.8 (**a**) Corpus luteal cyst: the cyst wall is lined by luteinized granulosa and theca interna cells. (**b**) Corpus luteal cyst: Higher magnification of the cyst wall

Endometriotic Cyst of Ovary

Image gallery: Figs. 6.9 and 6.10.

Definition: The cyst formation due to endometriosis of the ovary.

Epidemiology

- About 10% women in the reproductive age period is affected
- Common in reproductive age period
- Average age is 40 years
- More common in Caucasian women

Clinical features

- Often asymptomatic
- Chief complaints: Dysmenorrhea, pain in pelvic region, dyspareunia and infertility
- Acute abdominal pain due to rupture of cyst

Gross features

- Size: Variable, few cm to 15 cm
- Thick fibrous wall
- Reddish in colour
- Cut section: Thick chocolate coloured due to old haemorrhage, single

Histopathology

- Endometrial glands and stroma
- Areas of recent and old haemorrhage with pigment laden macrophages

- Endometrial glandular epithelium may show cytological atypia
- Decidual cells may be present

Immunohistochemistry

- Epithelial cells: positive for ER/PR
- Stroma: CD 10 positive

Differential Diagnosis

- Corpus luteal cyst
    - Corpus luteal cells present
    - No endometrial stroma
- Tubo-ovarian abscess
    - Foamy histiocytes may be present, but no endometrial glands or stroma
- Surface epithelial cystadenoma
    - Single to multiple layers of cuboidal cells
    - No endometrial glands or stroma

Prognosis

- Usually benign course
- Excision of the cyst is curable
- Long standing endometriosis may have 1% risk of development of clear cell carcinoma and endometrioid carcinoma
- Significant atypia in the glandular epithelial cells indicates the chance of the development of malignancy

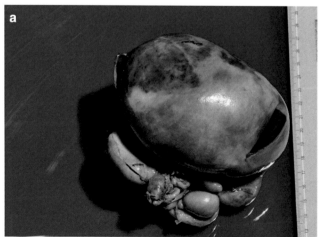 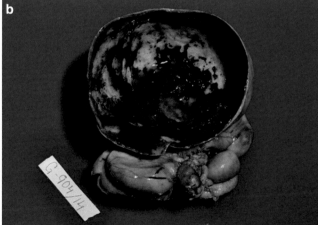

Fig. 6.9 (**a**) Gross picture of endometriotic cyst: The outer surface of the cyst is smooth. (**b**) Gross picture of endometriotic cyst: Large areas of haemorrhage

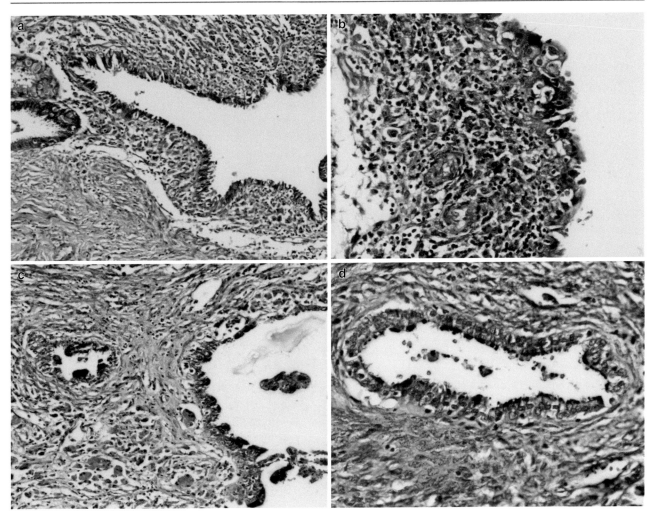

Fig. 6.10 (**a**) Endometriotic cyst of ovary: The cyst wall is lined by cuboidal cells. (**b**) Endometriotic cyst of ovary: Higher magnification of the same showing many pigment laden macrophages indicating old haemorrhage. (**c**) Endometriotic cyst of ovary: Endometrial glands in the ovarian stroma. (**d**) Endometriotic cyst of ovary: The endometrial glands in higher magnification

Non-Specific Inflammation

Image gallery: Fig. 6.11a–c.
  Common organisms: Mixed anaerobic bacteria.
  Risk factors

- Multiple sex partners
- Intrauterine contraceptive device use

Clinical features

- Pelvic pain
- Abnormal vaginal discharge or discharge per vagina
- Fever
- Various urinary problems

Gross features

- Enlarged unilateral or bilateral ovary often attached with fallopian tube
- Tubo-ovarian mass
- Shape: Distorted
- Surface is congested with exudates
- Adhesion with the neighbouring tissue

- Cut section: Unilocular to multiloculated solid cystic lesion

Histopathology

- Intense acute inflammatory cells
- Necrosis and foci of haemorrhage
- Chronic inflammatory cells consisting of lymphocytes, plasma cells and histiocytes in case of chronic inflammation
- In case of xanthogranulomatous inflammation: Abundant foamy histiocytes and chronic inflammatory cells present

Differential diagnosis

- Endometriosis
  – Presence of endometrial glands and stroma

Prognosis and therapy

- Identification of the organism followed by antibiotic therapy cures most of the patients
- Oophorectomy may be needed if the patient fails to respond by antibiotic therapy

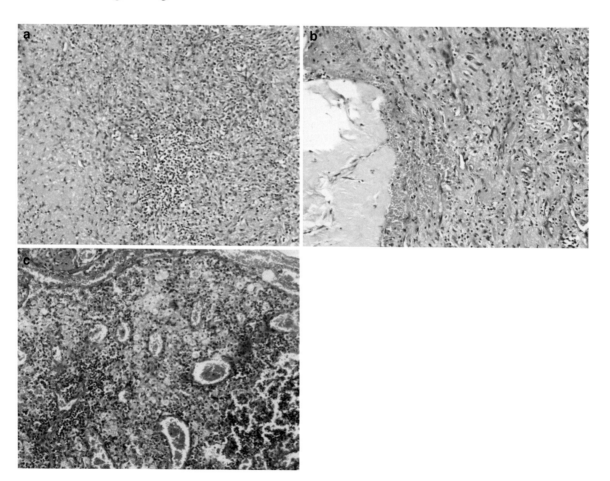

Fig. 6.11 (**a**) Non-specific inflammation: Diffuse chronic inflammatory cell infiltration. (**b**) Non-specific inflammation: The inflammatory cells are mainly composed of lymphocytes and plasma cells. (**c**) Xanthogranulomatous inflammation: Foamy histiocytes and inflammatory cells

Granulomatous Inflammation: Tuberculosis

Image gallery: Fig. 6.12.
  Epidemiology

- Ten percent of tuberculous infection of the female genital tract affects ovary
- Young women
- Mean age: 30 years

Clinical features

- Infertility

Histopathology

- Multiple epithelioid cells granulomas
- Multinucleated giant cells
- Necrosis

Ancillary studies

- Ziehl Neelsen stain: Positive for acid fast bacilli in case of tuberculosis
- Culture
- PCR

Treatment: Anti tubercular therapy.

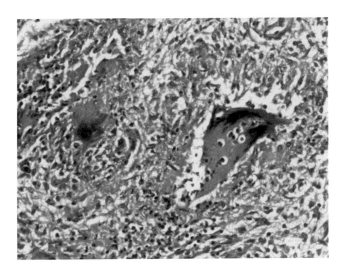

Fig. 6.12 Granulomatous inflammation in ovary: Epithelioid cell granulomas and giant cells

Ovarian Oedema

Image gallery: Fig. 6.13a, b.

Definition: This is a non-neoplastic condition of ovary characterized by massive oedema in the ovary.

Clinical features

- Mean age 21 years
- Unilateral involvement
- Chief complaints: Pain abdomen, menstrual irregularities

Gross features

- Enlarged ovary from few cm to 30 cm
- Shiny outer surface
- Thickened capsule
- Cut section: solid gelatinous

Histopathology

- Hypocellular, oedematous
- Extravasation of RBCs and fluid

- Foci of fibromatosis present: Oval to spindle cells in loose fascicles
- Isolated ovarian follicle may be seen

Differential diagnosis

- Fibroma of ovary with massive oedema
  - Normal ovarian stroma is pushed aside whereas in massive oedema the normal ovarian structure is entangled within it
- Ovarian neoplasms with oedema such as Krukenberg's tumour, sclerosing stromal tumour etc.

Prognosis and treatment

- Benign condition therefore conservative management is possible to keep the ovary.
- Wedge biopsy or frozen section may be helpful to diagnose the lesion.
- In case of failure of conservative management, oophorectomy is the treatment of choice.

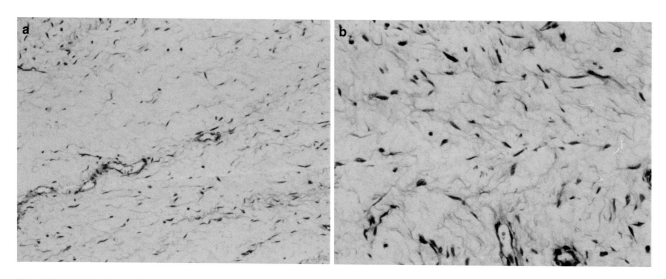

Fig. 6.13 (**a**) Ovarian oedema: Hypocellular and oedematous ovarian stroma. (**b**) Ovarian oedema: Widely scattered spindle cells in the pale coloured oedematous stroma

Stromal Hyperplasia and Stromal Hyperthecosis

Image gallery: Fig. 6.14a, b.

Definition

- Stromal hyperplasia: It is characterized by diffuse non-neoplastic proliferation of the stromal cells of the ovary.
- Stromal hyperthecosis: It is characterized by the additional presence of lutenized cells along with stromal hyperplasia.

Incidence

- It is a common lesion in post-menopausal women
- It occurs in 33% of the women in 60–70 year age

Clinical features

- Incidental
- Asymptomatic patient
- Androgenic excess: Virilization, acne
- Estrogenic excess: endometrial hyperplasia

- Obesity, hypertension, impaired glucose tolerance test

Gross features

- Bilateral enlarged ovary
- Diffuse or nodular enlargement
- Solid yellow to grey colour

Histopathology
Stromal hyperplasia

- Spindle shaped stromal cells arranged diffusely or in nodular fashion
- The cells have elongated nuclei with inconspicuous nucleoli

Stromal hyperthecosis

- Small nests of luteinized cells
  - Polygonal cells with abundant eosinophilic cytoplasm, centrally placed nuclei
- Atretic follicles may be seen
- Smooth muscle cells and hilus cells are also present

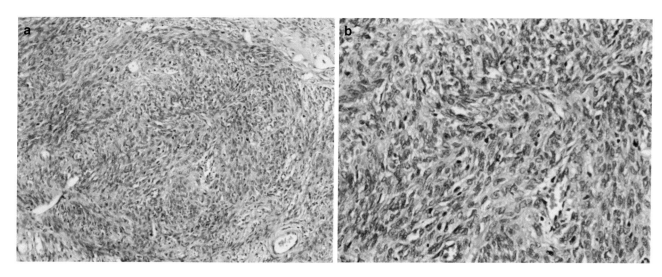

Fig. 6.14 (a) Stromal hyperplasia: Stromal cells arranged in nodular fashion. (b) Stromal hyperplasia: Spindle shaped with scanty cytoplasm and elongated nuclei

Suggested Reading

Chowdhury NN. Overview of tuberculosis of the female genital tract. J Indian Med Assoc. 1996;94(9):345–6. 361

Clement PB. The pathology of endometriosis: a survey of the many faces of a common disease emphasizing diagnostic pitfalls and unusual and newly appreciated aspects. Adv Anat Pathol. 2007;14(4):241–60.

Givens JR. Ovarian hyperthecosis. N Engl J Med. 1971;285(12):691.

Parker RL, Dadmanesh F, Young RH, Clement PB. Polypoid endometriosis: a clinicopathologic analysis of 24 cases and a review of the literature. Am J Surg Pathol. 2004;28(3):285–97.

Young RH, Scully RE. Fibromatosis and massive edema of the ovary, possibly related entities: a report of 14 cases of fibromatosis and 11 cases of massive edema. Int J Gynecol Pathol. 1984;3:153–78.

Classification of ovarian epithelial and mesenchymal tumours according to World Health Organization have been highlighted in Fig. 7.1 [1].

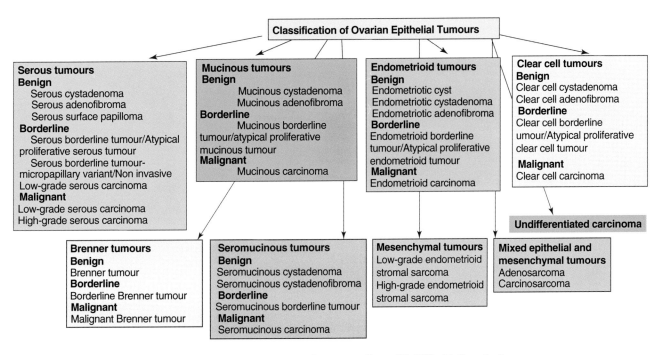

Fig. 7.1 Classification of epithelial and mesenchymal ovarian neoplasms according to World Health Organization

© Springer Nature Singapore Pte Ltd. 2019
P. Dey, *Color Atlas of Female Genital Tract Pathology*, https://doi.org/10.1007/978-981-13-1029-4_7

Serous Tumours

Serous Cystadenoma

Image gallery: Figs. 7.2, 7.3, 7.4, and 7.5
  Incidence

- The commonest benign surface epithelial tumour
- It constitutes 50% of all serous tumours
- Bilateral: 20%

Molecular genetics

- Polyclonal in nature, therefore these lesions are possibly nothing but hyperplastic inclusion cyst
- No KRAS/BRAF/P53 mutation

Clinical features

- Predominantly asymptomatic
- Occasionally: Pelvic mass. pain abdomen, vaginal bleeding

Gross features
Cystadenoma

- Cystic tumour
- More than 1–20 cm in diameter
- Unilocular or multilocular
- Thin translucent cyst wall
- Content: clear fluid

Cystadenofibroma

- In addition to cystic area solid fibrous component is present in variable amount

Histopathology

- Depending on the relative amount of cystic and solid fibrous component the terminology "cyst" of "fibroma" is used
- Lining of the cyst :
  - Cuboidal to columnar epithelial cells simulating fallopian tube lining cells
  - Usually the cells are ciliated
  - Scanty cytoplasm with monomorphic round nuclei
- Psammoma bodies may be present
- Cystadenofibroma shows collagenous stroma admixed with benign glands.
- Small papillary excrescences with monomorphic lining cells should be labelled as serous papilloma only.

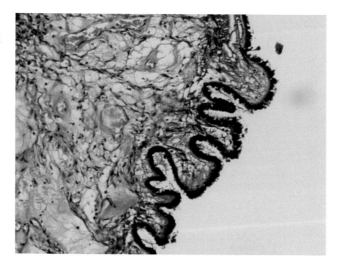

Fig. 7.3 Serous cystadenoma: the cyst is lined by single layer of cuboidal cells. The cells are ciliated here

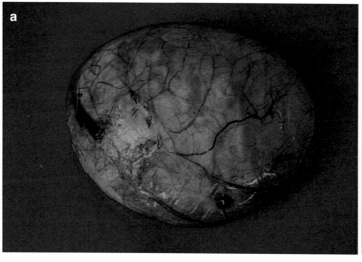 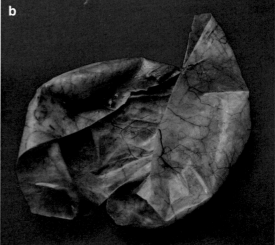

Fig. 7.2 (**a**) Gross picture of serous cystadenoma: cystic thin swelling with smooth shiny outer surface. (**b**) Gross picture of Serous cystadenoma: thin walled cyst

- Serous cystadenoma/ adnofibroma containing less than 10% area of borderline changes should be recognized as focal epithelial proliferation in a serous cystadenoma/ adnofibroma

Immunohistochemistry

- Positive: CK 7, WT 1, BER-EP4
- Negative: CK 20

Differential diagnosis

- Cortical inclusion cyst
  - Always less than 1 cm diameter in size
- Rete cysts
  - Hilar location
  - Proliferation of hilar cells
  - Cells with prominent cilia
- Endometriotic cyst
  - Presence of endometrial glands and stroma
- Mesonephric cyst
  - The wall of the cyst contains smooth muscle cells under the lining epithelium
- Hydrosalpinx
  - Operative history of swollen fallopian tube
- Mucinous cyst
  - Mucinous lining epithelium that are PAS positive

Prognosis and treatment

- Benign
- Simple cystectomy or salpingo oophorectomy is the treatment of choice

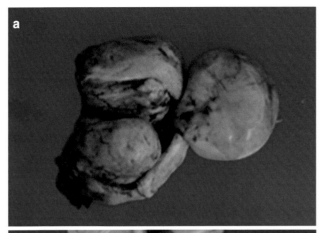

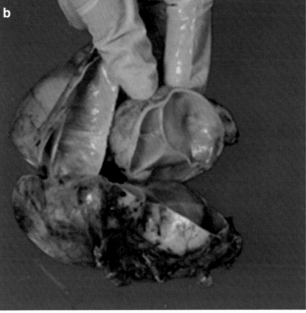

Fig. 7.4 (**a**) Gross picture of serous cyst adenofibroma: solid cystic growth. (**b**) Gross picture of serous cyst adenofibroma: cut section shows multiloculated cyst and solid area

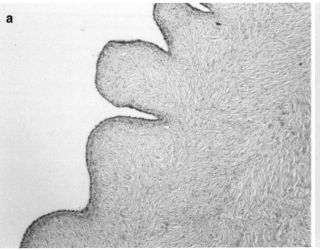

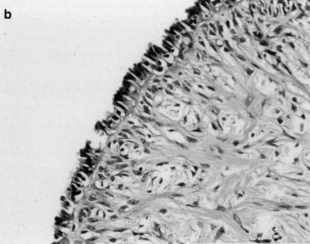

Fig. 7.5 (**a**) Serous cyst adenofibroma: thick fibrocollagenous wall. (**b**) Serous cyst adenofibroma: the lining of the cyst is formed by cuboidal epithelium

Serous Borderline Tumour

Image gallery: Figs. 7.6, 7.7, 7.8, and 7.9

Synonym: Atypical proliferative serous tumour, serous tumour of low malignant potential

Abbreviation: Serous borderline tumour (SBT)

Definition: The surface epithelial tumour that shows cellular atypia of the lining epithelial cells and proliferation without any underlying stromal invasion.

Epidemiology

- 10–15% of all serous epithelial tumours of ovary
- Bilateral: 25–30% cases
- Mean age: 45 years, lower than serous carcinomas

Molecular profile

- KRAS and BRAF mutation: Half of the cases
- These mutation is seen in the adjacent epithelial cells of the cyst wall of the borderline zone also

Clinical features

- Asymptomatic: majority of the patients
- Occasional: Pelvic mass and pain
- Raised serum CA-125 level

Gross features

- Variable size: several cm in diameter
- Cystic and partially solid
- Papillary excrescences may also be seen in the outer surface
- Cut section: Reddish to grey coloured papillary structures

Histopathology

- Papillae with hierarchical branching:
  - The large papillae divide and give rise to smaller papillae which again divide to produce much smaller papillae.
  - Papillary tufts are frequently detached from the tip and float in the cyst

- Tangentially cut papillae may simulate stromal invasion, however there will be no stromal reaction in such conditions
- Epithelial lining cells:
  - The lining epithelial cells of the papillae and cyst are cuboidal to columnar
  - Mild to moderate nuclear enlargement, pleomorphism and hyperchromasia present
  - The epithelial cells often show stratification
  - Low mitotic activity
- Psammoma body: 25% cases
- Lack of stromal invasion
- Microinvasion:

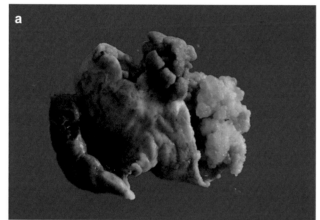

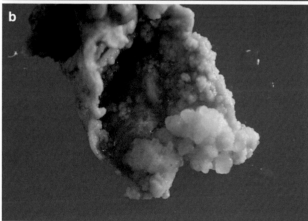

Fig. 7.6 (a) Gross picture of serous borderline tumour: partially solid tumour. (b) Gross picture of serous borderline tumour: cut section showing whitish polypoid growth

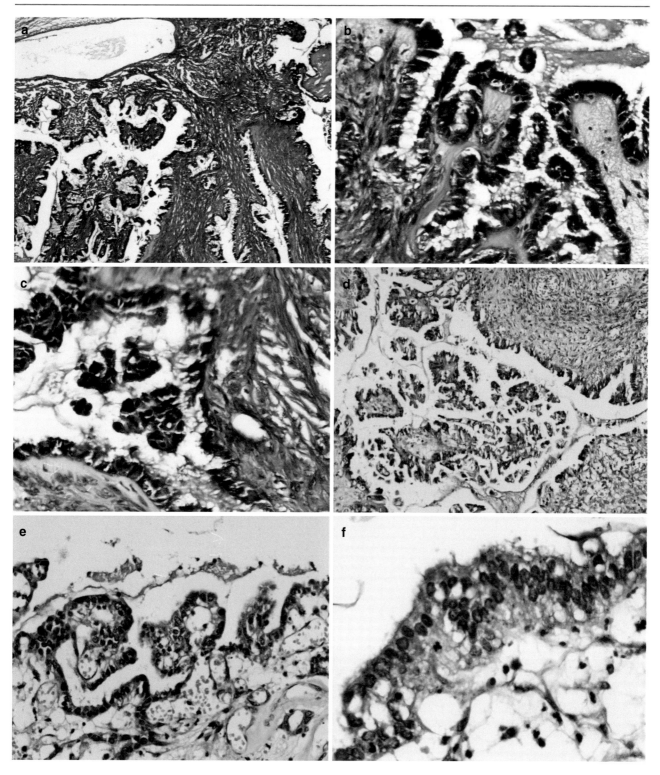

Fig. 7.7 (a) Serous borderline tumour: irregular branching papillae in a hierarchical manner. (b) Serous borderline tumour: the large papillae give rise to small papillae. (c) Serous borderline tumour: Multiple papillary structures. The micropapillae are detached. (d) Serous borderline tumour: branching and sub branching of papillae along with many detached micropapillae. (e) Serous borderline tumour: tufts of multi-layered cells. (f) Serous borderline tumour: the lining cells showing moderate nuclear enlargement and pleomorphism. (g) Serous border-line tumour: moderately enlarged nuclei with pleomorphism. (h) Serous borderline tumour, microinvasion: small groups of irregular glands in the stroma. The linear dimension of the invasive foci should be less than 5 mm

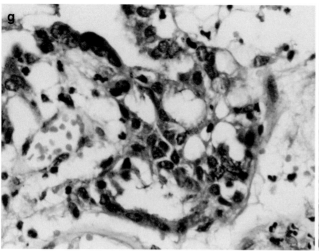 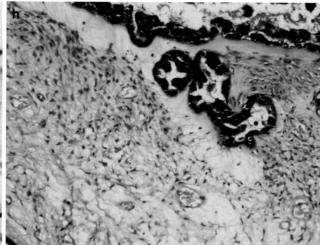

Fig. 7.7 (continued)

Usual eosinophilic type

- Variable frequency reported: 1% to as high as 25% of SBT
- Clusters of tumour cells in the stroma with abundant eosinophilic cytoplasm and having enlarged nuclei with prominent nucleoli
- The maximum linear dimension of the cells clusters is less than 5 mm diameter, and also less than 10 cm^2 area. However, the lesions may be multiple.
- The cells are negative for ER/PR and have low Ki 67 scoring

Microinvasive carcinoma

- Clusters of cells with irregular outline or micropapillae
- The group of cells are surrounded by clear space
- Cribriform appearance
- Desmoplastic reaction is often present around the cells
- The greatest dimension of the cluster is less than 5 mm
- D2-40 immunostaining demonstrated that this clear space is actually nothing but lymphatic space

Immunohistochemistry

- Positive: EMA, BER-EP4, CK 7, PAX 8, WT 1
- Negative: p53 and p16

Essential diagnostic criteria: see Box 7.1

Box 7.1 Essential Diagnostic Criteria of Serous Borderline Tumour
- Complex hierarchical branching papillary pattern present: large papillae divide into smaller papillae
- Nuclear atypia: cuboidal to columnar lining epithelial cells show mild to moderate nuclear enlargement and pleomorphism
- No stromal invasion
- Hobnail appearance frequently present
- If confluent growth present: it measures less than 5 mm area
- Positive for EMA, BER-EP4, CK 7, PAX 8, WT 1 and negative for p53 and p16
- K-RAS and BRAF mutations also noted
- Note: multiple sections needed to exclude invasive component

Differential diagnosis

- Benign serous tumours
  - Less than 10% area show borderline changes
- Serous adenocarcinoma
  - Definite stromal invasion present
- Struma ovarii wit papillary structure
  - Typical thyroid follicle present

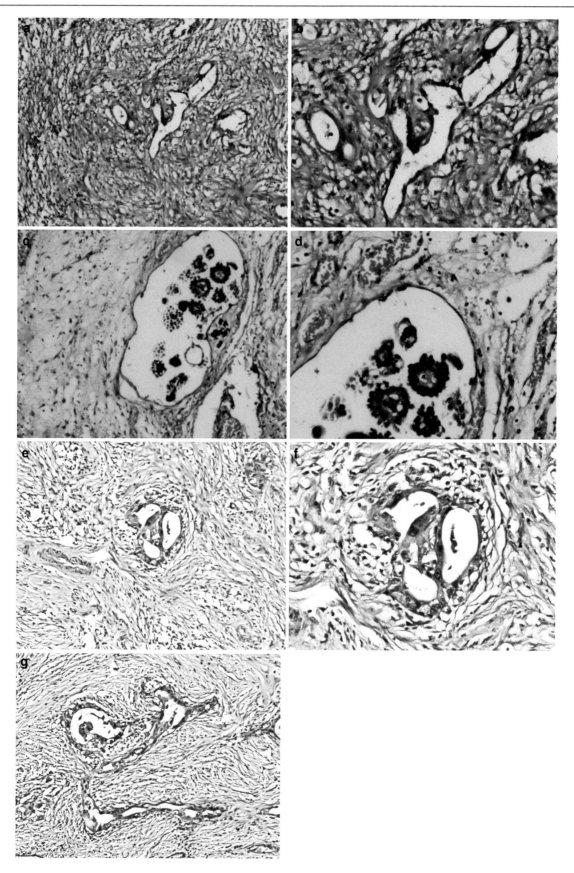

Fig. 7.8 (**a**) Peritoneal implant non-invasive: small gland surrounded by dense stroma. (**b**) Peritoneal implant non-invasive: Higher magnification of the same. (**c**) Peritoneal implant non-invasive: multiple papillae surrounded by dense fibrous stroma. (**d**) Peritoneal implant non-invasive: higher magnification of the same showing well circumscribed papillae from the surrounding tissue. (**e**) Invasive peritoneal implant: the glands within the stroma having irregular margin. (**f**) Invasive peritoneal implant: Higher magnification showing irregular margin of the glands. Note the surrounding lymphocytic infiltration around the glands. (**g**) Invasive peritoneal implant: the irregular glands with dense stromal reaction

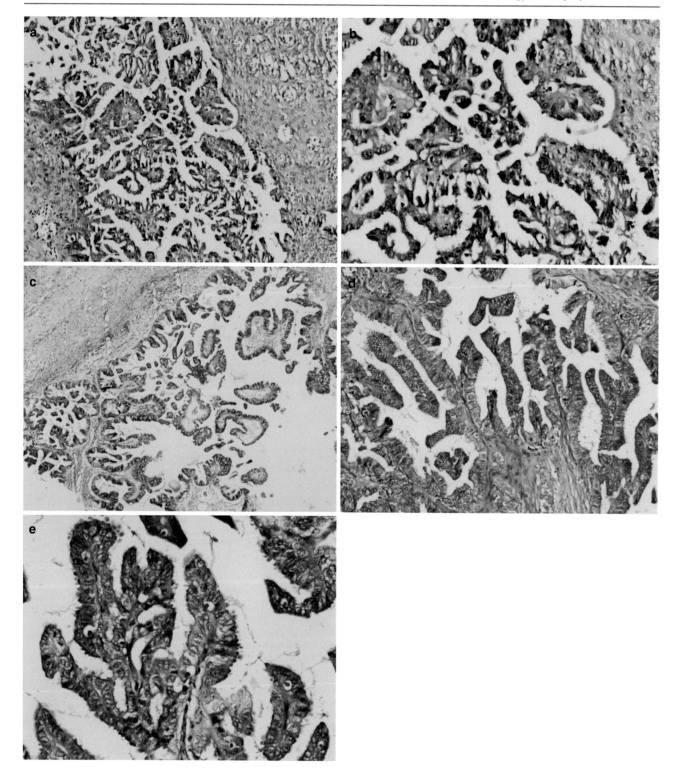

Fig. 7.9 (a) Serous borderline tumour, micropapillary variant: multiple complex and non-hierarchically branched papillae. (b) Serous borderline tumour, micropapillary variant: the complex branching papillae. (c) Serous borderline tumour, micropapillary variant: smaller papillae directly arising from the larger papillae. (d) Serous borderline tumour, micropapillary variant: the papillae are tall and thin. (e) Serous borderline tumour, micropapillary variant: the thin papillae with fibrovascular core. The papillae are lined by the cuboidal to columnar cells with moderately pleomorphic nuclei

Implants in SBT

- Peritoneal implants: 30–40% cases of SBT
- Classification of implants:
  - Non-invasive implant
    Epithelial type
    Desmoplastic type
  - Invasive implant
- Non-invasive implants:
  - Epithelial type
    Well circumscribed hierarchical branching papillae or single cell or tiny clusters of tumour cells with mild nuclear atypia
    Smooth transition with the surrounding stromal tissue
  - Desmoplastic type
    Papillary group, glands or small clusters or single cells with nuclear atypia surrounded by dense fibrous stroma
    Smooth transition with the surrounding stromal tissue
- Invasive implant
  - The papillae/glands/isolated clusters of cells within the stroma having irregular margin
  - Micropapillae formation
  - Island of cells surrounded by clear space
  - Overall 12% of SBT shows invasive implants
  - Higher chances of recurrence and more aggressive in behaviour

Pelvic Lymph Node Involvement in SBT

- Noted in 23% cases of SBT
- Sinusoidal spaces of lymph node is involved by the cluster of cells with abundant eosinophilic cytoplasm
- Not related with adverse prognosis

Prognosis

- SBT confined to ovary behaves as a benign fashion
- Five year survival is 95–100%
- Peritoneal non-invasive implants may have adhesion and recurrence
- No adverse prognosis in case of lymph nodal implants
- Death occur only in those cases that progress to low grade serous carcinoma

Treatment

- Total abdominal hysterectomy with bilateral salpingo oophorectomy in those patients who have completed their surgery
- Conservative treatment : Unilateral salpingo oophorectomy/ cystectomy in younger patients who want to complete family
- No adjuvant chemotherapy or radiotherapy is needed in non-invasive implants
- Doubtful role of adjuvant chemotherapy in case of invasive implants

Serous Borderline Tumour of Micropapillary Variant

Image gallery: Fig. 7.9a–e

Synonym: Non-invasive low grade serous carcinoma, serous borderline tumour of micropapillary variant

Abbreviation: Serous borderline tumour of micropapillary variant (SBT-MP)

Epidemiology

- It represent 14% of SBT
- Mean age 42 year

Molecular genetics

- Mutation of KRAS/BRAF
- Chromosomal 1p 36 loss
- Similar type of KRAS/BRAF mutation in both this tumour and Low grade serous carcinoma indicates that the former tumour is a precursor of the later tumour

Clinical features

- Asymptomatic
- Pelvic mass, abdominal pain

Gross features

- Solid and cystic
- Mean size: 8 cm in diameter
- Papillary excrescences may be present over the surface
- Cut section: cyst filled with fluid and also solid areas with papillae, no necrosis

Histopathology

- Multiple complex and non-hierarchically branched papillae
- The papillae are taller and more than five times tall than wide
- Scanty to almost no central fibrovascular core in the papillae
- Lining cells:
  - Columnar, cuboidal or hobnail type

  - Often ciliated
  - Significant nuclear atypia
  - Small and prominent nucleoli
  - Mitosis more than SBT
- Predominant cribriform arrangement of cells may be present
- At times there may be complete lack of papillae

Immunohistochemistry

- Positive: WT 1, CK 7, PAX 8, CAM 5.2, EMA
- Negative: p53

Diagnostic criteria: See Box 7.2

Box 7.2 Diagnostic Criteria of Serous Borderline Tumour of Micropapillary Variant

- Non-hierarchically branched papillae: multiple smaller papillae arise from the larger one directly
- Papillae are more than five times longer than wider
- Central core of papillae absent
- Hobnail appearance
- Frequent mitosis
- The area of confluent micropapillary change is more than 5mm diameter
- Micropapillary pattern consists of 10% of the tumour area
- Significant nuclear atypia
- *Immunohistochemistry*: positive for WT 1, CK 7, PAX 8, CAM 5.2, EMA

Prognosis and treatment

- SBT-MP is relatively more aggressive than the SBT
- These tumours are more commonly (27%) detected in advanced stage
- Stage I non-invasive low grade serous carcinoma has very good survival rate and it is almost similar than that in general population
- The treatment of SBT-MP is same as that of SBT

Serous Carcinoma of Ovary

Incidence

- 50% serous tumours benign
- 15% serous tumours borderline
- 35% serous tumours malignant

Bilateral: 70% of carcinomas

Low Grade Serous Carcinoma

Image gallery: Figs. 7.10, 7.11, and 7.12
Definition: This is an invasive serous epithelial tumour having mild cytological atypia.
Abbreviation: Low grade serous carcinoma (LGSC)
Epidemiology

- Uncommon and represents only 5–10% of serous carcinomas

Molecular genetics

- KRAS and BRAF mutation

Clinical features

- Lower age group than high grade serous carcinoma
- Predominantly asymptomatic
- Symptomatic: Mass abdomen or ascites

Gross features

- Variable in size
- Solid and cystic
- Papillary excrescences present

Histopathology

- Arrangement: papillae, glands, cribriform pattern and nests
- Invasion of the tumour in the deeper stroma
- Tumour cells are surrounded by clear space
- Individual tumour cells:
  - Cuboidal to columnar
  - Mildly pleomorphic nuclei with small nucleoli
- Low mitosis: Less than 3 per 10 HPF
- Frequent psammoma bodies
- Often SBT is present in other foci

Immunohistochemistry

- Same as BST
- Low Ki 67 scoring compared to high grade serous carcinoma

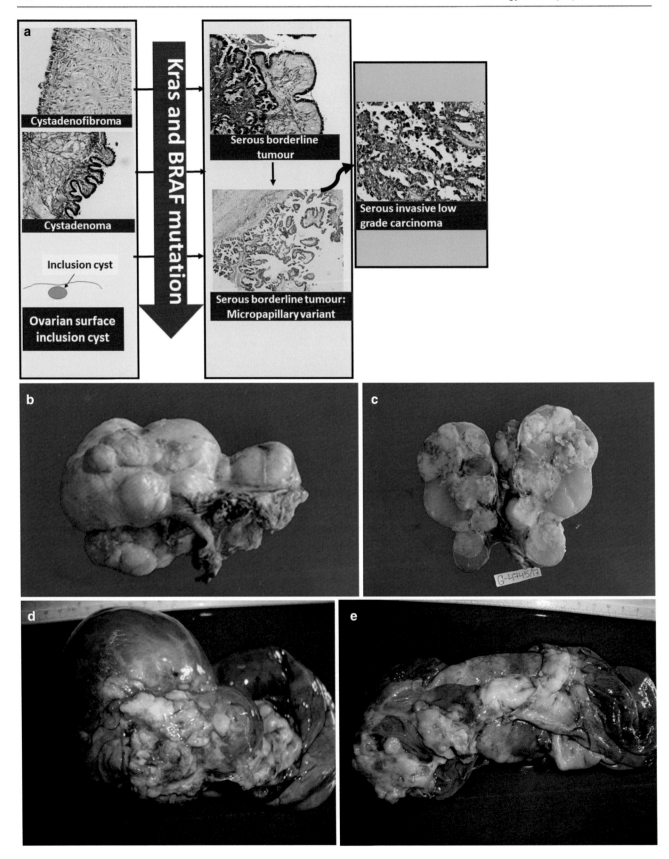

Fig. 7.10 (a) Pathogenesis of low grade serous carcinoma of ovary. (b) Gross picture of serous carcinoma: solid and partly cystic tumour. (c) Gross picture of serous carcinoma: cut section showing solid grey white areas with foci of cystic spaces containing thick material. (d) Gross picture of serous carcinoma: solid cystic tumour with capsular rupture. (e) Gross picture of serous carcinoma: cut section showing grey white fleshy growth. (f) Gross photograph of a high grade serous carcinoma showing solid grey white firm growth

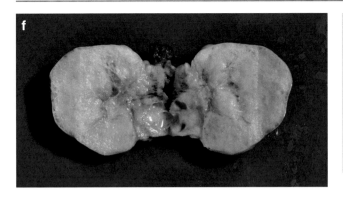

Fig. 7.10 (continued)

Key diagnostic features: see Box 7.3

Box 7.3 Key Diagnostic Features of Low Grade Serous Carcinoma
- Micropapillae, macropapillae and nests or single cells
- Definite stromal invasion

- Cuboidal to columnar tumour cells with mildly pleomorphic nuclei
- Frequent psammoma bodies
- Absence of necrosis
- Frequent foci of borderline serous tumour
- Immunohistochemistry: Positive for WT 1, CK 7, PAX 8, CAM 5.2, EMA
- Molecular genetics: KRAS and BRAF mutation

Prognosis

- Good in prognosis
- Five year survival: 85%

Treatment

- Total abdominal hysterectomy with bilateral salpingo oophorectomy
- Patients with Stage Ic or above: Adjuvant chemotherapy is recommended.
- Usually refractory to platinum based chemotherapy and the chemotherapy is not very much beneficial

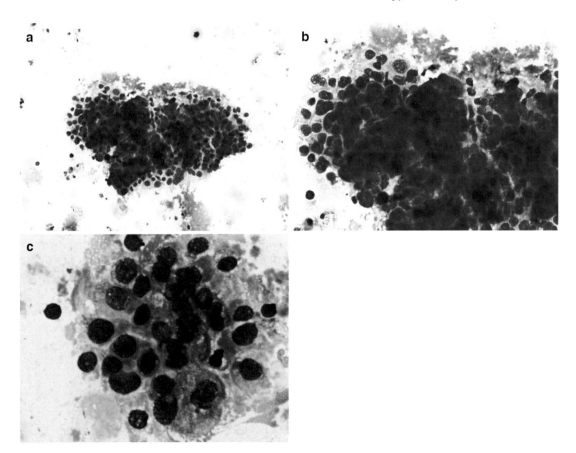

Fig. 7.11 (**a**) Cytology smear of serous carcinoma: Tight cohesive cluster of malignant cells. (**b**) Cytology smear of Serous carcinoma: Higher magnification of the same showing cells with moderate nuclear pleomorphism. (**c**) Cytology smear of Serous carcinoma: the individual cells show moderate amount of vacuolated cytoplasm and centrally placed pleomorphic nuclei having prominent nucleoli. (**d**) Ascitic fluid cytology smear and panel of immunohistochemistry on cell block preparation to confirm the ovarian origin of the tumour

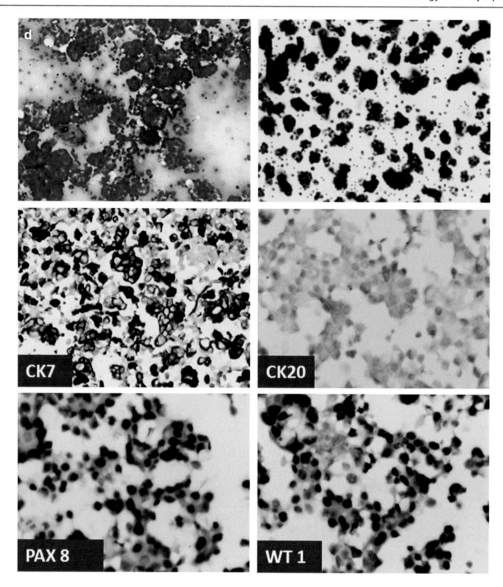

Fig. 7.11 (continued)

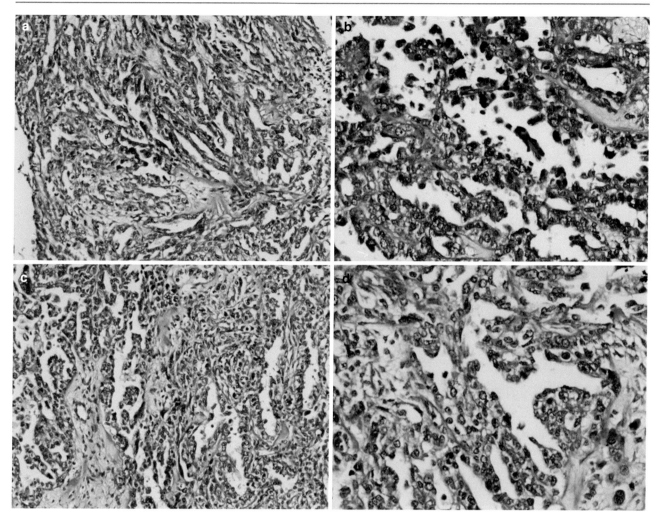

Fig. 7.12 (**a**) Low grade serous carcinoma: Tumour is composed of multiple papillae. (**b**) Low grade serous carcinoma: the papillae are lined by mildly pleomorphic tumour cells. (**c**) Low grade serous carci-noma: both glands and multiple papillae. (**d**) Low grade serous carci-noma: glands and cystic spaces

High Grade Serous Carcinoma

Image gallery: Figs. 7.13, 7.14, and 7.15

Definition: This is a type of serous carcinoma characterized by higher nuclear grade of the tumour cells.

Abbreviation: High grade serous carcinoma (HGSC)

Epidemiology

- It represents 50% of all ovarian carcinoma
- Common in sixth decade
- Mean age 63 year

- Higher incidence in western women

Genetic profile

- TP53 mutation occurs in almost all cases of HGSC
- BRCA 1 mutation in 50% cases
- Occasionally KRAS mutation
- Frequent DNA copy number alteration
  - DNA copy number gain or amplified areas contain CCNE1, AKT, NOTCH3, RSF1, and PIK3CA oncogenes

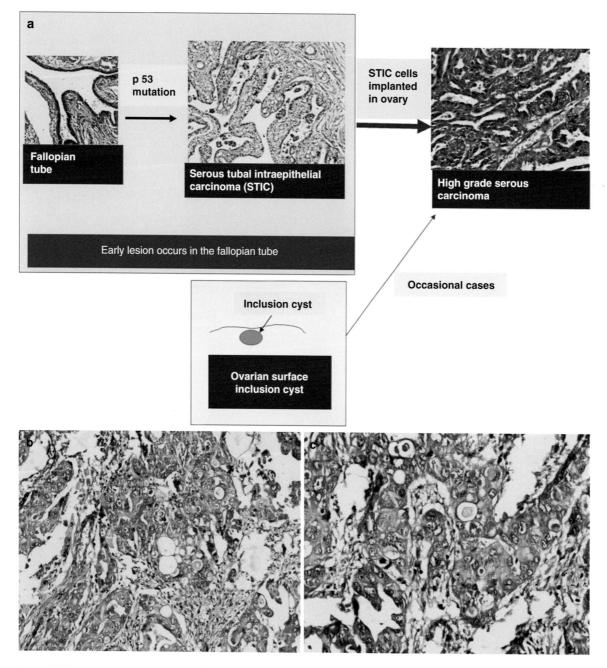

Fig. 7.13 (**a**) High grade serous carcinoma: possible pathogenesis. (**b**) High grade serous carcinoma. (**c**) High grade serous carcinoma: the tumour cells are mainly in solid sheets. (**d**) High grade serous carci-noma: the glands are lined by moderate to markedly pleomorphic cells with large prominent nucleoli. (**e**) High grade serous carcinoma: higher magnification showing markedly pleomorphic tumour cells

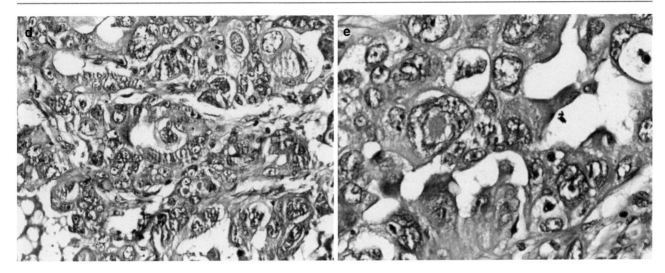

Fig. 7.13 (continued)

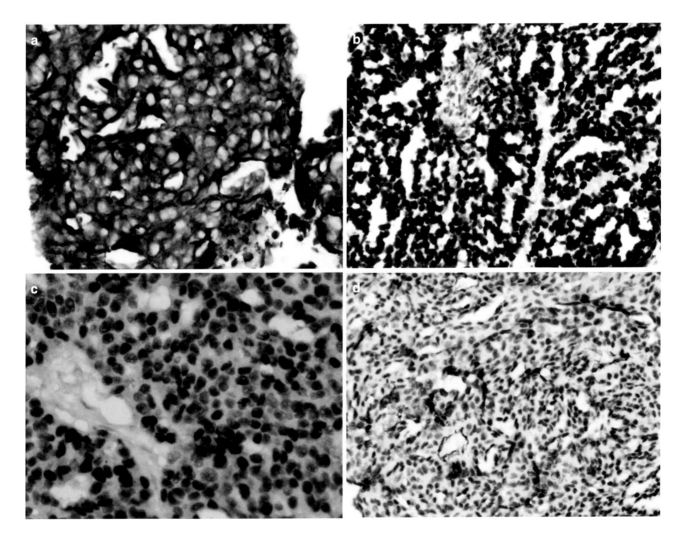

Fig. 7.14 (**a**) High grade serous carcinoma: strong cytoplasmic CK 7 positivity. (**b**) High grade serous carcinoma: nuclear positivity of p53. (**c**) High grade serous carcinoma: Nuclear positivity of Pax 8. (**d**) High grade serous carcinoma: nuclear positivity of wt1

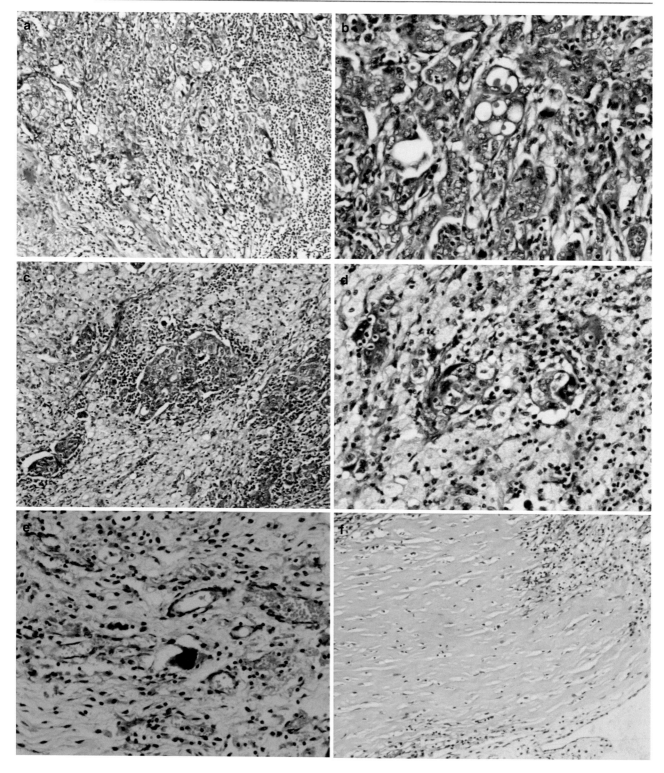

Fig. 7.15 (**a**) Chemotherapy response grade 1: diffuse sheets of viable tumour cells indicating no response. (**b**) Chemotherapy response grade 1: sheets of viable tumour cells, (**c**) Chemotherapy response grade 2: occasional clusters of viable tumour cells and dense inflammation indicating partial response. (**d**) Chemotherapy response grade 2: occasional viable tumours cells and foamy histiocytes, (**e**) Chemotherapy response grade 3: calcification and chronic inflammation. No viable tumour cells present indicating complete response. (**f**) Chemotherapy response grade 3: marked sclerosis

Note: Germ line mutation of BRCA 1 and BRCA 2 genes cause 50% risk of development in HGSC in normal healthy women

Clinical features

- Common symptoms: Abdominal pain, ascites, pelvic mass
- Gastrointestinal symptoms: Anorexia, nausea, quick satiety
- Pleural effusion
- High CA 125: More than 500 IU/ml

Gross features

- Variable size: 1–20 cm in diameter
- Solid and cystic
- Smooth shiny surface and papillary excrescences may be present
- Cut section: Grey white solid areas with haemorrhage and necrosis

Cytology

Fine needle aspiration cytology smears show:

- Clusters and discrete malignant cells
- The cells contain moderate amount of vacuolated cytoplasm
- Centrally placed moderately pleomorphic nuclei with prominent nucleoli

Histopathology

- Arrangement: predominantly solid sheets along with papillae, gland and nests
- Cells show high nucleo cytoplasmic ratio, moderate to marked nuclear pleomorphism
- Large and prominent nucleoli
- Mitosis: very high 20 to 30 per 10 HPF
- Necrosis present
- Desmoplastic stroma
- Psammoma body may be seen

Immunohistochemistry

- WT 1: strong nuclear positivity
- P 53: two types of pattern
  - Strong and diffuse nuclear stain that indicates missense mutation
  - Complete absence of stain that indicates nonsense mutation
- Positive : PAX 8, CK 7, EMA, BEREP4 and CDKN2A

Notes

- WT1, P53 and CDK 2NA positivity helps it to distinguish this tumour from endometrioid carcinoma of ovary which is negative for all these markers

Comparison of Immunohistochemistry between LGSC and HGSC: see Table 7.1
Key diagnostic features: see Box 7.4

Box 7.4 Key Diagnostic Features of High Grade Serous Carcinoma
- Mainly solid sheets of cells
- In addition, papillae and glands
- High mitotic rate
- Necrosis present
- Large cells with moderately pleomorphic nuclei having prominent nucleoli
- Strong nuclear positivity of WT 1 and p53
- In addition, positive for PAX 8, CK 7, EMA, BEREP4 and CDKN2A

Prognosis

- Prognosis depends mainly on the stage at the time of presentation
- About 80% patients present in advanced stage (stage III/IV)
- Five year survival of stage III/IV carcinoma: 50%
- Molecular markers have no accepted clinical value in prognosis

Treatment

- Stage I to IIa
- Total abdominal hysterectomy with bilateral salpingo oophorectomy along with omentectomy
- Peritoneal washing, peritoneal biopsy and thorough evaluation of the retroperitoneal area
- The role of adjuvant chemotherapy is controversial
- Advanced disease stage IIb to IIIc
- Debulking surgery followed by adjuvant chemotherapy
- Platinum-based chemotherapy

Table 7.1 Comparison of immunohistochemistry between LGSC and HGSC

Immunohistochemistry	LGSC	HGSC
P53	Negative	Positive
PAX-8	Positive	Positive
WT 1	Positive	Positive
CDK2NA	Negative	Positive
CK7	Positive	Positive
CK 20	Negative	Negative

Mucinous Tumours of Ovary

Table 7.2 shows the relative incidences of mucinous neoplasm of ovary.

Table 7.2 Incidence of mucinous tumours of ovary

Incidence of mucinous tumours of ovary	
All type of mucinous tumour	15% of ovarian tumour
Mucinous adenoma	75%
Mucinous borderline tumour	10%
Mucinous adenocarcinoma	15%

Mucinous Cystadenoma and Mucinous Adenofibroma

Image gallery: Figs. 7.16 and 7.17

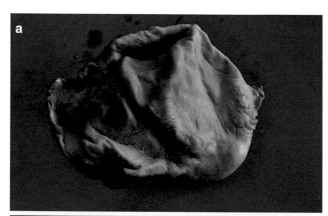

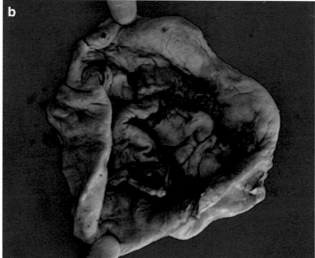

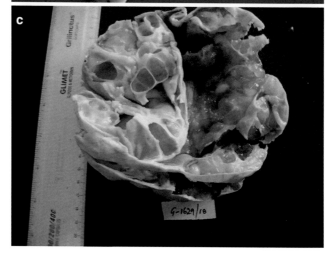

Fig. 7.16 (**a**) Gross picture of mucinous cystadenoma: shiny smooth outer surface of the cyst. (**b**) Mucinous cystadenoma: the cyst is thin walled with multiple folds in the inner surface. (**c**) Mucinous cystadenoma: multiloculated cysts filled with mucoid material

Epidemiology

- It represent 75–80% mucinous neoplasm of ovary
- Usually unilateral
- Mucinous adenofibroma is uncommon

Genetic profile

- KRAS mutation: 55% cases

Clinical features

- Common in the reproductive age period
- Mean age 50 year
- Usually asymptomatic
- Pelvic or abdominal pain
- Mass in pelvis

Gross features

- Cystic mass
- Variable size: Few cm to 25 cm diameter
- Average: 10 cm
- Shiny smooth outer surface
- Cut section: contains mucinous material, multilocular or uncommonly unilocular, thin walled

Histopathology

- Amount of fibrous material determines the designation of mucinous cystadenoma or adenofibroma. Adenofibroma contains more fibrous component.
- The tumour contains many cysts and glands
- Lining: Mucus secreting columnar cells
- Paneth cells or intestinal goblet cells may be present
- Mucinous material may be extravasated and may cause granulomatous reaction
- Occasional areas may show papillae
- Focal nuclear enlargement and pleomorphism may be present in less than 10% area
- Brenner and dermoid cyst: 10% cases

Differential diagnosis

Serous cystadenoma
- Serous columnar/cuboidal lining

Mucinous borderline tumour
- Stratification
- Mild to moderate nuclear atypia
- Papillae formation
- More than 10% area shows cellular atypia

Prognosis

- Benign tumour
- Complete excision of the lesion by either cystectomy of oophorectomy is the treatment of choice

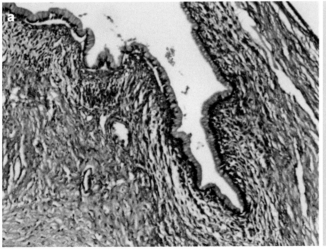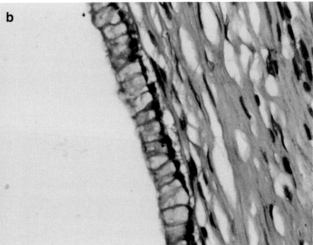

Fig. 7.17 (**a**) Mucinous cystadenoma: the fibrocollagenous wall of the cyst is lined by mucus secreting columnar epithelium. (**b**) Mucinous cystadenoma: higher magnification showing tall columnar cells with basally placed nuclei

Borderline Mucinous Tumours

Image gallery: Figs. 7.18 and 7.19

Definition: This tumour is characterized by proliferation of atypical mucinous epithelial cells that is more than the benign mucinous neoplasms in absence of any stromal invasion.

Abbreviation: Mucinous borderline tumour (MBT)

Epidemiology

- It constitutes of 15% of all ovarian mucinous tumours
- Represents 70% of all borderline tumours of ovary in Asian countries
- Mainly occurs in the reproductive age period
- Mean age: 45 years

Genetic profile

- KRAS mutation (50–75%)
- No germline mutation of BRCA 1 and BRC1 2

Clinical features

- Asymptomatic
- Abdominal pain
- Mass in pelvis

Gross features

- Almost always unilateral
- Variable size,
- Mean diameter: 8–10 cm
- Cystic with smooth surface
- Cut section:
  – Multiloculated cysts
  – Solid areas may be present
  – Contains mucinous material

Histopathology

- Cysts and glands are lined by mucinous epithelium
- Tall columnar mucin secreting epithelial cells
- Stratification of the epithelial cells: Less than three layer
- Complex papillary infolding of the lining epithelium
- Nuclei show mild to moderate enlargement and pleomorphism
- Prominent nucleoli
- Goblet cells, Paneth cells and neuroendocrine cells in intestinal type of MBT
- Endocervical type mucinous cells in endocervical MBT
- Mitotic activity is more than that of benign counterpart
- Often associated with pseudomyxoma ovarii (20% cases)

Key diagnostic features: See Box 7.5

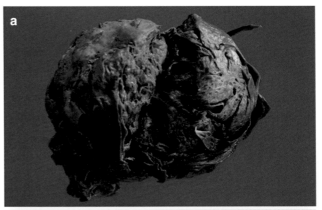
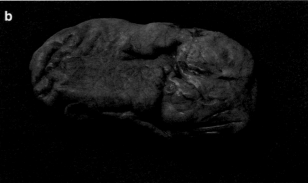
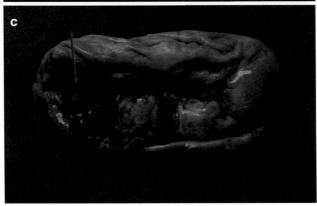

Fig. 7.18 (**a**) Borderline mucinous tumour: predominantly solid tumour with focal cystic changes. (**b**) Borderline mucinous tumour: outer surface is bosselated. (**c**) Borderline mucinous tumour: solid area with foci of haemorrhage (see *arrow*)

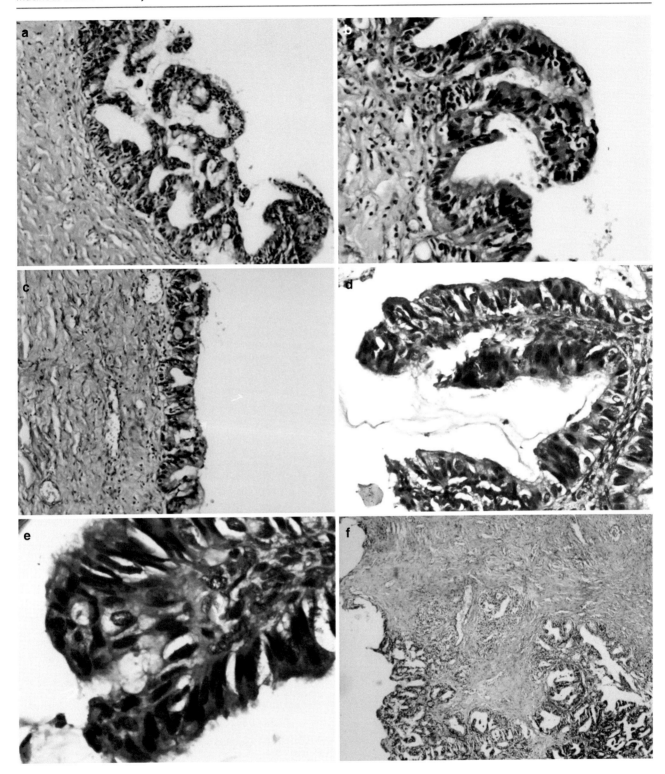

Fig. 7.19 (**a**) Borderline mucinous tumour: complex papillary infolding of the lining epithelium. (**b**) Borderline mucinous tumour: the piling of the epithelial cells form small tufts. Note the nuclear enlargement and pleomorphism of the cells. (**c**) Borderline mucinous tumour: tall columnar mucin secreting epithelial cells showing nuclear pleomorphism. (**d**) Borderline mucinous tumour with intraepithelial carcinoma: the foci of the tumour show marked nuclear pleomorphism. (**e**) Borderline mucinous tumour with intraepithelial carcinoma: higher magnification showing severely pleomorphic nuclei. (**f**) Borderline mucinous tumour with microinvasion: Stromal microinvasion present. (**g**) Borderline mucinous tumour with microinvasion: stromal microinvasion is less than 5 mm in linear extension. (**h**) Borderline mucinous tumour with microinvasion: higher magnification of the area of microinvasive foci

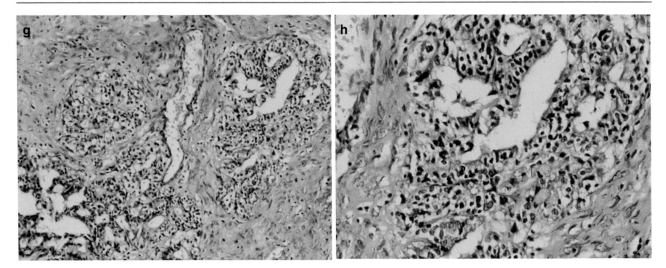

Fig. 7.19 (continued)

MBT with intraepithelial carcinoma

- MBT that shows foci with marked nuclear pleomorphism of the epithelial cells

MBT with microinvasion

- Foci of microinvasion that is less than 5 mm in the linear extension or 10^2 mm area.
- Number of the foci of tumour area is not important
- Stromal microinvasion is noted in 1/3rd of MBT

Immunohistochemistry

- CK 7: Positive
- CK 20: Usually negative
- CDX 2: Variably positive
- PAX 8: Positive (60%)

Differential diagnosis

- Mucinous adenocarcinoma
  - Cribriform pattern
  - Complex glandular arrangement
  - Marked nuclear atypia
- Cystadenoma
  - Focal areas may show atypia, however this constitutes less than 10% tumour volume

Prognosis

- Majority cases present in stage I and they have excellent prognosis
- No death occurs due to the disease itself

Treatment

- Unilateral salpingo-oophorectomy is the treatment of choice

Mucinous Adenocarcinoma

Image gallery: Figs. 7.20, 7.21, 7.22, and 7.23

Definition: This is a surface epithelial malignancy of ovary lined by intestinal type of cells with intracytoplasmic mucin having significant cytological atypia and shows stromal invasion.

Epidemiology

- Uncommon and represents about 10% of mucinous tumour of ovary
- It constitutes 5% of all ovarian carcinomas

Genetic profile

- KRAS mutation present
- Similar type of mutation as seen in MBT

Clinical features

- Elderly female commonly affected
- Mean age: 45 years
- Usually asymptomatic
- Patient may have pain abdomen, alteration of bowel and bladder functions

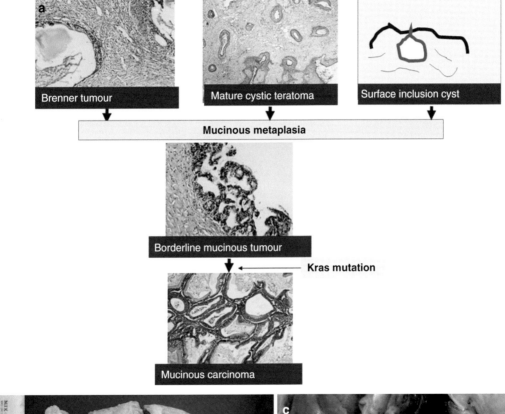

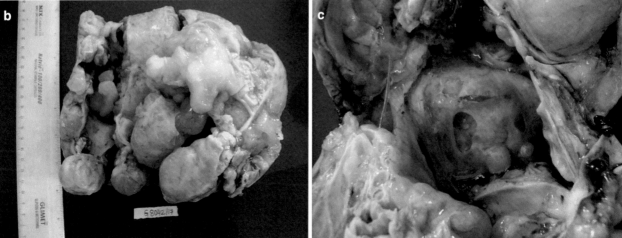

Fig. 7.20 (**a**) Probable pathogenesis of mucinous carcinoma of ovary. (**b**) Gross picture of mucinous carcinoma: the tumour is predominantly solid and partly cystic. (**c**) Gross picture of mucinous carcinoma: cut section showing solid areas, small cysts and foci of haemorrhage

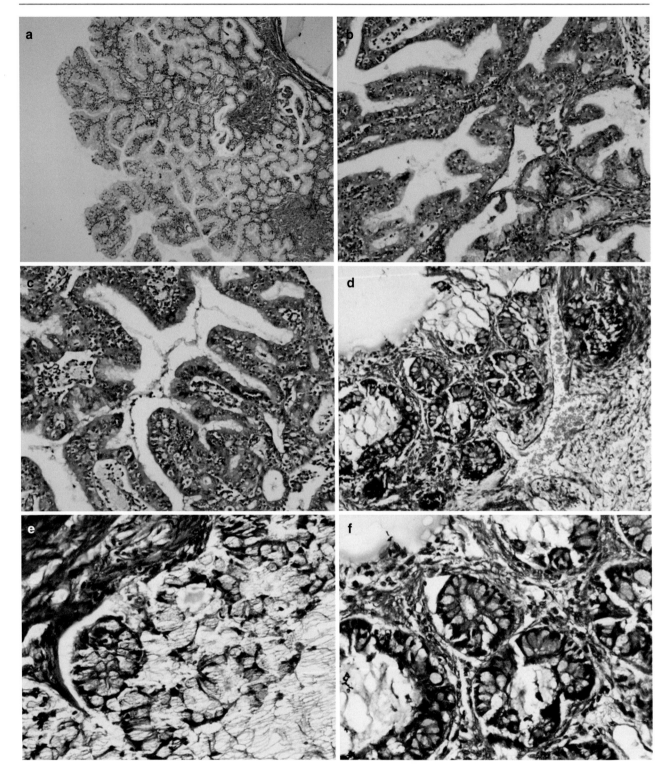

Fig. 7.21 (**a**) Mucinous carcinoma: complex architectural pattern of the gland along with crowding of the glands. (**b**) Mucinous carcinoma: complex branching of the glands. (**c**) Mucinous carcinoma. the papillae are lined by tall columnar mucin secreting cells. (**d**) Mucinous carcinoma: multiple glands invading deep in the stroma. (**e**) Mucinous carcinoma: the mucin secreting glands are floating in the extracellular mucin. (**f**) Mucinous carcinoma: The lining cells of the glands are tall columnar mucin secreting. (**g**) Mucinous carcinoma: The cribriform arrangement of the glands. (**h**) Mucinous carcinoma: the glands within the lymphatic spaces. (**i**) Mucinous carcinoma: higher magnification of the same

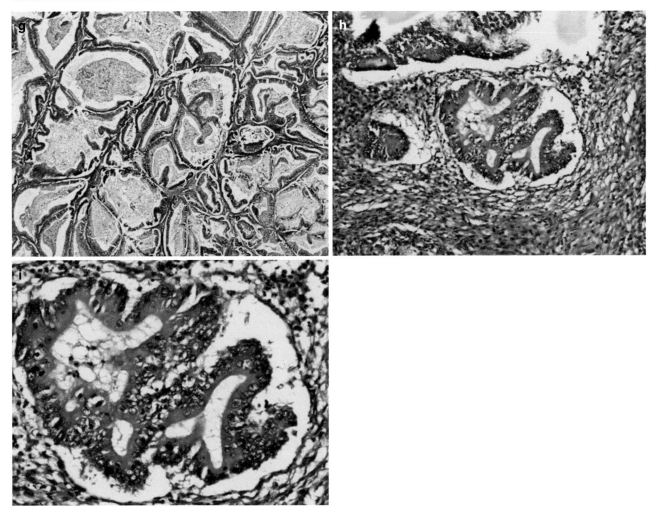

Fig. 7.21 (continued)

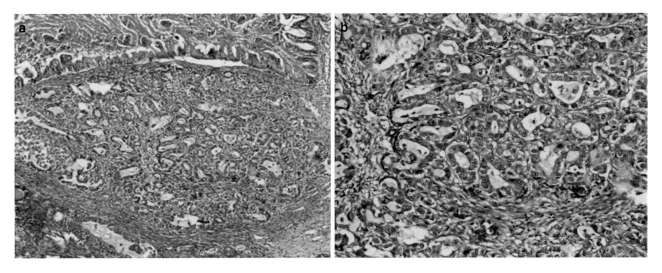

Fig. 7.22 (**a**) Mucinous carcinoma: confluent growth pattern indicating invasion. (**b**) Mucinous carcinoma: confluent cribriform arrangement in invasion

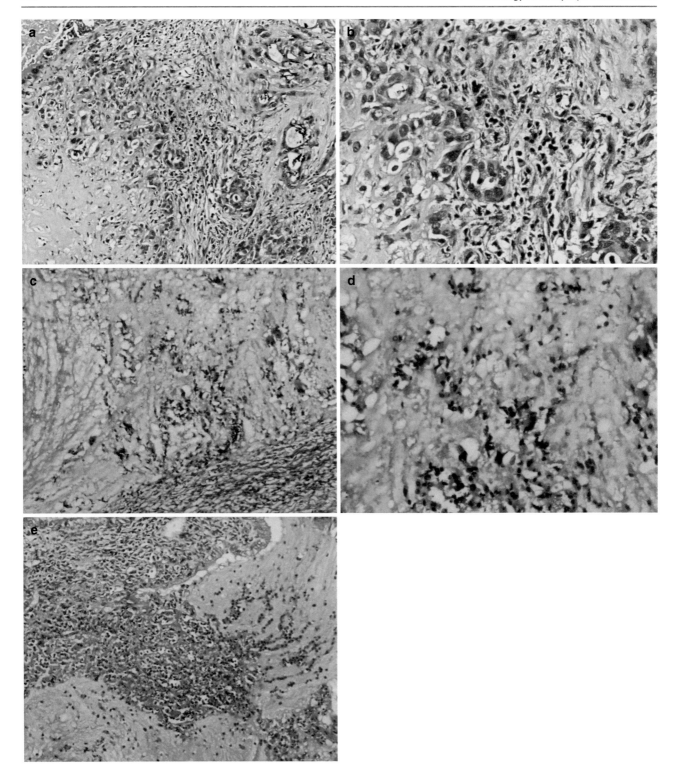

Fig. 7.23 (**a**) Mucinous carcinoma: Infiltrating invasive growth. (**b**) Mucinous carcinoma: infiltrating invasive growth in higher magnification. Note the tiny glands and individual cells are infiltrating in the stroma. (**c**) Mucinous carcinoma: carcinoma cells floating cells in mucin. (**d**) Mucinous carcinoma: higher magnification showing floating cells in mucin. (**e**) Mucinous carcinoma: areas of necrosis in the tumour

- CA 125 is not much raised

Gross features

- Unilateral: 95%
- Large multiloculated cyst
- Size: variable, usually more than 10 cm in diameter, mean size 15 cm
- Solid-cystic mass
- Cut section: Contains mucinous fluid, firm and fleshy areas along with multiple cysts, areas of haemorrhage and necrosis
- Cyst may be adhered with the neighbouring structure due to rupture

Histopathology

- Admixture of borderline and benign areas may be present
- Multiple glands and cysts
- Complex architectural pattern of the gland along with crowding
- Glands lined by mucin secreting epithelial cells that are tall columnar having moderate amount of cytoplasm with moderately pleomorphic nuclei
- Brisk mitotic activity
- Goblet cells are frequently seen

Invasion

Expansile or confluent invasion

- Common
- Confluent architecturally complex glands
- Cribriform appearance
- No intervening stroma in between the glands
- Marked cytological atypia

Destructive or infiltrating type

- Irregular clusters, nests, single cell or glands in the stroma
- Desmoplastic stromal reaction
- Often clear space around the tumour cells

Immunohistochemistry

- CK7: Strong positive
- CK 20: Negative
- CDX 2: Weak positive

- Beta catenin: Negative
- MUC 5AC and MUC 2: Positive

Key diagnostic features: see Box 7.6

Box 7.6 Key Diagnostic Features of Mucinous Adenocarcinoma
- Multiple glands and cysts
- Complex architectural pattern of the gland along with crowding
- Glands lined by mucin secreting epithelial cells that are tall columnar with mild to moderate nuclear pleomorphism
- Definite evidence of stromal invasion:
  - Cribriform appearance of complex glandular architecture
  - Destructive stromal invasion by irregular clusters of cells
- Presence of goblet cells
- Positive for CK 7, PAX-8, and MUC 5AC and MUC 2
- Negative for CK 20, ER/PR, WT 1 and Beta catenin

Differential diagnosis

- Metastatic mucinous adenocarcinoma
  - History of primary mucinous tumour in other site
  - Size: Less than 10 cm
  - Bilateral tumour
  - Invasive or destructive infiltration of tumour cells in the stroma
  - Hilar lymphovascular growth
  - Extravasated mucin in the stroma
  - Absence of associated Brenner tumour or teratoma
  - Strongly positive CK 20, CDX 2, and beta catenin

Prognosis and treatment

- Prognosis mainly depends on stage of the tumour
- Good in prognosis as the majority patients present in stage I
- Five year survival of stage I carcinoma: 98%
- Confluent type of invasion recurs less than destructive invasive
- Total abdominal hysterectomy with bilateral salpingo oophorectomy is adequate
- Adjuvant platinum based chemotherapy is less effective

Mucinous Tumours with Mural Nodules

Definition: Mural nodule of a mucinous tumour is characterized by distinct nodular structure in the wall of the mucinous neoplasm.

Gross features

- Size: Microscopic to several cm
- Solid, reddish brown
- Single to multiple

Types:

1. Sarcoma like nodule
   a. Usually multiple
   b. Well circumscribed
   c. Many multinucleated giant cells and histiocytes
   d. Other types: Predominant spindle cells with pleomorphism
   e. Weakly positive cytokeratin
   f. Strongly positive vimentin
2. Sarcomatous nodule
   a. Rhabdomyosarcoma: Large rhabdoid cells
   b. Fibrosarcomas: Herringbone pattern
   c. Undifferentiated pleomorphic sarcoma
   d. Strong positive : Cytokeratin and vimentin
3. Anaplastic carcinoma type
   a. Single or multiple
   b. Sheets of polygonal epithelial cells or spindle cells
   c. Moderate to marked nuclear atypia
   d. Strong positive : Cytokeratin and EMA

Mucinous Neoplasm of Ovary with Pseudomyxoma Peritonei

Image gallery: Figs. 7.24, 7.25, 7.26, and 7.27

Definition: Pseudomyxoma peritonei is characterized by ascites containing mucinous material or peritoneal nodule in association with low grade mucinous tumour along with collection of extracellular mucin.

Etiology:

- Most cases are developed from primary appendicular neoplasm such as appendicular adenoma, villous adenoma or mucinous carcinoma
- Ovary is secondarily involved

Types

- Disseminated peritoneal adenomucinosis (DPAM)
- Peritoneal mucinous carcinomatosis (PMCA)

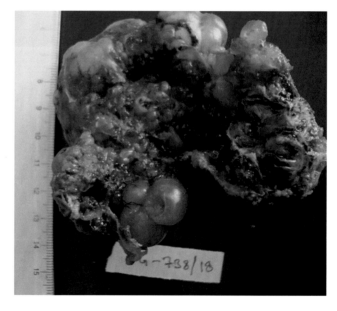

Fig. 7.24 Pseudomyxoma: gross photograph showing thick mucinous material in the omentum

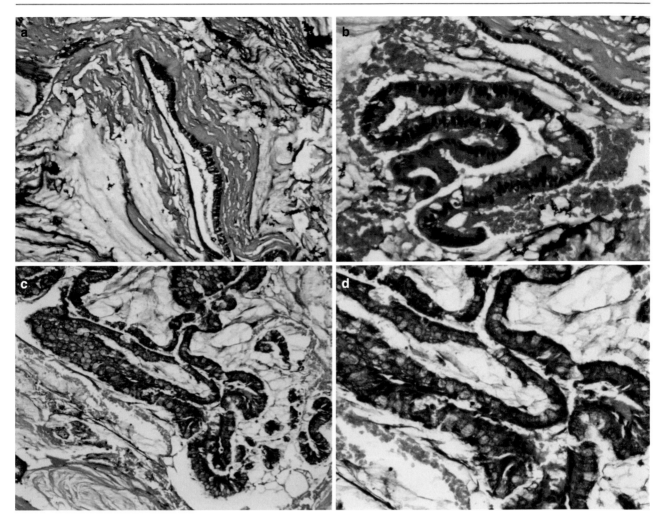

Fig. 7.25 (**a**) Pseudomyxoma: mucinous material and glands within the ovarian stroma. (**b**) Pseudomyxoma: involved ovary showing mucinous glands with bland looking columnar cells. (**c**) Pseudomyxoma in omentum: large areas of pool of mucin with mucinous glands. (**d**) Pseudomyxoma in omentum: benign looking mucinous glands in pool of mucin

Disseminated peritoneal adenomucinosis (see Table 7.3)

- Primary site: Primary site is invariably in appendix
- Histopathology
  - Scanty cellularity
  - Cells embedded in abundant mucinous material
  - Cells show minimal nuclear atypia and rare mitotic activity
- Lymph nodal and organ involvement are rare

Peritoneal mucinous carcinomatosis

- Primary site: Appendix, small and large intestine
- Histopathology
  - Moderately cellular
  - Cells are embedded in mucinous material
  - Proliferating mucin secreting glands
  - Significant nuclear atypia
- Lymph nodal and organ involvement are common

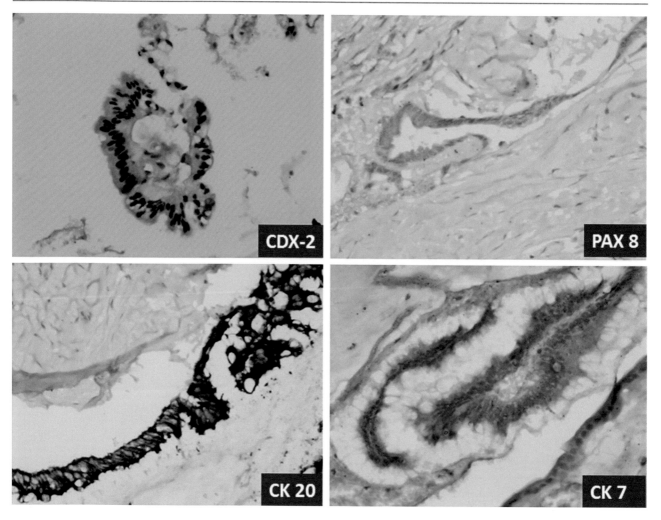

Fig. 7.26: Strong nuclear positivity of CDX 2 and membranous positivity of CK 20 indicate the primary site as gastrointestinal tract

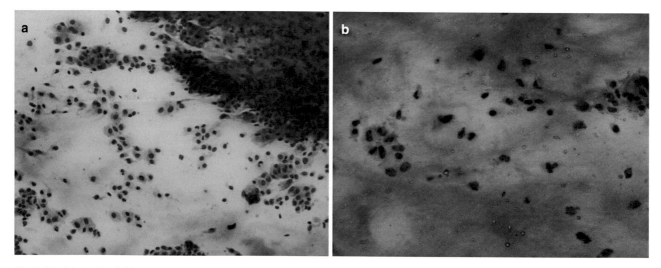

Fig. 7.27 (**a**) Ascitic fluid cytology of Pseudomyxoma: the scattered epithelial cells in the mucinous background. (**b**) Ascitic fluid cytology of Pseudomyxoma: the tumour cells are benign looking with moderate amount of cytoplasm and round monomorphic nuclei. (**c**) Ascitic fluid cytology of Pseudomyxoma: the discrete benign looking tumour cells in thin bluish mucinous material

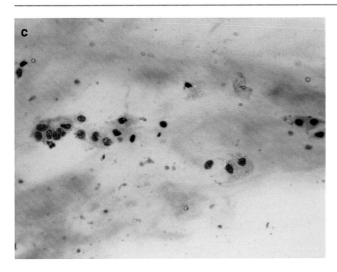

Table 7.3 Distinguishing features between disseminated peritoneal adenomucinosis (DPAM) versus peritoneal mucinous carcinomatosis (PMCA)

Features	PMCA	DPAM
Cellularity	Moderately cellular	Scanty
Nuclear pleomorphism	Present	Almost monomorphic
Mitosis	Present	Almost nil
Organ involvement	Frequent involvement of parenchyma	Rarely involved
Primary organ	Mainly appendix	Colon, small intestine and appendix

Fig. 7.27 (continued)

Endometrioid Tumours

Endometriotic Cyst

Described in previous chapter

Endometrioid Cystadenoma and Adenofibroma

Epidemiology

- Very rare
- It represents only 1% surface epithelial tumours

Clinical features

- Mean age: 55 year
- No specific clinical features

Gross features

- Variable size: Few cm to 10 cm in diameter
- Smooth outer surface
- Cut section: Solid cystic lesion, honeycomb appearance

Histopathology

- Fibrous stroma
- Multiple tubules and glands
- Glands are lined by endometrioid type of tall columnar epithelium which is often ciliated
- Squamous differentiation may be seen

Prognosis

- Benign

Endometrioid Borderline Tumour

Epidemiology

- Rare neoplasm
- Incidence: 0.2% of surface epithelial neoplasms of ovary

Clinical features

- Mean age: 50 year
- Mass in lower abdomen

Gross features

- Size: Mean size is 10 cm
- Predominantly solid and partly cystic
- Cut section: Cyst contains fluid, haemorrhage and necrotic foci

Histopathology

- Tubular and cystic endometrial glands surrounded by dense stromal tissue
- Glands are often crowded and show architectural complexity
- Lining epithelial cells are proliferative
- The cells show mild nuclear atypia
- Squamous metaplasia may be noted

Prognosis

- Benign in course

Endometrioid Carcinoma

Image gallery: Figs. 7.28, 7.29, 7.30, 7.31, and 7.32
Epidemiology

- It constitutes 15–20% of all ovarian carcinoma
- Commonly seen in perimenopausal and postmenopausal patient: 5th and 6th decades of life
- Mean age: 56 year
- Frequently associated with endometriosis: 42% cases

Clinical features

- Predominantly asymptomatic
- May have pelvic mass and pain abdomen
- Frequently elevated CA 125 level (80%)

Gross features

- Bilateral: 17%
- Size: Variable in size, 10–20 cm, Mean size: 15 cm
- Solid-cystic neoplasm
- Cut section: friable, soft fleshy with areas of haemorrhage and necrosis

Histopathology

- Pattern: Gland, tubules, villoglandular, adenoid cystic, and cribriform arrangement of the tumour cells
- Lining of the gland:
  - Single to multi-layered
  - Cuboidal to columnar cells
  - Non-mucin secreting cells
  - Mild to moderate nuclear atypia depending on the grade of tumour
- Invasion
  - Confluent pattern: Confluent glands with crowding and little intervening stroma occupying more than 5 mm. It is more common.
  - Destructive pattern: Foci of irregularly shaped glands, cell clusters or single cells surrounded by the desmoplastic stroma.
- Squamous differentiation:
  - 30% cases
  - Benign looking squamous cells
  - Spindle shaped cells may be adjacent to the squamous cells
- Different types of cells in the endometrioid carcinoma
  - Oxyphil cells: Large cell, polygonal appearance, abundant cytoplasm containing eosinophilic granules, central round nuclei having prominent nucleoli

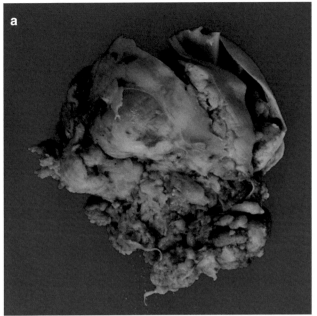

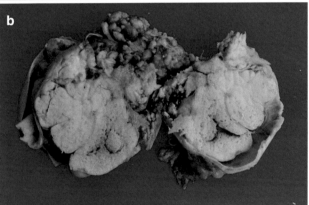

Fig. 7.28 (**a**) Endometrioid carcinoma: solid-cystic neoplasm. (**b**) Endometrioid carcinoma: cut section showing solid tumour with foci of necrosis

  - Mucin containing cells
  - Ciliated cell: Lining epithelial cells of the gland show cilia
- Morphologic pattern
  - Microglandular or sex cord stromal type pattern
    Tubular gland
    Rosette-like glands simulating Call-Exner bodies
    This pattern resembles granulosa cell tumour
  - Sertoli Leydig cell pattern
    Solid tubular structure
    Hollow tubules
    Paired cell arrangement
    Stromal luteinized cells
- Grading of endometrioid carcinoma: Same as that of uterine endometrial carcinoma

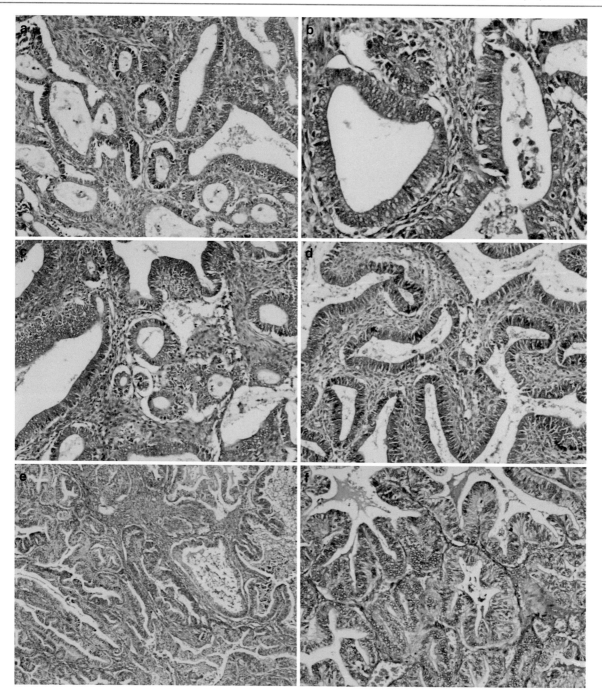

Fig. 7.29 (a) Endometrioid carcinoma: Multiple variable shaped endometrial looking glands. (b) Endometrioid carcinoma: The glands are lined by moderately pleomorphic columnar cells. (c) Endometrioid carcinoma: Glands showing multi-layered lining epithelium. (d) Endometrioid carcinoma: Branching dilated glands. (e) Endometrioid carcinoma: complex branching glands along with small papillary structures. (f) Endometrioid carcinoma: papillary infolding of the glands. (g) Endometrioid carcinoma: foci of squamous differentiation. (h) Endometrioid carcinoma, squamous differentiation: higher magnification showing polyhedral benign squamous cells

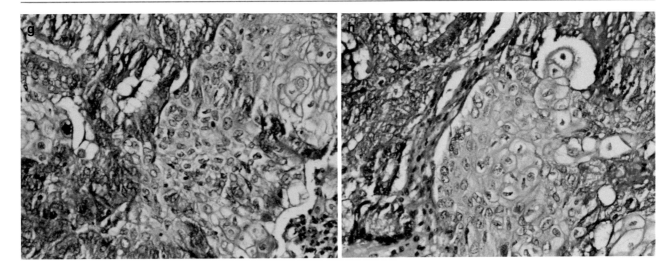

Fig. 7.29 (continued)

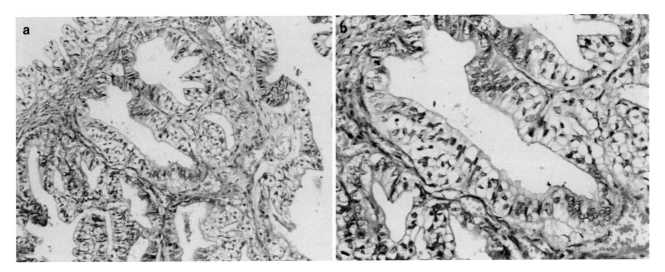

Fig. 7.30 (**a**) Endometrioid carcinoma, secretory type: Secretory changes in the glandular lining cells. (**b**) Endometrioid carcinoma, secretory type: the glandular lining cells showing both supra and sub nuclear vacuolation

– Nuclear grade is probably more important as majority of the endometrioid carcinoma is of low grade

Immunohistochemistry
Positive: CK 7, B 72.3, ER, PR
Negative: WT 1, p 16
Molecular genetics

- Somatic mutation of CTNNB1 (38%): This gene encodes b-catenin
- PTEN mutation (21% case)
- Promoter methylation of MLH 1: Resulting microsatellite instability (19% cases)

Key diagnostic features: see Box 7.7

Box 7.7 Key Diagnostic Features of Endometrioid Carcinoma
- Predominantly glandular arrangement and in addition villoglandular, adenoid cystic, and cribriform arrangement seen
- Cuboidal to columnar cells with Mild to moderate nuclear atypia
- Squamous differentiation in 1/3rd of cases
- Stromal invasion : destructive or confluent
- Other types:
  – Microglandular or sex cord stromal type pattern
  – Sertoli Leydig cell pattern

> - Secretory changes mimicking early secretory endometrium
> - Oxyphil variant
> - *Immunohistochemistry*: Tumour cells are positive for CK 7,
> - B 72.3, ER, PR: Negative for WT 1, p 16

Differential diagnosis

- Sertoli Leydig cell tumour (see Table 7.4)
  - Young patient around 25 year
  - Virilizing features may be seen
  - No squamous metaplasia
  - No foci of endometriosis
  - Positive for inhibin and negative for EMA
- Clear cell carcinoma
  - Always higher nuclear grade
  - Hobnail appearance present
- Metastatic colonic carcinoma
  - Bilateral
  - Dirty necrosis
  - Garland like arrangement
  - CK 7 negative and CK 20 positive cells
  - CDX 2 positive
- High grade serous adenocarcinoma versus poorly differentiated endometrioid carcinoma; It is often difficult to differentiates these two entities and immunohistochemistry may be helpful in this aspect (see Table 7.5)

Prognosis

- Mainly depends on the stage of the tumour
- Five year survival: 78%

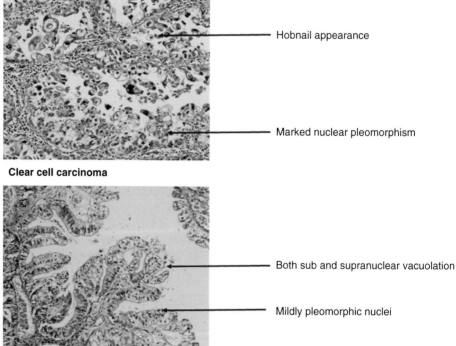

Clear cell carcinoma — Hobnail appearance

— Marked nuclear pleomorphism

Secretory type endometrioid carcinoma — Both sub and supranuclear vacuolation

— Mildly pleomorphic nuclei

Fig. 7.31 Distinguishing features of secretory type endometrioid carcinoma from clear cell carcinoma

Fig. 7.32 Distinguishing features of endometrioid carcinoma from sertoli Leydig cell tumour

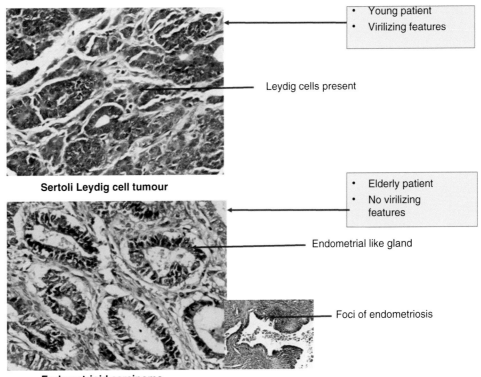

- Young patient
- Virilizing features

Leydig cells present

Sertoli Leydig cell tumour

- Elderly patient
- No virilizing features

Endometrial like gland

Foci of endometriosis

Endometrioid carcinoma

Table 7.4 Distinguishing features between endometrioid carcinoma versus sex cord stromal tumour

Features	Sertoli Leydig cell tumour	Endometrioid carcinoma
Age	Young patient, around 30 years	Peri or postmenopausal patient
Virilizing effect	Often present	Absent
Squamous metaplasia	Absent	Often present
Endometriosis	Absent	Often present
Luminal mucin	Absent	Often present
Immunohistochemistry	Positive for inhibin and calretinin	Positive for EMA, ER/PR

Table 7.5 Distinguishing features between endometrioid carcinoma versus high grade serous adenocarcinoma

Antibody	Endometrioid carcinoma	High grade serous adenocarcinoma
WT 1	Negative	Positive
P53	Usually negative	Positive
CDK2NA	Often positive	Usually negative

Clear Cell Tumours of Ovary

Image gallery: Figs. 7.33 and 7.34

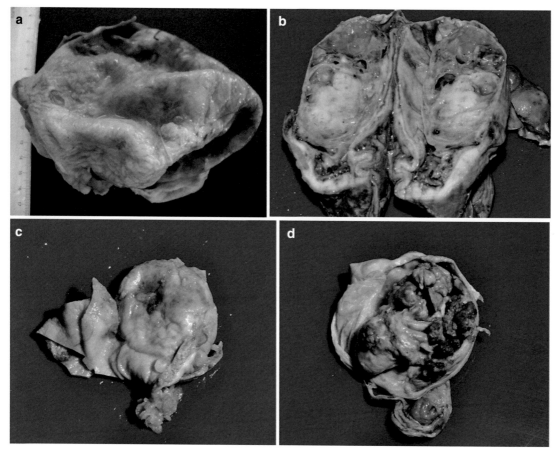

Fig. 7.33 (**a**) Clear cell carcinoma: thick wall cyst with foci of solid areas. (**b**) Clear cell carcinoma: solid grey white tumour with areas of thick gelatinous material. (**c**) Clear cell carcinoma: shiny outer surface with areas of discolouration due to haemorrhage. (**d**) Clear cell carcinoma: Solid cystic grey white tumour with areas of necrosis and haemorrhage

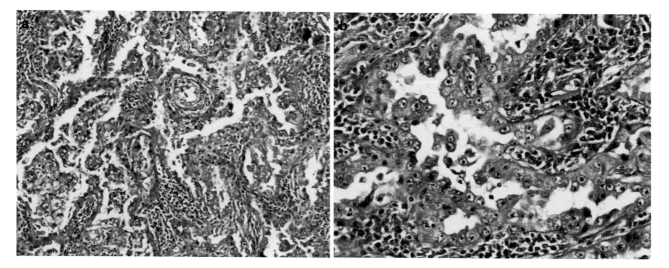

Fig. 7.34 (**a**) Clear cell carcinoma: complex branched papillae. (**b**) Clear cell carcinoma: the papillae lined by moderately pleomorphic nuclei with large prominent nucleoli. (**c**) Clear cell carcinoma: solid pattern. (**d**) Clear cell carcinoma: solid group of cells with abundant clear cytoplasm and central pleomorphic nuclei. (**e**) Clear cell carcinoma: Higher magnification showing glands and solid cluster of cells. (**f**) Clear cell carcinoma: hobnail appearance of the glandular epithelial cells. (**g**) Clear cell carcinoma: multiple groups of cells separated by fibrous setae. Note the detached tips of the cells giving hobnail appearance. (**h**) Clear cell carcinoma: clear cells with centrally placed moderately pleomorphic nuclei

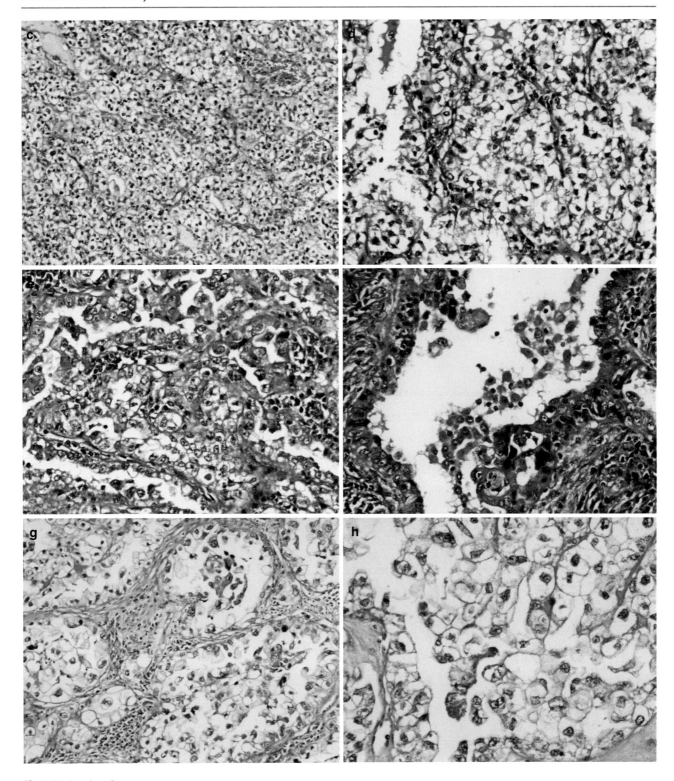

Fig. 7.34 (continued)

Clear Cell Adenoma and Adenofibroma

Epidemiology

- Extremely uncommon : Less than 1%
- Only few case reports are present

Clinical features

- Asymptomatic
- Incidentally detected

Gross features

- Solid-cystic tumour
- Size: 2–15 cm, mean 12 cm diameter
- Outer surface smooth and lobulated
- Cut section: Honeycomb appearance

Histopathology

- Stroma is fibrocollagenous
- Multiple glands lined by flattened cells with bland mono-morphic nuclei
- No mitotic activity
- Endometriotic foci may be present

Prognosis

- Benign in course

Clear Cell Borderline Tumour

Epidemiology

- Very rare
- Only 0.2% of all ovarian epithelial neoplasm
- Less than 1% of all borderline neoplastic lesions of ovary
- Mean age is 60–68 years

Clinical features

- Asymptomatic
- Incidentally detected

Gross features

- Same as that of cystadenoma or adenofibroma

Histopathology

- Multiple glands
- Focal crowding present
- Glandular epithelium shows cuboidal or hobnail type of cells
- Epithelial cells have mild nuclear enlargement and pleomorphism
- Stratification of the lining cells of the glands
- Focal endometriosis may be present

Prognosis

- Overall all the reported cases had benign course

Clear Cell Carcinoma

Epidemiology

- It constitutes of 8% of all ovarian carcinoma
- It develops from endometriosis in 70% cases
- Often associated with Lynch syndrome

Clinical features

- Mean age 57 year, also occurs in younger patient
- Paraneoplastic hypercalcemia: 10% cases
- Thromboembolism: 46%
- Features of endometriosis

Gross features

- Mainly unilateral
- Variable size: few cm to 30 cm
- Mean size: 15 cm
- Solid-cystic
- Cut section: solid fleshy area with haemorrhage and necrosis

Histopathology

- Pattern: Papillary, tubulocystic and solid sheet
- Papillary pattern
  - Complex branched papillae
  - Central fibrovascular core, often hyalinised
  - Lining: Clear cell or hobnail type of cells
- Tubulocystic pattern
  - Variable sized tubules and cysts
  - Lining: Cuboidal to columnar cells, hobnail cells
- Solid pattern
  - Sheets of polygonal cells
  - Clear cytoplasm
  - Centrally placed hyperchromatic nuclei having prominent nucleoli
- Clear cell contain glycogen: PAS positive and diastase sensitive
- Eosinophilic hyaline globules
- Psammoma body
- Endometriosis is often present (30–50% cases)

Immunohistochemistry

- Positive: CK 7, EMA
- Negative: Alpha fetoprotein, p53

Molecular genetics

- BRAF mutation: 6% cases
- ARID1A mutation: 57% cases
- PTEN mutation: 20% cases
- P53 Mutation: 8% cases

Key diagnostic features: see Box 7.8

Box 7.8 Key Diagnostic Features of Clear Cell Carcinoma
- Papillary, tubulocystic and solid sheets of cells
- Complex branched papillae with central fibrovascular core
- Usually small and regular papillae
- Papillae lined by clear cells
- Hobnail appearance
- Solid sheets of clear cells with centrally placed hyperchromatic nuclei having prominent nucleoli
- Cells are PAS positive and diastase sensitive (containing glycogen)
- Eosinophilic hyaline globules and Psammoma body
- Immunohistochemistry: positive for CK 7 and EMA

Note: All clear cell carcinomas are high grade

Differential diagnosis (Fig. 7.35)

- Yolk sac tumour (see Table 7.6)
  - Young patient
  - Raised alpha feto protein
  - Schiller–Duval body bodies
- Serous adenocarcinoma
  - Papillae are irregular and broad
  - Highly pleomorphic nuclei
  - High mitotic index
- Juvenile granulosa cell tumour
  - Young patient
  - Call Exner bodies
  - Absent hobnail cells and clear cells
  - Positive for inhibin
- Dysgerminoma (Table 7.7)
  - Solid sheets of cells may simulate clear cell carcinoma
  - Young age

– Group of cells separated by fibroconnective tissue that are infiltrated by lymphocytes
– Positive for placental leucocyte alkaline phosphatase
• Endometrioid carcinomas with secretory changes
    – No hobnail appearance
    – No hyaline globules

Prognosis

• It depends on the FIGO staging
• Early stage (stage I) have good prognosis
• Five year survival:
    – Stage I: 69%

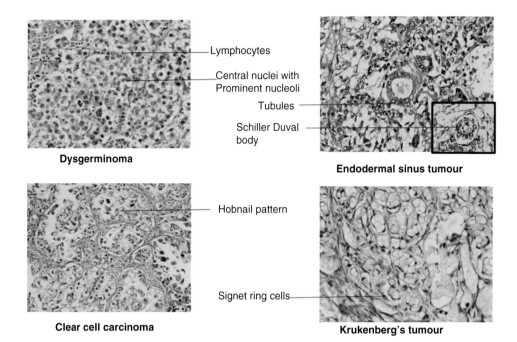

Fig. 7.35 Differential diagnosis of clear cell carcinoma

Table 7.6 Distinguishing features between clear cell carcinoma versus yolk sac tumour

Features	Clear cell carcinoma	Yolk sac tumour
Age	Elderly patient	Young patient
Serum alpha fetoprotein	Normal	Raised
Papillae	Complex branching papillae with central hyalinised fibrovascular core	Festoon like pattern
Hobnail appearance	Present	Absent
Schiller–Duvall bodies	Absent	Present

Table 7.7 Distinguishing features between clear cell carcinoma versus dysgerminoma

Features	Clear cell carcinoma	Dysgerminoma
Age	Elderly patient	Young patient
Cell morphology	Polygonal cells with abundant clear cytoplasm	Predominantly round cells with eosinophilic cytoplasm
Tubulocystic pattern	Present	Absent
Lymphocytes in between the group of cells	Absent	Present
Epithelioid cell granuloma	Absent	Present

Brenner Tumour

Image gallery: Figs. 7.36 and 7.37
Epidemiology

- It constitutes 5% of all benign epithelial tumours
- Age range of the patient: 4th to 6th decade
- Mean age: 55 year

Clinical features

- Asymptomatic, incidentally detected

Gross features

- Variable size: Microscopic to 20 cm in diameter
- Unilateral, only 10% bilateral
- Smooth bosselated
- Cut section: Solid tumour, grey white, small cysts may be seen
- Associated mucinous neoplasm in 25% cases

Histopathology

- Arrangement: Islands, cord, and nests of the tumour cell
- Nest of cells may have central lumen like structure
- Microcystic spaces
- Tumour cells:
    - Transitional cells: Cells with abundant clear cytoplasm, centrally placed nuclei with coffee bean like nuclear grooving
    - Mucinous cells
    - Ciliated cells
- Calcification may be seen
- Brenner tumour with extensive mucinous change : Mixed Brenner and mucinous neoplasm

Immunohistochemistry

- Positive: CK 7, uroplakin, thrombomodulin, S100 and GATA 3
- Negative: CK 20

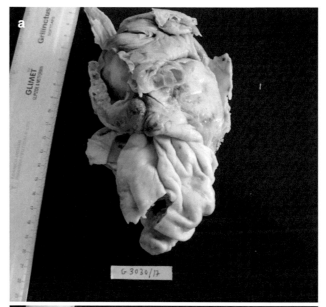

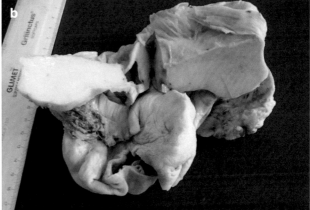

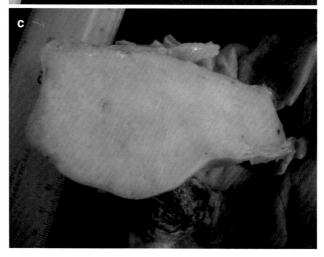

Fig. 7.36 (**a**) Brenner tumour: smooth outer surface with thin walled cyst. (**b**) Brenner tumour: partly solid and partly cystic tumour on cut section. (**c**) Brenner tumour: solid grey white area of the tumour

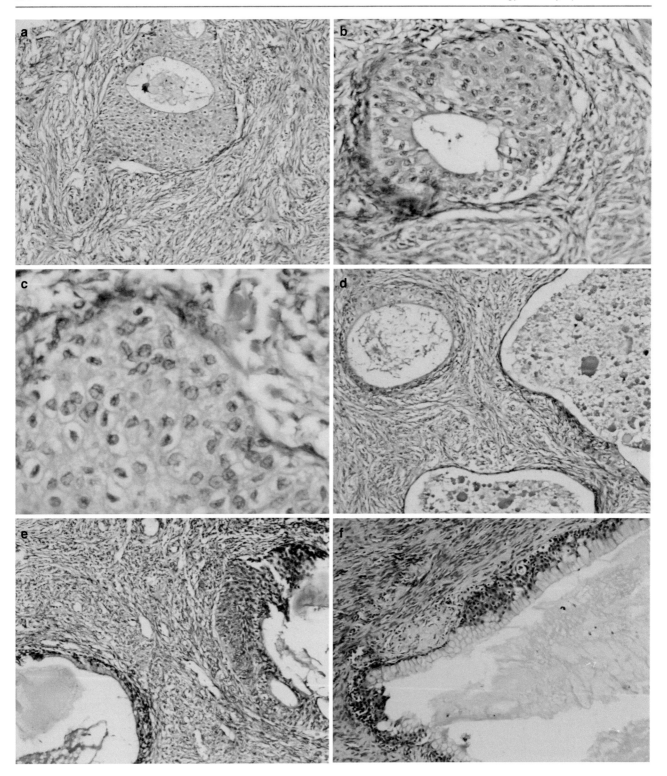

Fig. 7.37 (**a**) Brenner tumour: nests of transitional cells. (**b**) Brenner tumour: the nest of cells with central lumen like structure. (**c**) Brenner tumour: many cells show deep longitudinal nuclear groove. (**d**) Brenner tumour: microcystic spaces. (**e**) Brenner tumour: occasional microcys-tic spaces are lined by mucus secreting cells. (**f**) Brenner tumour: mucinous metaplasia in the tumour. (**g**) Brenner tumour: the tall columnar mucus secreting cells in higher magnification

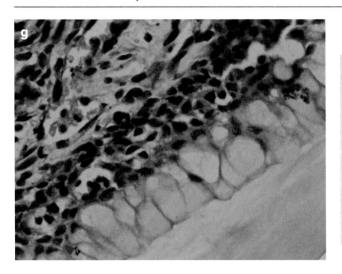

Fig. 7.37 (continued)

Key diagnostic features: see Box 7.9

Box 7.9 Key Diagnostic Features of Brenner Tumour
- Predominantly arranged as nests and cords
- Nest may show central lumen like structure
  - Predominantly transitional cells with abundant clear cytoplasm,
  - Coffee bean like nuclear grooving
  - Mucinous and ciliated cells
- Immunohistochemistry: Positive for CK 7, uroplakin, thrombomodulin, S100 and GATA 3; No expression of CK 20

Borderline Brenner Tumour

Image gallery: Fig. 7.38a–c

Synonym: Proliferating Brenner tumour, Brenner tumour of low malignant potential

Epidemiology

- It accounts for only 3.5% of all Brenner tumour
- Older female
- Mean age: 59 years

Clinical features

- Pain abdomen
- Pelvic mass

Gross features

- Unilateral
- Mean size 14 cm, usually larger than benign Brenner tumour
- Well circumscribed
- Mainly solid tumour and partly cystic

Histopathology

- Arrangement: Nests, cystic and papillary
- The papillae arise from the cyst wall
- Lining of the papillae is made of transitional cells with mild to moderate nuclear atypia
- Multiple nests of transitional cells in the stroma. The nest are more closely spaced and relatively large than the benign counterpart
- Variable mitosis
- Frequent mucinous metaplasia present
- Benign Brenner component is also present

Prognosis

- Benign in behaviour

Key diagnostic features: see Box 7.10

Box 7.10 Key Diagnostic Features of Borderline Brenner Tumour
- Large nests and more closely arranged
- Transitional cells show mild to moderate nuclear atypia
- Increased mitotic activity
- No evidence of invasion

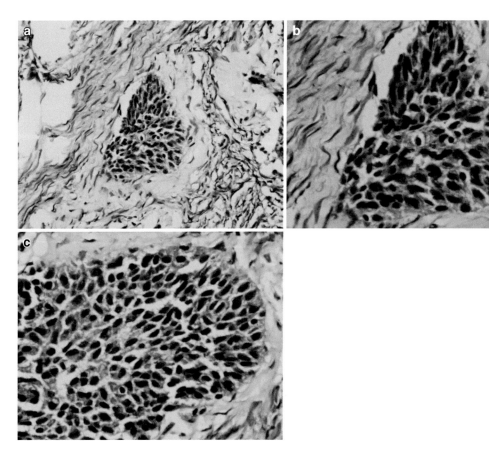

Fig. 7.38 (**a**) Borderline brenner tumour: Irregular nest of tumour cells. (**b**) Borderline brenner tumour: the cells show moderate nuclear atypia. (**c**) Borderline brenner tumour: The margin of the nest does not show infiltration in the stroma. Note the moderate nuclear pleomorphism of the tumour cells

Malignant Brenner tumour

Image gallery: Fig. 7.39a–d
Epidemiology

- It constitutes 5% of all Brenner tumour
- Age group: 50–70 year
- Mean age: 63 year

Clinical features

- Vague abdominal pain and pelvic mass

Gross features

- Predominantly unilateral
- Only 16% bilateral
- Variable size, usually large
- Mean size: 15–20 cm
- Solid and partly cystic
- Cyst shows friable and polypoid area
- Areas of haemorrhage and necrosis
- Rarely the tumour may be totally solid

Histopathology

- Large nests of tumour cells with irregular outline
- The irregular cords of cells are surrounded by desmoplastic stroma
- The thick papillae with fibrovascular core often arise on the cyst wall
- The lining cells resemble transitional cell carcinoma of the urinary bladder
- The individual cells are large polygonal with moderately pleomorphic nuclei
- Mitotic activity is frequent
- Benign Brenner tumour component is often present

Immunohistochemistry
Positive: CK, WT1, p16 and EMA
Negative: CK 20 (urothelial carcinoma of bladder is positive for CK 20)

Molecular genetics

- PIK3CA mutation in exon 9

Key diagnostic features: see Box 7.11

Box 7.11 Key Diagnostic Features of Malignant Brenner Tumour
- Desmoplastic stromal reaction around the nests of tumour cells
- Nests are large and irregular
- Large polygonal tumour cells with moderately pleomorphic nuclei
- High mitotic activity
- The presence of benign Brenner tumour component

Note: In absence of benign Brenner tumour component one should always keep the possibility of HGSC and endometrioid carcinoma

---

Differential diagnosis

- Urothelial cell carcinoma (Transitional cell carcinoma)
  - The absence of benign or borderline Brenner component
- Serous adenocarcinoma with necrosis
  - Difficult to differentiate with malignant Brenner in absence of benign counterpart of Brenner
- Undifferentiated carcinoma
  - Absent urothelial like cell morphology

Prognosis

- Most of the malignant Brenner tumour present in early stage
- Good in prognosis
- Five year survival of stage I: 88%

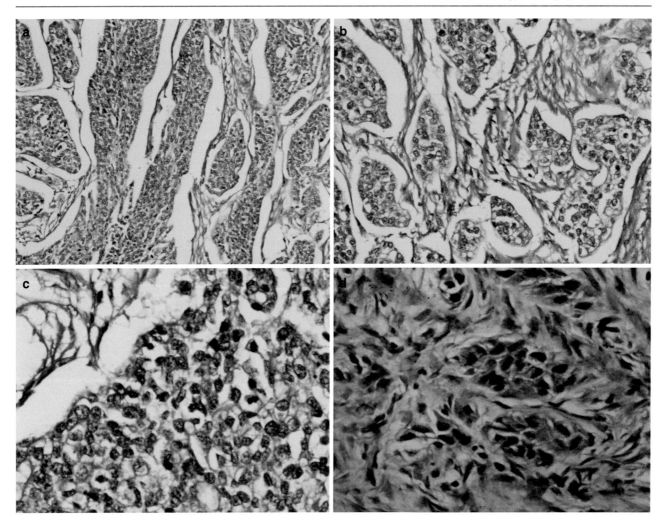

Fig. 7.39 (**a**) Malignant Brenner tumour: variably sized nests of tumour cells. (**b**) Malignant Brenner tumour: The group of cells are separated by the fibrous septae. (**c**) Malignant Brenner tumour: the cells showing moderate nuclear pleomorphism. (**d**) Malignant Brenner: Small islands of the cells with irregular margin indicating stromal infiltration

Undifferentiated Carcinoma

Image gallery: Fig. 7.40a, b
    Incidence: Less than 5% of ovarian carcinomas
    Clinical feature

- Post-menopausal patient
- Mean age around 55 years
- Complaints: same as other ovarian carcinoma

Gross

- Solid mass
- Areas of haemorrhage and necrosis

Histopathology

- Solid sheets of cells
- Large cells with scanty cytoplasm
- Moderately pleomorphic, vesicular nuclei
- High mitosis

Immunohistochemistry

- Positive: CK 7, B72.3 and EMA

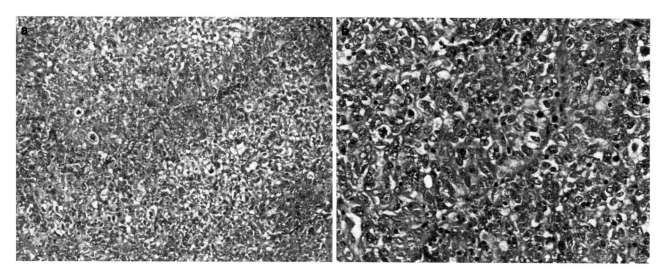

Fig. 7.40 (**a**) Undifferentiated carcinoma: Diffuse sheet of tumour cells. (**b**) Undifferentiated carcinoma: Large cells with scanty cytoplasm having enlarged moderately pleomorphic nuclei

Carcinosarcoma

Image gallery: Figs. 7.41 and 7.42
  Epidemiology

- Rare in ovary
- Only 1% of all malignant ovarian tumour
- Elderly patient
- 60–80 year age group
- Mean age: 65 year

Synonym: Malignant mixed Müllerian tumour, metaplastic carcinoma
  Clinical features

- Non-specific symptoms, same as other ovarian tumours

Gross features

- One third tumours are bilateral
- Variable size, usually large
- Mean diameter 14 cm
- Usually solid tumour
- Areas of haemorrhage and necrosis present

Histopathology

- Both carcinoma and sarcoma components present
- Carcinoma: Commonly high grade endometrioid and serous carcinoma, other types are clear cell carcinoma, squamous carcinoma and mucinous adenocarcinoma
- Sarcoma component
  - Homologous: Leiomyosarcoma and endometrial stromal sarcoma
  - Heterologous: Chondrosarcoma, rhabdomyosarcoma, osteosarcoma, liposarcoma

Immunohistochemistry

- Immunological markers are not really helpful for the diagnosis

- Heterologous elements can be confirmed by the immunohistochemistry
- Carcinoma part is positive for PAX 8 and WT1

Molecular genetics

- Mutation of p53 and also CDKN2A

Differential diagnosis

- *Immature teratoma*
  - Patients are usually young
  - Different germ layers are present
  - Immature neural elements such as rosettes are present

Prognosis

- Overall poor prognosis as most of them present in advanced stage
- Five year survival only 30%
- Median survival: 20 months

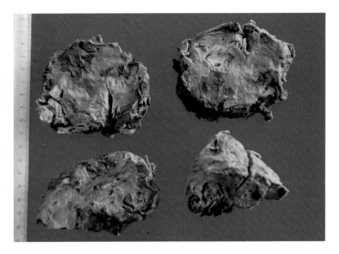

Fig. 7.41 Gross picture of carcinosarcoma: Solid firm tumour with foci of haemorrhage

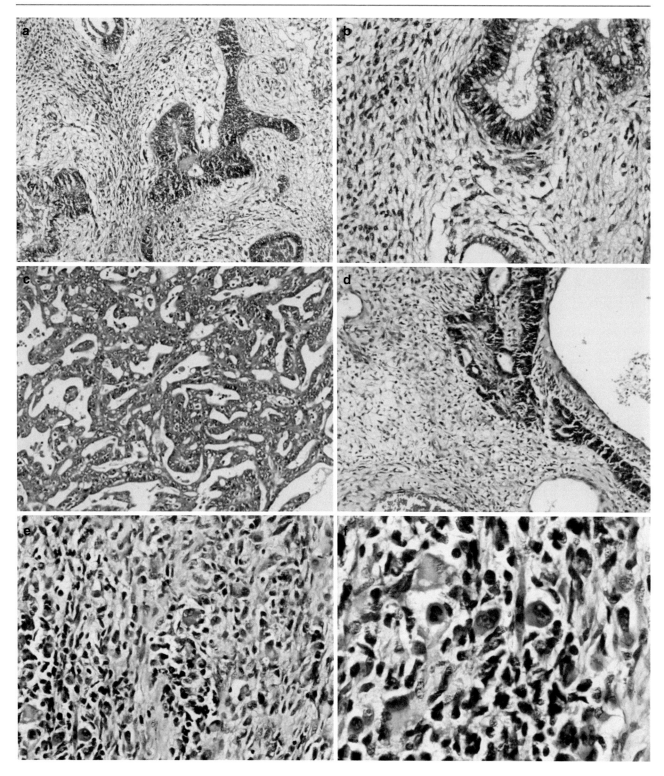

Fig. 7.42 (**a**) Carcinosarcoma: Both adenocarcinoma and sarcoma component. (**b**) Carcinosarcoma: Adenocarcinoma component showing glands lined by moderately pleomorphic nuclei. The sarcoma part is made of spindle cells with moderately pleomorphic nuclei. (**c**) Carcinosarcoma: Serous carcinoma component. (**d**) Carcinosarcoma: Endometrioid carcinoma and homologous sarcoma component. (**e**) Carcinosarcoma: Rhabdoid differentiation of the sarcoma part. (**f**) Carcinosarcoma: Higher magnification showing rhabdoid cells with moderate deep pink cytoplasm and round pleomorphic nuclei. (**g**) Carcinosarcoma: Osteosarcoma component showing bony material and malignant bone cells. (**h**) Carcinosarcoma: Malignant osteoid cells. (**i**) Carcinosarcoma: Chondrosarcoma element

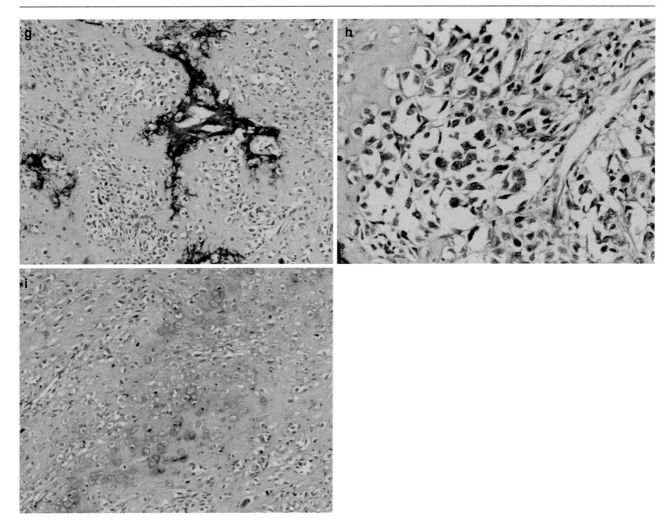

Fig. 7.42 (continued)

Adenosarcoma

Image gallery: Fig. 7.43a–c
  Synonym: Low grade Müllerian adenosarcoma
  Incidence: Rare
  Clinical features

- Mean age: 55 year
- Non-specific symptoms

Gross feature

- Unilateral
- Solid tumour

Histopathology

- Biphasic tumour
- Many benign endometrioid glands
- The glands are surrounded by stromal tissue
- The stroma shows oval to spindle cells with mild to moderately pleomorphic nuclei
- Mitosis is frequent

Immunohistochemistry

- Stromal cells are positive for CD 10, ER/PR

Prognosis

- Bad prognosis relative to endometrial adenosarcoma

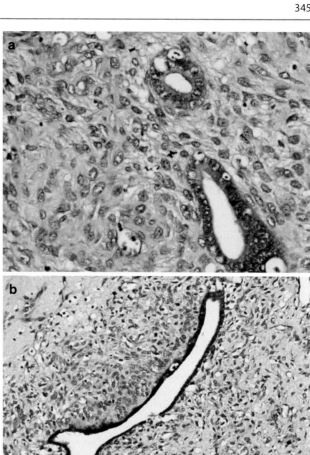
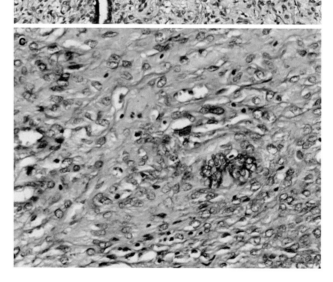

Fig. 7.43 (**a**) Adenosarcoma: Multiple benign looking glands are surrounded by oval to spindle cells with frequent mitotic activity. (**b**) Adenosarcoma: Condensed sarcoma element around the benign gland. (**c**) Adenosarcoma: Large pleomorphic stromal cells

Mesenchymal Tumours

Endometrial Stromal Sarcoma from Endometriosis

Image gallery: Fig. 7.44a–c
Epidemiology

- Rare tumour in ovary
- Only case reports available
- Age range: 10–70

Clinical features

- Pelvic mass
- Abdominal pain
- Back pain

Gross features

- Unilateral (75%)
- Usually more than 10 cm diameter
- Solid-cystic
- Yellowish soft tumour
- Areas of haemorrhage

Histopathology

- Endometriotic foci present
- Sheets of oval to spindle cells resembling endometrial stromal cells
- Thick walled small vessels present
- Storiform fibrosis may be present

Immunohistochemistry

- Positive: CD 10

Molecular genetics

- Translocation t (7:17) (p21: q15): fusion of JAZF1- SUZ12

Differential diagnosis

- Adenosarcoma
    - Predominantly spindle shaped stromal cells with more abundant well distributed glands
- Granulosa cell tumour
    - Lack of any endometriotic foci
    - Nuclear grooving present
    - Positive Calretinin and negative CD 10 immunostaining

Prognosis

- FIGO staging of the tumour is the most important prognostic factors
- Most of the cases present in advanced stage

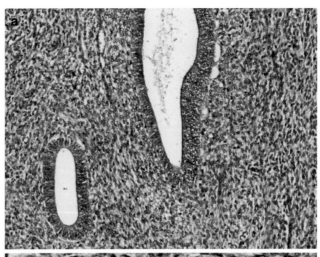
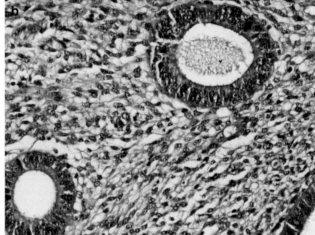
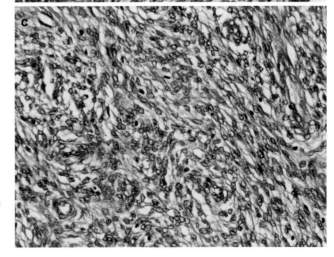

Fig. 7.44 (**a**) Endometrial stromal sarcoma from endometriosis: Endometrial glands surrounded by round to oval cells resembling endometrial stromal cell. (**b**) Endometrial stromal sarcoma from endometriosis: The tumour cells are oval to spindle shaped. (**c**) Endometrial stromal sarcoma from endometriosis: The tumour cells are arranged in sheets and small fascicles

Neuroendocrine Carcinoma of Ovary

Large cell Neuroendocrine Tumour of Ovary (LCNET)

Image gallery: Fig. 7.45a–c
  Epidemiology

- Primary large cell neuroendocrine tumours of ovary is very rare
- Majority of the cases are associated with other surface epithelial neoplasms of ovary

Clinical features

- Nonspecific clinical features as seen in other ovarian carcinomas
- Paraneoplastic syndrome

Gross features

- Predominantly unilateral and solid

Histopathology

- Nests, trabeculae or sheets of cells
- Large cells with moderate amount of cytoplasm
- Nuclei show coarse chromatin

Immunohistochemistry

- Positive: Chromogranin, synaptophysin and CD 56

Prognosis

- Poorer prognosis than the other epithelial carcinomas in same stage

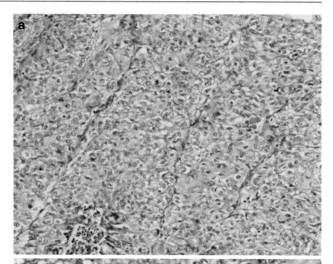
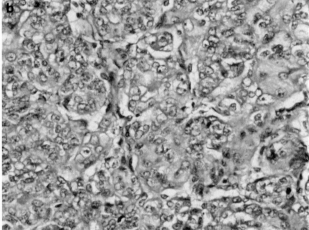
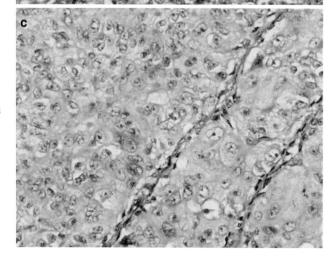

Fig. 7.45 (**a**) Large cell neuroendocrine tumour: Nests of tumour cells. (**b**) Large cell neuroendocrine tumour: small nests of cells separated by thin fibrous band. The individual cells are large with abundant cytoplasm. (**c**) Large cell neuroendocrine tumour: Tumour cells with abundant cytoplasm, indistinct cell margin and large nuclei having prominent nucleoli

Small Cell Type of Neuroendocrine Carcinoma

Image gallery: Fig. 7.46a, b
  Epidemiology

- Commoner than large cell neuroendocrine tumour

  Clinical features

- Elderly patient
- Same as that of LCNET
- Absence of hypercalcemia

  Histopathology

- Diffuse sheets of cells
- Small round cells
- Round nuclei with fine granular chromatin

  Immunohistochemistry
  Positive: CD 56, NSE
  Negative: CK, EMA

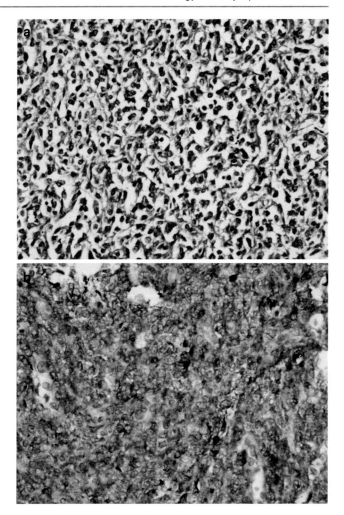

Fig. 7.46 (**a**) Small cell carcinoma: Nests of small cells with hyperchromatic nuclei. (**b**) Small cell carcinoma: the cells showing strong cytoplasmic CD 56 positivity

Seromucinous Carcinoma

Image gallery: Fig. 7.47a–c

Definition: This is a type of ovarian carcinoma that consists of both serous and also endocervical type of mucinous epithelial components.

Incidence: An uncommon tumour

Clinical features

- The mean age is around 45 years
- Lower abdominal mass

Gross features

- Average size of the tumour is about 12 cm diameter
- Both cystic and solid areas present
- Papillae seen

Histopathology

- Tumour contains serous carcinoma elements
- Papillary excrescence and cribriform growth pattern
- Endocervical type mucinous epithelium
- Mitosis present in variable quantity

Prognosis

- Till uncertain as less number of cases reported till now, however prognosis is favourable in stage I disease

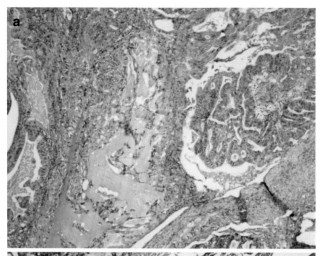
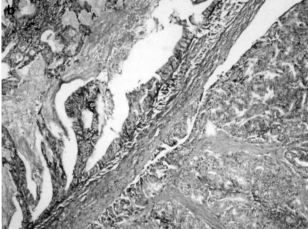
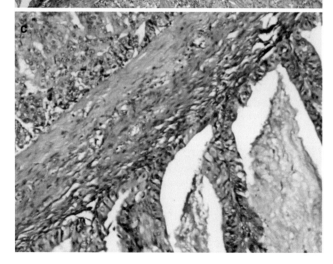

Fig. 7.47 (**a**) Seromucinous carcinoma: Both serous and mucinous component present. (**b**) Seromucinous carcinoma: Tall mucin secreting tumour cells forming papillary structure. (**c**) Seromucinous carcinoma: Upper left corner shows serous component and other areas show multiple papillary structures lined by mucinous epithelium

Reference

1. Kurman RJ, Carcangiu ML, Herrington S, Young RH. WHO classification of tumours of female genital reproductive organs. 4th ed. Lyon: International Agency for Research on Cancer; 2014.

Selected References

Acs G. Serous and mucinous borderline (low malignant potential) tumours of the ovary. Am J Clin Pathol. 2005;123(Suppl):S13–57.

Arnogiannaki N, Grigoriadis C, Zygouris D, Terzakis E, Sebastiadou M, Tserkezoglou A. Proliferative Brenner tumour of the ovary. Clinicopathological study of two cases and review of the literature. Eur J Gynaecol Oncol. 2011;32(5):576–8.

Atienza-Amores M, Guerini-Rocco E, Soslow RA, Park KJ, Weigelt B. Small cell carcinoma of the gynecologic tract: a multifaceted spectrum of lesions. Gynecol Oncol. 2014;134(2):410–8.

Brown J, Frumovitz M. Mucinous tumours of the ovary: current thoughts on diagnosis and management. Curr Oncol Rep. 2014;16(6):389.

Burks RT, Sherman ME, Kurman RJ. Micropapillary serous carcinoma of the ovary. A distinctive low-grade carcinoma related to serous borderline tumours. Am J Surg Pathol. 1996;20(11):1319–30.

Cantrell LA, Van Le L. Carcinosarcoma of the ovary a review. Obstet Gynecol Surv. 2009;64(10):673–80.

Czernobilsky B, Silverman BB, Mikuta JJ. Endometrioid carcinoma of the ovary. A clinicopathologic study of 75 cases. Cancer. 1970;26(5):1141–52.

De Cecio R, Cantile M, Collina F, Marra L, Santonastaso C, Scaffa C, Botti G, Losito NS. Borderline Brenner tumour of the ovary: a case report with immunohistochemical and molecular study. J Ovarian Res. 2014;7:101.

del Carmen MG, Birrer M, Schorge JO. Carcinosarcoma of the ovary: a review of the literature. Gynecol Oncol. 2012;125(1):271–7.

DePriest PD, Banks ER, Powell DE, van Nagell JR Jr, Gallion HH, Puls LE, Hunter JE, Kryscio RJ, Royalty MB. Endometrioid carcinoma of the ovary and endometriosis: the association in postmenopausal women. Gynecol Oncol. 1992;47(1):71–5.

Diaz-Padilla I, Malpica AL, Minig L, Chiva LM, Gershenson DM, Gonzalez-Martin A. Ovarian low-grade serous carcinoma: a comprehensive update. Gynecol Oncol. 2012;126(2):279–85.

Dietel M, Hauptmann S. Serous tumours of low malignant potential of the ovary. Diagnostic pathology. Virchows Arch. 2000;436(5):403–12.

Fischerova D, Zikan M, Dundr P, Cibula D. Diagnosis, treatment, and follow-up of borderline ovarian tumours. Oncologist. 2012;17(12):1515–33.

Fujiwara K, Shintani D, Nishikawa T. Clear-cell carcinoma of the ovary. Ann Oncol. 2016;27(Suppl 1):i50–2.

Gezginç K, Karatayli R, Yazici F, Acar A, Çelik Ç, Çapar M, Tavli L. Malignant Brenner tumour of the ovary: analysis of 13 cases. Int J Clin Oncol. 2012;17(4):324–9.

Glasspool RM, McNeish IA. Clear cell carcinoma of ovary and uterus. Curr Oncol Rep. 2013;15(6):566–72.

Hart WR. Borderline epithelial tumours of the ovary. Mod Pathol. 2005a;18(Suppl 2):S33–50.

Hart WR. Mucinous tumours of the ovary: a review. Int J Gynecol Pathol. 2005b;24(1):4–25.

Kaldawy A, Segev Y, Lavie O, Auslender R, Sopik V, Narod SA. Low-grade serous ovarian cancer: a review. Gynecol Oncol. 2016;143(2):433–8.

Khunamornpong S, Settakorn J, Sukpan K, et al. Mucinous tumour of low malignant potential ("borderline" or "atypical proliferative" tumour) of the ovary: a study of 171 cases with the assessment of intraepithelial carcinoma and microinvasion. Int J Gynecol Pathol. 2011;30:18–230.

Kondi-Pafiti A, Kairi-Vassilatou E, Iavazzo C, Vouza E, Mavrigiannaki P, Kleanthis C, Vlahodimitropoulos D, Liapis A. Clinicopathological features and immunoprofile of 30 cases of Brenner ovarian tumours. Arch Gynecol Obstet. 2012;285(6):1699–702.

Lee KR, Scully RE. Mucinous tumours of the ovary: a clinicopathologic study of 196 borderline tumours (of intestinal type) and carcinomas,including an evaluation of 11 cases with pseudomyxoma peritonei. Am J Surg Pathol. 2000;24:1447–64.

McKenney JK, Balzer BL, Longacre TA. Patterns of stromal invasion in ovarian serous tumours of low malignant potential (borderline tumours): a reevaluation of the concept of stromal microinvasion. Am J Surg Pathol. 2006a;30:1209–21.

McKenney JK, Balzer BL, Longacre TA. Lymph node involvement in ovarian serous tumours of low malignant potential (borderline tumours): pathology, prognosis, and proposed classification. Am J Surg Pathol. 2006b;30:614–24.

Michael H, Roth LM. Invasive and noninvasive implants in ovarian serous tumours of low malignant potential. Cancer. 1986;57(6):1240–7.

Naik JD, Seligmann J, Perren TJ. Mucinous tumours of the ovary. J Clin Pathol. 2012;65(7):580.

Oliva E, Egger JF, Young RH. Primary endometrioid stromal sarcoma of the ovary: a clinicopathologic study of 27 cases with morphologic and behavioral features similar to those of uterine low-grade. Am J Surg Pathol. 2014;38(3):305–15.

Perren TJ. Mucinous epithelial ovarian carcinoma. Ann Oncol. 2016;27(Suppl 1):i53–7.

Prat J. Ovarian tumours of borderline malignancy (tumours of low malignant potential): a critical appraisal. Adv Anat Pathol. 1999;6(5):247–74.

Ramalingam P. Morphologic, immunophenotypic, and molecular features of epithelial ovarian cancer. Oncology. 2016;30(2):166–76.

Ronnett BM, Yan H, Kurman RJ, et al. Patients with pseudomyxoma peritonei associated with disseminated peritoneal adenomucinosis have a significantly more favorable prognosis than patients with peritoneal mucinous carcinomatosis. Cancer. 2001;92:85–91.

Scully RE. Small cell carcinoma of hypercalcemic type. Int J Gynecol Pathol. 1993;12(2):148–52.

Shakuntala PN, Uma Devi K, Shobha K, Bafna UD, Geetashree M. Pure large cell neuroendocrine carcinoma of ovary: a rare clinical entity and review of literature. Case Rep Oncol Med. 2012;2012:120727.

Shappell HW, Riopel MA, Smith Sehdev AE, Ronnett BM, Kurman RJ. Diagnostic criteria and behavior of ovarian seromucinous (endocervical-type mucinous and mixed cell-type) tumours: atypical proliferative (borderline) tumours, intraepithelial, microinvasive, and invasive carcinomas. Am J Surg Pathol. 2002;26(12):1529–41.

Sinha R, Sundaram M. Endometrial stromal sarcoma from endometriosis. J Minim Invasive Gynecol. 2010;17(5):541–2.

Smith Sehdev AE, Sehdev PS, Kurman RJ. Noninvasive and invasive micropapillary (low-grade) serous carcinoma of the ovary: a clinicopathologic analysis of 135 cases. Am J Surg Pathol. 2003;27(6):725–36.

Vang R, Shih IM, Kurman RJ. Ovarian low-grade and high-grade serous carcinoma: pathogenesis, clinicopathologic and molecular biologic features, and diagnostic problems. Adv Anat Pathol. 2009;16(5):267–82.

Voutsadakis IA. Large cell neuroendocrine carcinoma of the ovary: a pathologic entity in search of clinical identity. World J Clin Oncol. 2014;5(2):36–8.

Classification of sex cord tumours of ovary according to World Health Organization is highlighted in Fig. 8.1.

Fig. 8.1 World health organization's classification of ovarian sex cord tumour

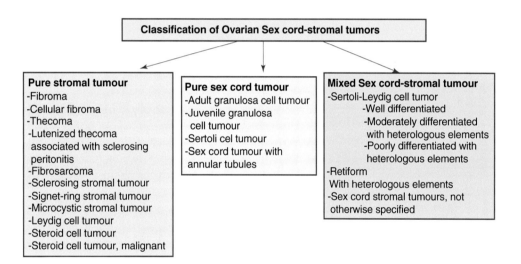

Classification of Ovarian Sex cord-stromal tumors

Pure stromal tumour
-Fibroma
-Cellular fibroma
-Thecoma
-Lutenized thecoma
 associated with sclerosing
 peritonitis
-Fibrosarcoma
-Sclerosing stromal tumour
-Signet-ring stromal tumour
-Microcystic stromal tumour
-Leydig cell tumour
-Steroid cell tumour
-Steroid cell tumour, malignant

Pure sex cord tumour
-Adult granulosa cell tumour
-Juvenile granulosa
 cell tumour
-Sertoli cel tumour
-Sex cord tumour with
 annular tubules

Mixed Sex cord-stromal tumour
-Sertoli-Leydig cell tumor
        -Well differentiated
        -Moderately differentiated
         with heterologous elements
        -Poorly differentiated with
         heterologous elements
-Retiform
 With heterologous elements
-Sex cord stromal tumours, not
 otherwise specified

© Springer Nature Singapore Pte Ltd. 2019
P. Dey, *Color Atlas of Female Genital Tract Pathology*, https://doi.org/10.1007/978-981-13-1029-4_8

Pure Sex Cord Tumour

Granulosa Cell Tumour

Image gallery: Figs. 8.2, 8.3, 8.4, 8.5, 8.6, 8.7, and 8.8

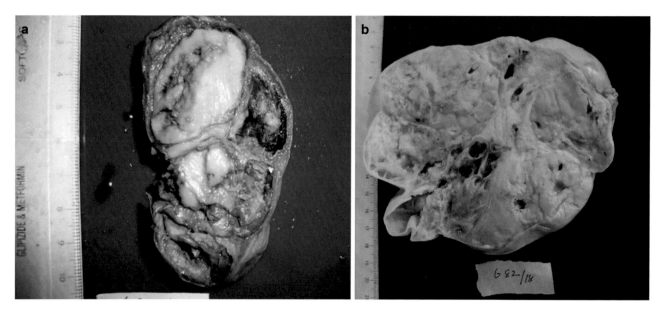

Fig. 8.2   (**a**) Gross picture of granulosa cell tumour: cut section showing solid grey to yellow in colour with areas of necrosis. (**b**) Gross picture of granulosa cell tumour: cut section showing solid yellowish areas

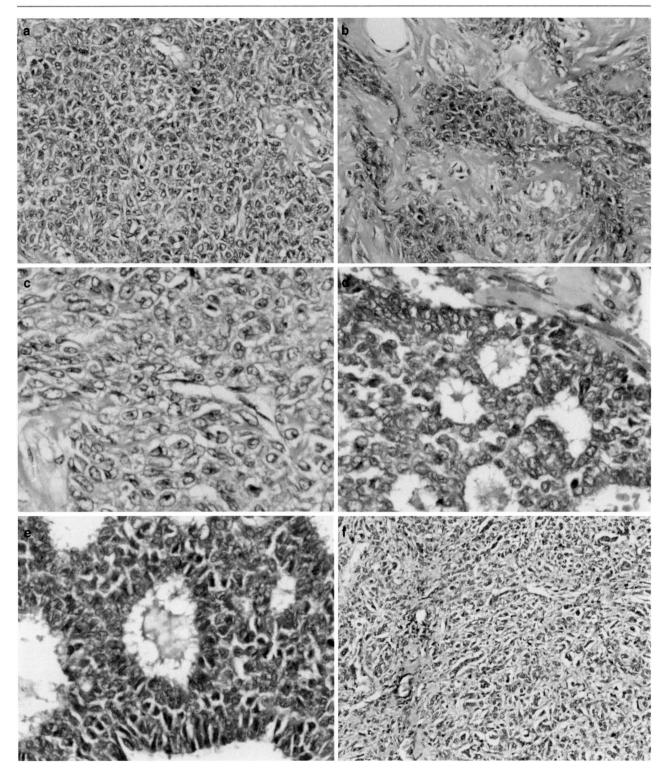

Fig. 8.3 (**a**) Granulosa cell tumour: diffuse sheet of tumour cells. (**b**) Granulosa cell tumour: figure: granulosa cell tumour: fibrotic areas. (**c**) Granulosa cell tumour: deep longitudinal nuclear groove. (**d**) Granulosa cell tumour: the gland like arrangement of cells with central pinkish material in Call Exner body. (**e**) Granulosa cell tumour: higher magnification of Call Exner body showing the gland like arrangement of the cells. Note the absent basement membrane as we see in the gland. (**f**) Granulosa cell tumour: ribbon like arrangement of the tumour cells. (**g**) Granulosa cell tumour: the cells are arranged in small and long ribbon. (**h**) Granulosa cell tumour, reticular pattern: the rows of tumour cells in between the clear spaces. (**i**) Granulosa cell tumour: macrofollicular pattern showing multiple large follicles

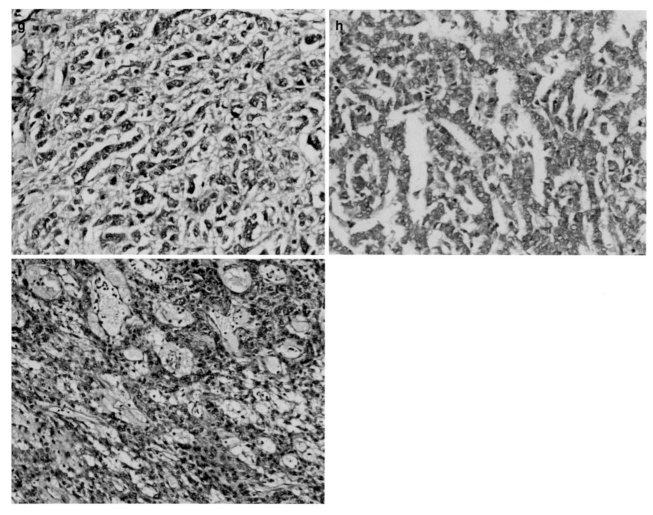

Fig. 8.3 (continued)

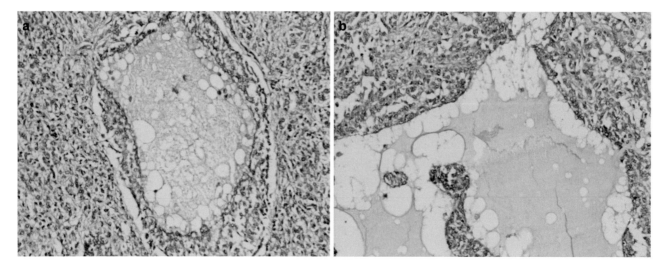

Fig. 8.4 (**a**) Granulosa cell tumour, cystic pattern: large cystic spaces. (**b**) Granulosa cell tumour, cystic pattern: the cystic spaces are lined by the tumour cells

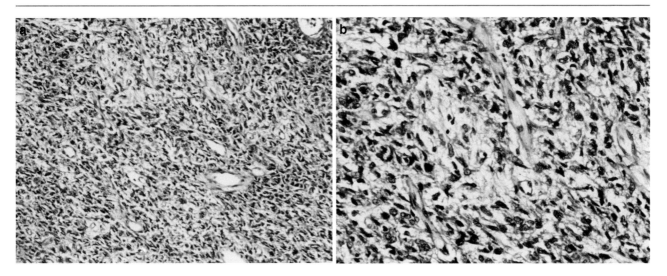

Fig. 8.5 (**a**) Granulosa cell tumour, sarcomatoid area: oval to spindle cells in interwoven small bundles. (**b**) Granulosa cell tumour, sarcomatoid area: the tumour showing oval to spindle cells with moderately pleomorphic nuclei giving sarcoma like appearance

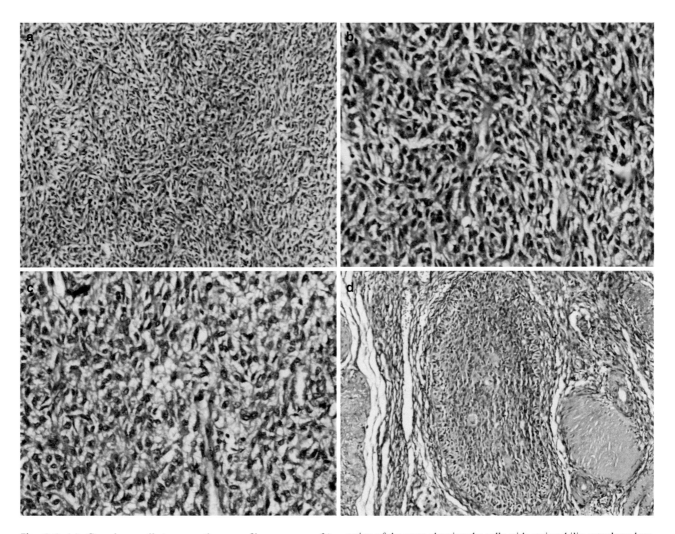

Fig. 8.6 (**a**) Granulosa cell tumour: thecoma fibroma area. (**b**) Granulosa cell tumour, thecoma fibroma area: the small fascicles of the cells. (**c**) Granulosa cell tumour, thecoma fibroma area: higher magnifi- cation of the same showing the cells with eosinophilic cytoplasm hav- ing elongated nuclei. (**d**) Granulosa cell tumour: incidentally detected microscopic foci of the tumour

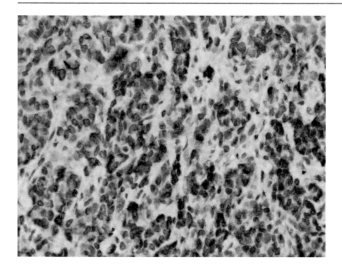

Fig. 8.7 Granulosa cell tumour: the tumour cells showing cytoplasmic inhibin positivity

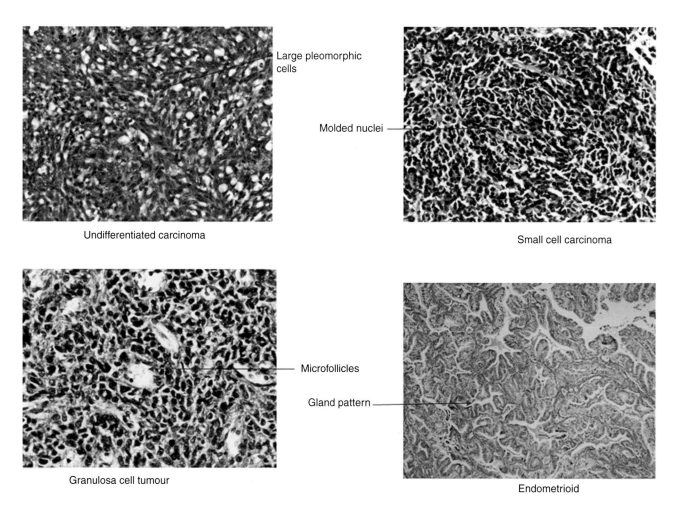

Fig. 8.8 Differential diagnosis of granulosa cell tumour

Adult Granulosa Cell Tumour

Abbreviation: Adult granulosa cell tumour (AGCT)
  Epidemiology

- Represents 1% of all ovarian neoplasms
- Constitutes 95% of granulosa cell tumours of ovary
- About 5% cases may have endometrial carcinoma

Clinical features

- Elderly patient, usually postmenopausal
- Mean age 50 years
- Abdominal mass or pain abdomen
- Abnormal vaginal bleeding due to excess oestrogen
- Virilization, hirsutism at times due to androgenic effect

Gross features

- Unilateral : 95%
- Variable size: Microscopic to large (25 cm)
- Mean size: 12 cm
- Predominantly solid and partly cystic
- Cut section: Yellowish, small cysts, areas of haemorrhage

Histopathology

- Arrangement: Diffuse, microfollicular, macrocystic, tubular, insular, trabecular
- Tumour cells
  - Round to oval and occasionally spindle shaped
  - Scanty cytoplasm
  - Monomorphic pale nuclei with evenly dispersed fine chromatin
  - Longitudinal nuclear groove
  - Inconspicuous nucleoli
- Other types of cells
  - Bizarre cells: Cells with bizarre hyperchromatic large nuclei
  - Hepatocyte: Occasionally hepatocyte like cells in small nests or acini
  - Luteinized cells: Luteinized granulosa cells contain abundant eosinophilic granular cytoplasm
  - Theca cells: Present
- Mitosis: Less than 5 per 10 HPF
- Different patterns

- Diffuse sheet
  The commonest pattern
  Cells are diffusely arranged
- Microfollicular
  Characteristic Call Exner bodies present: Granulosa cells are arranged around the central eosinophilic material
  Call Exner body is the hall mark of granulosa cell tumour
- Macrocystic
  Multiple large variable sized cysts
  Cysts are lined by granulosa cells
- Trabecular
  Bands of granulosa cells in a fibrous stroma
- Insular
  Small nests of granular cells in between the fibrous stroma
- Tubular
  Many solid and hollow tubules are present

Immunohistochemistry

- Tumours cells are positive for inhibin, calretinin, WT 1 and CD 56. The cells are also positive for vimentin, serodiagnostic factor 1 (SF 1) and FOXL2.
- Negative : EMA and CK7

Molecular genetics

- Point mutation of FOXL2 gene (more than 90% cases)
- Trisomy 12 and 14
  Diagnostic key features: See Box 8.1

Box 8.1 Diagnostic key features of adult granulosa cell tumour

- Tumour cells are arranged in diffuse, microfollicular, macrocystic, tubular, insular, trabecular pattern
- Round to oval tumour cells with monomorphic nuclei having nuclear groove
- Characteristic Call Exner bodies present
- Mitosis is usually scanty
- In addition, hepatocyte like cells, theca cells and luteinized cells may be present
- Immunohistochemistry: Positive for inhibin, calretinin, FOXL2, WT 1 and CD 56
- Molecular genetics: Point mutation of FOXL2 gene

Differential diagnosis (Fig. 8.8)

- Undifferentiated carcinoma
  - Nuclear pleomorphism more
  - Higher mitotic count
  - No nuclear groove
  - Negative for inhibin and calretinin
- Endometrial stromal sarcoma
  - Typical vascular pattern
  - No nuclear groove
  - Reticulin stain: The reticulin fibres encircles around individual tumour cells
  - Negative for inhibin
- Follicular cyst
  - Large follicular cysts may be confused with cystic AGCT
  - The cyst is lined by luteinized cells
- Small cell carcinoma
  - Presence of hypercalcemia
  - Lack of typical cytomorphology of AGCT
  - High mitotic rate
  - Negative inhibin and calretinin stain
- Endometrioid carcinoma
  - The presence of acini, microfollicles and diffuse sheets of cells may be confused with AGCT
  - The foci of squamous differentiation is a helpful clue for endometrioid carcinoma
  - In addition, the absent cytomorphological features of AGCT may also help in diagnosis

Prognosis

- FIGO staging is the most important prognostic factors
- Stage I 10 year survival: 85%
- High potential to recurrence and overall recurrence rate is 30%
- Recurrence may occur after 5 year
- Large size (more than 5 cm), bilaterality, and mitosis more than 5 per 10 HPF are bad prognostic indicators

Treatment

- Early stage: Salpingo-oophorectomy in
- Advanced stage: Tumour reductive surgery followed by chemotherapy

Juvenile Granulosa Cell Tumour

Image gallery: Fig. 8.9
  Abbreviation: Juvenile granulosa cell tumour (JGCT)
  Epidemiology

- 10% of all ovarian neoplasms in younger patient
- 5% of all granulosa cell tumour

Clinical features

- Average age: 15 year
- About 97% patients are below 30 year age
- Young patient: Isosexual pseudoprecocity due to excess estrogen
- Older children: Abnormal uterine bleeding
- Overall: pelvic pain, mass lower abdomen
- Gross features: Same as that of adult GCT

Histopathology

- Arrangement: Diffuse sheet of cells and macrofollicles
- Variable sized follicles within the diffuse sheet of cells
- The follicles are lined by the granulosa cells and central lumen is filled with eosinophilic material
- The tumour cells are round with abundant eosinophilic cytoplasm
- Nuclei are round hyperchromatic
- No nuclear grooving
- Frequent mitotic activity (2 to 30 per 10 HPF)
- Rarely adult GCT component may be admixed

Morphological distinguishing features of AGCT versus JGCT are highlighted in the Table 8.1
  Immunohistochemistry: Same as that of AGCT
  Molecular genetics

- Usually no mutation of FOXL2 gene

Key diagnostic features: See box 8.2

Box 8.2 Key diagnostic features of Juvenile granulosa cell tumour
- Diffuse sheet of cells, nodules and macrofollicles
- Round with abundant eosinophilic cytoplasm having round hyperchromatic nuclei
- Marked nuclear pleomorphism
- Absent nuclear grooves
- Very high mitotic rate

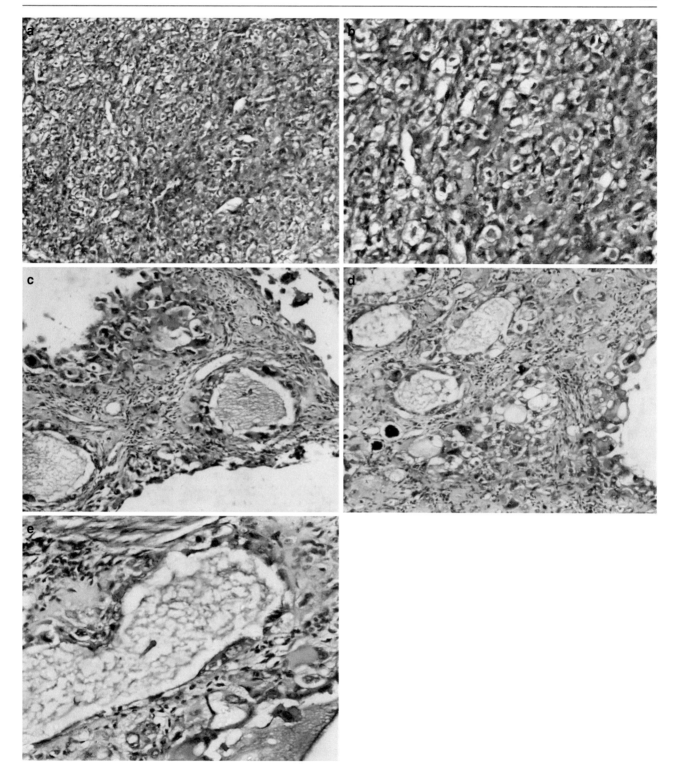

Fig. 8.9 (**a**) Granulosa cell tumour, juvenile type: diffuse sheets of moderately pleomorphic tumour cells. (**b**) Granulosa cell tumour, juvenile type: the tumour cells showing moderate amount of cytoplasm and large pleomorphic nuclei. (**c**) Granulosa cell tumour, juvenile type: multiple macrofollicles. (**d**) Granulosa cell tumour, juvenile type: diffuse sheet and macrofollicles. (**e**) Granulosa cell tumour, juvenile type: the large follicles are lined by moderately pleomorphic tumour cells

Table 8.1 Morphological distinguishing features of AGCT versus JGCT Box 8.1

Features	Juvenile granulosa cell tumour	Adult granulosa cell tumour
Nuclear pleomorphism	Significant	Monomorphic
Nuclear groove	Absent	Present
Cytoplasm	Abundant eosinophilic	Scanty
Mitosis	Usually high	Low
Microfollicles	Absent	Present
Call Exner body	Infrequent	Frequent

Differential diagnosis

- Adult granulosa cell tumour: Discussed above
- Yolk sac tumour
  - Presence of Schiller–Duval bodies
  - High alpha fetoprotein level
  - Negative for inhibin stain
- Small cell carcinoma of the hypercalcemic type
  - Hypercalcemia
  - Frequent extra ovarian spread
  - No microfollicles
  - Scanty cytoplasm
  - Negative for inhibin and positive for CD 56

Prognosis

- Presents in early stage so good in prognosis
- Unlike AGCT, this JGCTs recur early

Treatment

- Stage I: Unilateral salpingo oophorectomy with staging
- Advanced stage: total abdominal hysterectomy with bilateral salpingo-oophorectomy followed by combination chemotherapy

Sertoli Cell Tumour

Image gallery: Fig. 8.10

  Incidence: Rare, only 4 % of sex cord stromal tumour
  Clinical features

- It occurs in any age, usually in reproductive age period
- Complaints: Pain abdomen, and bleeding per vagina

Gross features:

- Unilateral tumour
- Average 8–9 cm diameter
- Solid, yellowish on cut section

Histopathology

- Multiple well-formed tubules
- Cuboidal to columnar cell lining
- Monomorphic nuclei
- Mitosis is infrequent

  Immunohistochemistry: Positive for WT 1, calretinin and inhibin
  Prognosis:

- Usually benign and is limited to ovary.
- Rarely malignant: Criteria more than 5 mitosis per 10 high power field, nuclear pleomorphism, and necrosis

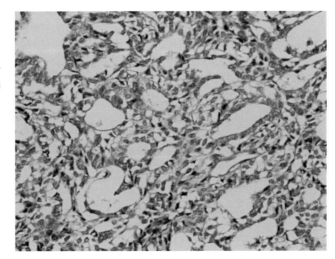

Fig. 8.10 Sertoli cell tumour: closely packed tubule formed by sertoli cells

Pure Stromal Tumour

Thecoma
Image gallery: Fig. 8.11a–f

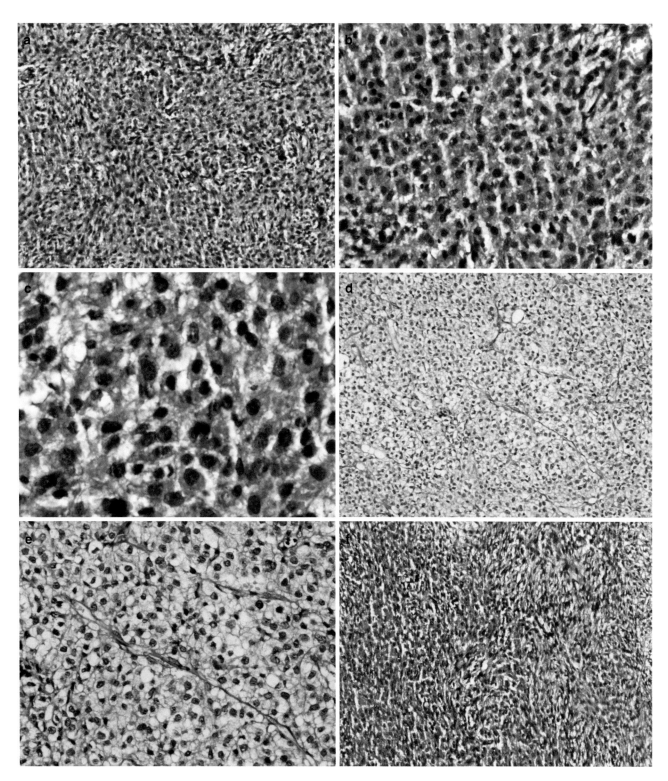

Fig. 8.11 (**a**) Thecoma: diffuse sheet of cells. (**b**) Thecoma: the tumour cells with eosinophilic cytoplasm and central monomorphic nuclei. (**c**) Thecoma: higher magnification showing better morphology of the same. (**d**) Thecoma: nests of tumour cells. (**e**) Thecoma: groups of polyhedral cells with abundant clear cytoplasm. (**f**) Fibroma thecoma: both fibroma and thecoma areas. (**g**) Differential diagnosis of thecoma

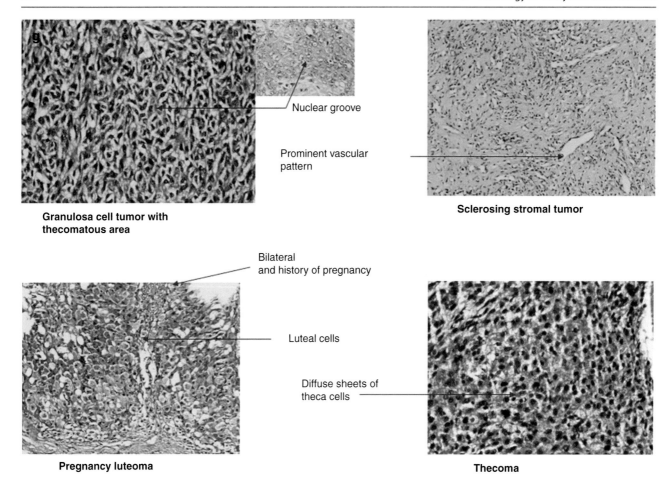

Granulosa cell tumor with thecomatous area

Nuclear groove

Prominent vascular pattern

Sclerosing stromal tumor

Bilateral and history of pregnancy

Luteal cells

Diffuse sheets of theca cells

Pregnancy luteoma

Thecoma

Fig. 8.11 (continued)

Epidemiology

- It represents only 1% of all ovarian neoplasms

Clinical features

- Elderly patient
- Mean age 59 year
- Presents with pelvic mass
- Abnormal uterine bleeding due to excess estrogenic effect
- Associated endometrial adenocarcinoma in 20% cases

Gross features

- Mainly unilateral (about 95%)
- Variable size: 1–10 cm diameter

- Solid yellowish
- Occasionally focal cystic changes, haemorrhage and necrosis may be present

Histopathology

- Diffuse sheets of cells
- Individual tumour cells are round to spindle shaped
- Cells contain abundant pale vacuolated cytoplasm with central monomorphic nuclei
- Usually no cytological atypia or mitotic activity
- Rarely pleomorphic degenerative nuclei are seen
- Uncommonly thecoma may show extensive calcification

Immunohistochemistry: Calretinin and inhibin positive
Key diagnostic features: See Box 8.3

Box 8.3 Key diagnostic features of thecoma
- Diffuse sheets of tumour cells
- Round to spindle cells with abundant pale cytoplasm
- Absence of nuclear atypia and mitosis
- Areas of fibromatous component may be seen
- Immunohistochemistry: Calretinin and inhibin positive

Differential diagnosis (Fig. 8.11g)

- Adult granulosa cell tumour
  - Nuclear groove present
  - Reticulin fibre condensation around the group of cells instead of individual cells
- Fibroma
  - Predominantly spindle cells in fascicles
  - Scanty cytoplasm
- Sclerosing stromal tumour
  - Relatively younger patient
  - Prominent vascular pattern
- Pregnancy luteoma
  - Bilateral involvement of ovary
  - Multiple

Prognosis and treatment

- Benign tumour
- Unilateral salpingo-oophorectomy is the treatment of choice

Fibroma
Image gallery: Figs. 8.12, 8.13, and 8.14
Epidemiology

- It constitutes 4% of all ovarian neoplasm
- Fibroma occurs in fourth to fifth decade
- Mean age 48 years

Clinical features

- Mostly symptomatic
- Patients may present with pelvic mass
- Characteristically associated with
  - Meigs' syndrome: Ascites and pleural effusion
  - Gorlin's syndrome (basal cell nevus syndrome): Basal cell carcinoma, mesenteric cyst, dura mater calcification

Gross features

- Unilateral (90%)
- Variable size: 1–20 cm
- Mean size: 6 cm
- Solid
- Cut section: Firm, yellow, occasionally whorled appearance
- Calcification may be seen
- In case of torsion: Haemorrhage and necrosis

Histopathology

- Arrangement: Intersecting fascicles and storiform pattern
- Oval to spindle cells with scanty cytoplasm
- Rarely cytoplasmic hyaline globules may be seen
- Spindle shaped nuclei with bland chromatin
- Usually cellular however occasional fibroma may show oedema and low cellularity
- Mitotic count is usually low to absent
- Sex cord differentiation may be seen in less than 10% area
- Variants:
  - Mitotically active: Mitosis 4 to 19 per 10 HPF, however no nuclear atypia is seen
  - Cellular fibroma: Densely cellular fibroma

Immunohistochemistry

- Positive for vimentin, inhibin and calretinin
- Negative for SMA and CD 10

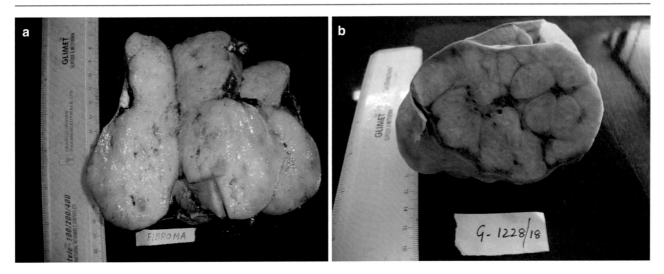

Fig. 8.12 (**a**) Gross picture of fibroma: solid grey white tumour. (**b**) Gross picture of fibroma: at times cut section of the tumour may show whorled appearance resembling leiomyoma

Molecular genetics

- Loss of heterozygosity at 19p13.3 and 9q22.3

Key diagnostic features: See Box 8.4

Box 8.4 Key diagnostic features of fibroma
- Intersecting fascicles and storiform pattern of tumour cells
- Oval to spindle cells with scanty cytoplasm and bland chromatin
- Usually scanty mitosis
- Cellular fibroma may have increased mitotic activity (more than 3 per 10 HPF)
- Immunohistochemistry: Calretinin and inhibin positive

Differential diagnosis (Fig. 8.15)

- Stromal hyperplasia
  - Bilateral
  - Absence of collagenous stroma
- Massive ovarian oedema
  - Normal ovarian follicles and corpus luteum may be included in the pathological area
- Fibrosarcomas
  - Cellular atypia along with more than 4 mitosis per 10 HPF

Prognosis and treatment

- Benign tumour
- Unilateral salpingo oophorectomy is the treatment of choice

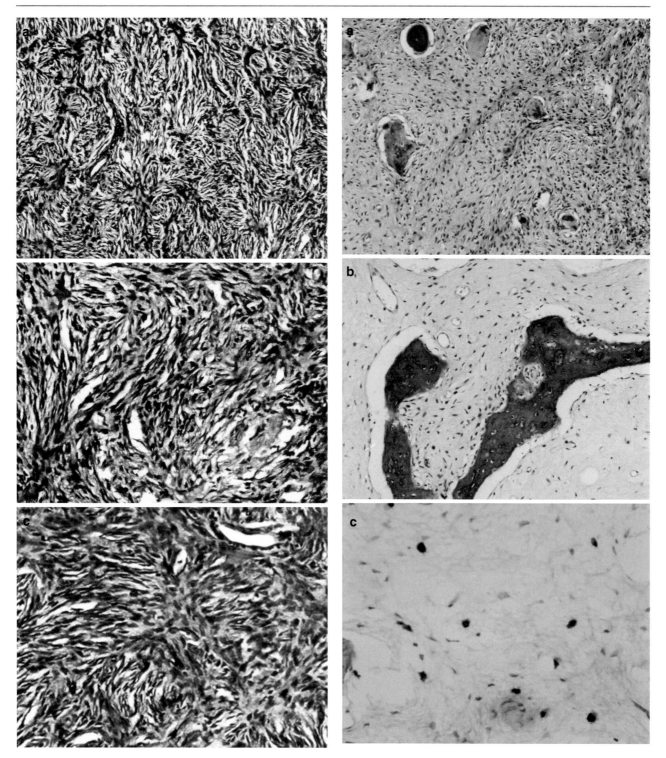

Fig. 8.13 (**a**) Fibroma: multiple interwoven small fascicles of tumour cells. (**b**) Fibroma: interwoven fascicles. (**c**) Fibroma: the spindle shaped tumour cells with elongated nuclei

Fig. 8.14 (**a**) Fibroma: focal areas of bone formation. (**b**) Fibroma: large bony trabeculae. (**c**) Fibroma with bone formation: the fibroma cells are positive for calretinin

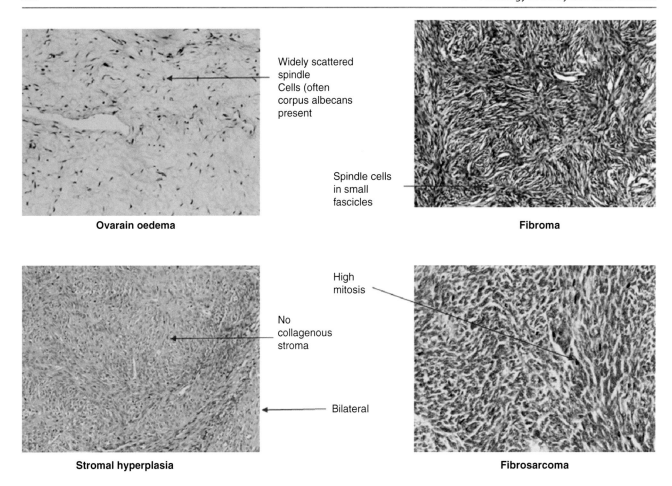

Fig. 8.15 Differential diagnosis of fibroma of ovary

Fibrosarcoma

Image gallery: Fig. 8.16a–c

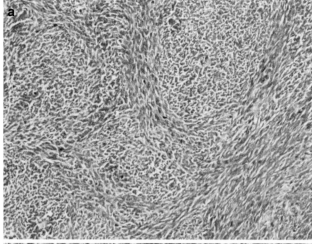

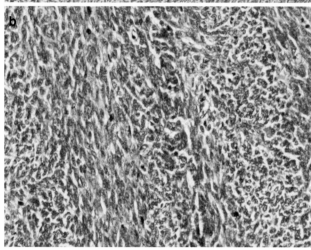

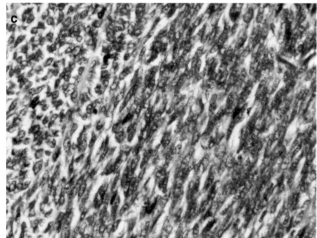

Fig. 8.16 (**a**) Fibrosarcoma: whorled fascicles. (**b**) Fibrosarcoma: interwoven bundles of tumour cells. (**c**) Fibrosarcoma: frequent mitotic activity present

Epidemiology

- Rare tumour
- Commonest sarcoma of ovary

Clinical features

- It occurs in sixth to seventh decade of life
- Mean age: 58 year
- Mass in pelvis or pain abdomen

Gross features

- Unilateral
- Large, Average size is 17 cm
- Solid
- Cut section: grey white

Histopathology

- Arrangement: Herringbone pattern
- Oval to spindle cells with scanty eosinophilic cytoplasm
- Nuclei are spindle shaped with moderately pleomorphic
- Mitotic activity: more than 4 per 10 HPF

Diagnostic criteria

- Significant nuclear pleomorphism: Essential feature
- High mitosis: <4 per 10 HPF
- Tumour necrosis

Molecular genetics

- Trisomy 12

Differential diagnosis

- Mitotically active cellular fibroma
- No nuclear pleomorphism

Prognosis

- Highly aggressive neoplasm with poor prognosis

Sclerosing Stromal Tumour

Image gallery: Figs. 8.17 and 8.18

Epidemiology

- Rare neoplasm
- Only 2% of all sex cord tumours

Clinical features

- Young patients
- Mean age 27 years
- Abdominal pain, pelvic mass, menstrual disturbances
- Virilization is uncommon

Gross features

- Unilateral
- Variable size: 1–15 cm
- Cut section: Solid and yellowish

Histopathology

- Pseudolobular pattern: Alternate cellular and hypocellular areas
- Cellular area: It consists of round to spindle shaped cells with bland nuclei.
  - Round cells: They contain eosinophilic cytoplasm which may be vacuolated. Nuclei are monomorphic and round and often eccentric. The cells often simulate signet ring cells.
  - Spindle cells: They contain scanty cytoplasm and spindle shaped nuclei.
- Hypocellular area: Dense collagenous stroma or myxomatous or oedematous area
- Characteristic branched thin walled blood vessels
- Low mitotic activity

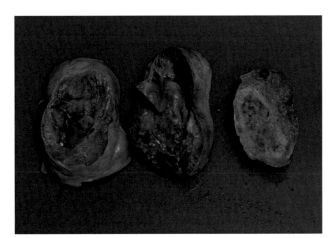

Fig. 8.17 Gross picture of sections of the sclerosing stromal tumour showing greyish solid areas

Immunohistochemistry

- Positive: Calretinin, infrequently inhibin, vimentin and CD 34
- Negative: CK and EMA

Molecular genetics: Trisomy 12

Key diagnostic features: See Box 8.5

Box 8.5 Key diagnostic features of Sclerosing stromal tumour

- Pseudolobular pattern of alternate cellular and hypocellular areas
- Bland looking round to spindle shaped cells
- Round cells have eosinophilic vacuolated cytoplasm with monomorphic round nuclei giving signet ring cell appearance
- Spindle cells contain scanty cytoplasm with spindle shaped nuclei
- Branched thin walled blood vessels
- Low mitotic count
- *Immunohistochemistry*: Calretinin and inhibin positive

Differential diagnosis

- Fibroma
  - Predominantly spindle shaped cells may simulates fibroma
  - It occurs in much elderly patient
  - No pesudolobular pattern
  - No branched thin walled vessels
- Krukenberg's tumour
  - The vacuoles in the signet ring cells in Krukenberg's tumour contain mucin whereas the vacuoles in sclerosing stromal tumour contains lipid
  - This tumour is positive for CK and EMA
- Luteinized thecoma
  - Absent pesudolobular pattern
  - No branched thin walled blood vessels

Prognosis

- Benign in behaviour

Treatment

- Unilateral oophorectomy

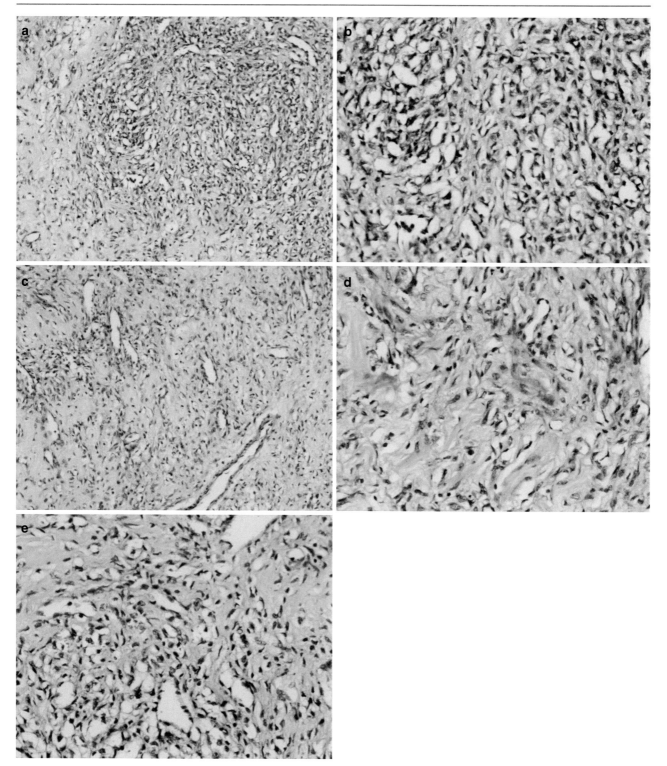

Fig. 8.18 (**a**) Sclerosing stromal tumour: alternate cellular and hypo-cellular areas. (**b**) Sclerosing stromal tumour: both round cells and spindle cells in the vascularized stroma. (**c**) Sclerosing stromal tumour: many branching thin walled blood vessel in the tumour. (**d**) Sclerosing stromal tumour: spindle cells within the dense collagenous stroma. (**e**) Sclerosing stromal tumour: vascular channels within the collagenous stroma

Steroid Cell Tumour

It comprises of

- Steroid cell tumour
- Stromal luteoma
- Leydig cell tumour

Steroid Cell Tumour: Not Otherwise Specified

Image gallery: Fig. 8.19a, b

Epidemiology

- Rare tumour
- Only 1% of all sex cord tumours and 0.1% of all ovarian tumours

Clinical features

- Usually seen in postmenopausal patient
- Average age is 45 year
- Usually asymptomatic
- Androgenic manifestation: Virilization and hirsutism (50% cases)
- Estrogenic manifestation: Abnormal vaginal bleeding
- Rarely Cushing's syndrome

Gross features

- Unilateral
- Variable size: 1–30 cm, mean diameter 8 cm

- Solid
- Cut section: yellow to brown colour

Histopathology

- Arrangement: Diffuse sheet, nest, or cord
- The group of tumour cells are separated by thin fibrous septa
- Individual cells are large polygonal with abundant eosinophilic to vacuolated cytoplasm
- Cell have central round monomorphic nuclei

Immunohistochemistry

- Positive: Inhibin, calretinin

Prognosis

- About 30% tumours are malignant in nature
- The features suggestive of malignant behaviours
  - Mitosis: More than 2 per 10 HPF
  - Large size: More than 7 cm diameter
  - Nuclear atypia: Significant
  - Haemorrhage and necrosis: Present

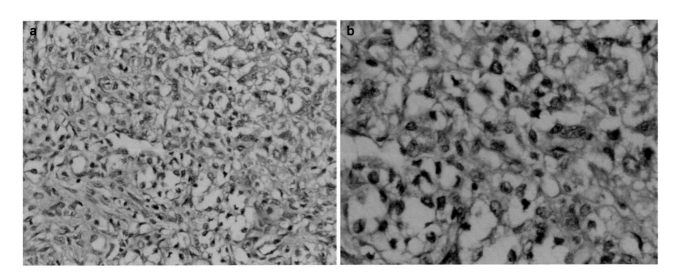

Fig. 8.19 (a) Steroid cell tumour: diffuse sheet of tumour cells. (b) Steroid cell tumour: the polygonal tumour cells with abundant clear cytoplasm and central round nuclei

Stromal Luteoma

Epidemiology

- It represents 25% of steroid cell tumours

Clinical features

- Elderly patient
- Common complaints:
  - Oestrogen excess: Abnormal vaginal bleeding
  - Androgenic excess: Virilization

Gross features

- Unilateral (95%)
- Small 0.5–2 cm in diameter
- Solid
- Well circumscribed, grey white to yellow

Histopathology

- Arrangement: diffuse sheets, cords or nests of cells
- Polygonal cells with abundant eosinophilic granular cytoplasm that often contains lipochrome pigment
- Central round monomorphic nuclei with single prominent nucleoli
- Surrounding tissue shows stromal hyperthecosis

Immunohistochemistry

- Positive: Inhibin, calretinin

Differential diagnosis

- *Pregnancy luteoma*
  - Young patient with history of pregnancy
  - Multifocal
- *Stromal hyperthecosis*
  - Small in size less than 0.5 cm
- Luteinized thecoma
  - Stroma is fibromatous

Prognosis and treatment

- Benign tumour
- Unilateral oophorectomy is adequate treatment

Leydig Cell Tumour

Epidemiology

- It represents 19% of all steroid cell tumours
- When the tumour is located in the hilum of ovary then it is known as hilus cell tumour
- When the tumour is located within the parenchyma of ovary then it is known as leydig cell tumour of non-hilus cell type

Clinical features

- Often presents as androgenic manifestation
- Mean age: 58 year

Hilus Cell Type of Leydig Cell Tumour

Gross features

- Unilateral
- Located in the hilum of ovary
- Reddish brown, solid

Histopathology

- Well circumscribed tumour
- Diffuse sheets of tumour cells
- Round to polygonal cells
- Cells contain abundant eosinophilic cytoplasm with central monomorphic round nuclei
- The nuclei of the cells are often aggregated together and provides a important clue in diagnosis
- Reinke crystals in the cytoplasm in 50% cases

Leydig Cell Tumour of Non-Hilus Cell Type

Location: In the parenchyma of ovary

Histopathology: Same as that of hilus leydig cell tumour

Prognosis and treatment

- Benign in nature
- Unilateral oophorectomy

Mixed Sex Cord Stromal Tumour

Sertoli Leydig Cell Tumour

Image gallery: Figs. 8.20, 8.21, 8.22, 8.23, 8.24, and 8.25
   Abbreviation: Sertoli Leydig cell tumour (SLCT)
   Epidemiology

- Rare tumour
- Less than 0.5% of all ovarian neoplasms
- It occurs in wide age group from 10 to 80 year, however 3/4th of the patients are below 30 year age
- Mean age 25 year

Clinical features

- Non-specific: abdominal pain, pelvic mass
- Androgenic manifestation in 30–40% cases: Hirsutism, frontal baldness, deep voice, acne
- Estrogenic manifestation or raised alpha-fetoprotein level in occasional cases

Gross features

- Unilateral (about 95%)
- Usually large 2–30 cm
- Mean 15 cm diameter
- Cut section: Solid tumour, partly cystic area may be seen, yellowish
- Cystic areas are more common in tumour containing heterologous elements

Histopathology
The following types of tumours are present

- Well differentiated sertoli Leydig cell tumour
  - Multiple nodules or lobules in low powered examination
  - Predominantly tubules interspersed in connective tissue stroma
  - Both hollow and solid tubules are present
  - Hollow tubules are usually small or occasionally cystically dilated and resembles endometrioid carcinoma
  - Solid tubules are small round clusters with irregular margin
  - Lining of the tubules are cuboidal cells with scanty cytoplasm. Nuclei are bland looking monomorphic round shape.
  - Sertoli cells have abundant vacuolated cytoplasm with centrally placed small round nuclei
  - Leydig cells are also present as nests or in cords
- Intermediately differentiated sertoli Leydig cell tumour
  - Multiple lobules of cells

- The cells are arranged as nests, cord, or occasional tubules
- Microcysts are also seen
- The individual tumour cells are small with scanty cytoplasm having round or angulated hyperchromatic nuclei.
- Occasionally nuclei are bizarre in look
- Mitosis: Relatively high, about 5 per 10 HPF
- Leydig cells are also present
- Poorly differentiated sertoli Leydig cell tumour
  - Multiple fascicles of oval to spindle cells
  - The cells have scanty cytoplasm and spindle shaped hyperchromatic nuclei
  - High mitotic activities: 10–20 per 10 HPF
  - Occasional small tubules of sertoli cells may be present
  - Leydig cells are usually absent
- Retiform sertoli Leydig cell tumour
  - Arrangement: Slit like tubules, small cysts and papillae
  - Tubules : Elongated, irregularly branched spaces
  - Cysts and tubules may contain eosinophilic material
  - Lining cells are small cuboidal with scanty cytoplasm and small round nuclei
  - Small hyalinised papillary structures may also be seen
- Sertoli Leydig cell tumour with heterologous component
  - Mucinous epithelium: Usually benign gastrointestinal type, occasionally borderline changes may be present
  - Heterologous stromal element: Cartilaginous, skeletal muscle or rhabdomyosarcoma elements

Immunohistochemistry

- Positive for inhibin, calretinin, CD 56, SF-1, WT 1. The tumour cells also express FOXL2.
- Heterologous element:
  - Mucosal epithelium is positive for CK and EMA
  - Connective tissue: Positive for vimentin
  - Hepatocytes: Positive for alpha fetoprotein

Key diagnostic features: See Box 8.6

Box 8.6 Key diagnostic features of Sertoli Leydig cell tumour
- Multiple nodules or lobules of tumour cells
- Many solid and hollow tubules
- Amount of tubules depends on the differentiation

- The tubules are lined by cuboidal cells with scanty cytoplasm
- Mild to moderate nuclear atypia depending on the grade
- Mitosis low to high
- Poorly differentiated tumour shows multiple fascicles of oval to spindle cells with very high mitosis (>10 per 10 HPF)
- Sertoli Leydig cell tumour with heterologous component shows cartilaginous, skeletal muscle or rhabdomyosarcoma elements
- Retiform sertoli Leydig cell tumour shows slit like tubules, small cysts and papillae
- Immunohistochemistry: inhibin, calretinin, CD 56, SF-1, WT 1. and FOXL2

Differential diagnosis

- Endometrioid carcinoma
  - Elderly age group
  - Often shows squamous metaplastic components
  - Lumen of the glands contain mucinous material
  - Fibrous stromal tissue
  - Negative for inhibin and calretinin
- Krukenberg's tumour
  - Bilateral tumour
  - Signet ring cells containing mucin
  - Markedly atypical cells present
- Carcinosarcoma
  - Elderly patient
  - High grade carcinomatous area

- Malignant stromal elements
- Cartilage are malignant (chondrosarcoma)
- Yolk sac tumour
  - Typical Schiller Duval bodies present
  - Slit like spaces are lined by highly malignant cells
  - Alpha feto protein level in serum is high
- Teratoma
  - The presence of squamous and neuroectodermal elements
- Dysgerminoma
  - Lymphocytes in the connective tissue stroma
  - Individual tumour cells show large nuclei with prominent nucleoli

Prognosis

- Other than stage of the tumour prognosis depends on the grade of tumour
- Well differentiated SLCT are all benign
- Poorly differentiated SLCT, retiform type of SLCT and tumour with heterologous elements are all malignant in nature
- The malignant tumour recurs within one year (60% cases)

Treatment

- It depends on stage and degree of differentiation and intention to keep fertility
- Stage I tumours: unilateral salpingo-oophorectomy
- Advanced stage tumours with poor differentiation : Total abdominal hysterectomy with bilateral salpingo-oophorectomy followed by chemotherapy

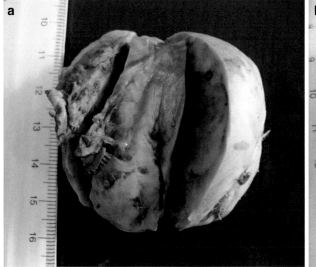 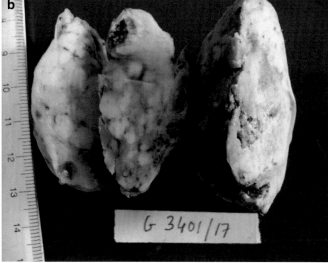

Fig. 8.20 (**a**) Sertoli Leydig cell tumour: solid tumour with smooth outer surface. (**b**) Sertoli Leydig cell tumour: cut section showing grey white and yellowish solid areas

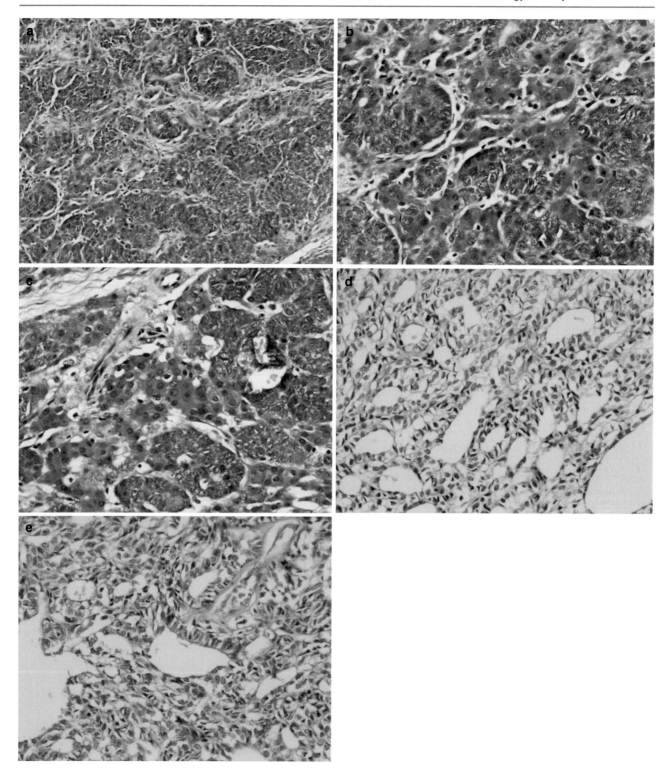

Fig. 8.21 (a) Sertoli Leydig cell tumour: multiple nests of sertoli cell with interspersed Leydig cells. (b) Sertoli Leydig cell tumour: Sertoli cells with admixed intervening Leydig cells. (c) Sertoli Leydig cell tumour: clusters of Leydig cells with abundant eosinophilic cytoplasm. (d) Sertoli Leydig cell tumour, well differentiated: multiple well-formed tubules. (e) Sertoli Leydig cell tumour, well differentiated: multiple hollow tubules

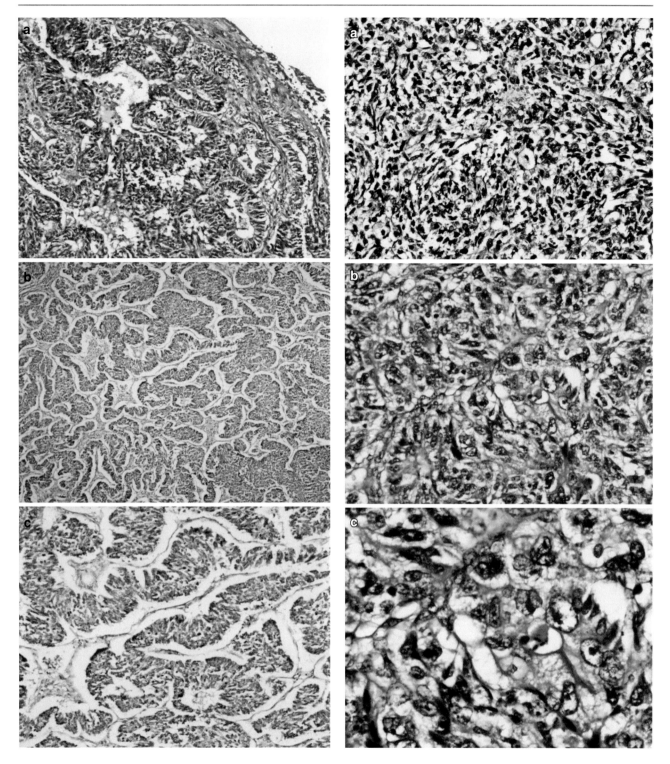

Fig. 8.22 (**a**) Sertoli Leydig cell tumour, intermediate differentiation: hollow tubules and solid clusters of sertoli cells. (**b**) Sertoli Leydig cell tumour, intermediate differentiation: multiple solid groups of immature sertoli cells. (**c**) Sertoli Leydig cell tumour, intermediate differentiation: large nests and cords of immature sertoli cells

Fig. 8.23 (**a**) Sertoli Leydig cell tumour, poor differentiation: diffuse sheet of sertoli cells. (**b**) Sertoli Leydig cell tumour, poor differentiation: cells showing moderate to marked nuclear pleomorphism. (**c**) Sertoli Leydig cell tumour, poor differentiation: higher magnification of the same showing nuclear pleomorphism

Fig. 8.24 (**a**) Sertoli Leydig cell tumour, spindle cell type: spindle cells in small fascicles. (**b**) Sertoli Leydig cell tumour, spindle cell type: the tumour cells have moderately pleomorphic oval to spindle shaped nuclei. (**c**) Sertoli Leydig cell tumour, spindle cell type: foci of Leydig cells present

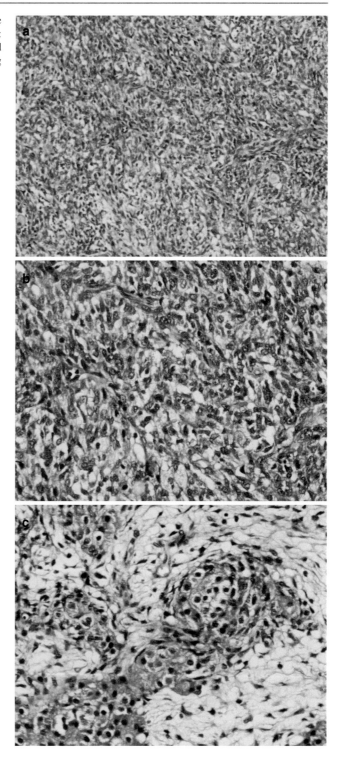

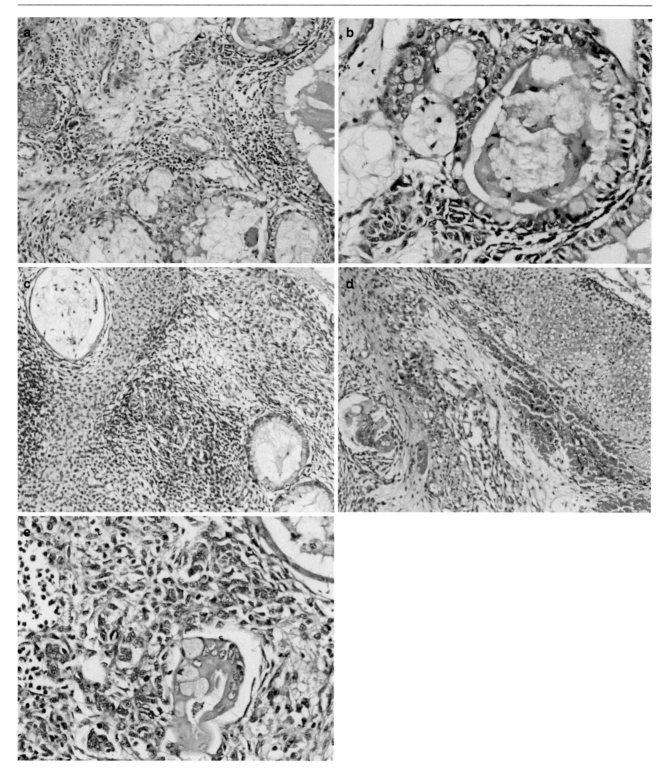

Fig. 8.25 (**a**) Sertoli Leydig cell tumour, mucinous metaplasia: multiple foci showing mucinous glands. (**b**) Sertoli Leydig cell tumour, mucinous metaplasia: the glands are lined by mucin secreting epithelial cells. (**c**) Sertoli Leydig cell tumour, mucinous and cartilaginous metaplasia: large areas showing cartilaginous metaplasia with focal mucinous metaplasia. (**d**) Sertoli Leydig cell tumour with cartilaginous metaplasia: pale blue cartilaginous area. (**e**) Sertoli Leydig cell tumour with osseous metaplasia: bony area

Gynandroblastoma

Definition: This type of sex cord tumour consists of both granulosa cell tumour and sex cord stromal tumour.

> *Epidemiology*: Very rare
>
> *Histopathology*

- The minor component is at least 10% of the volume of tumour

Suggested Reading

Atram M, Anshu SS, Gangane N. Sclerosing stromal tumour of the ovary. Obstet Gynecol Sci. 2014;57(5):405–8.

Bennett JA, Oliva E, Young RH. Sclerosing stromal tumours with prominent luteinization during pregnancy: a report of 8 cases emphasizing diagnostic problems. Int J Gynecol Pathol. 2015;34:357–62.

Burandt E, Young RH. Thecoma of the ovary: a report of 70 cases emphasizing aspects of its histopathology different from those often portrayed and its differential diagnosis. Am J Surg Pathol. 2014;38(8):1023–32.

Dal Cin P, Pauwels P, Van den Berghe H. Fibrosarcoma versus cellular fibroma of the ovary. Am J Surg Pathol. 1998;22(4):508–10.

Geetha P, Nair MK. Granulosa cell tumours of the ovary. Aust N Z J Obstet Gynaecol. 2010;50(3):216–20.

Haroon S, Idrees R, Fatima S, Memon A, Kayani N. Ovarian steroid cell tumour, not otherwise specified: a clinicopathological and immunohistochemical experience of 12 cases. J Obstet Gynaecol Res. 2015;41(3):424–31.

Hayes MC, Scully RE. Ovarian steroid cell tumour (not otherwise specified): a clinicopathological analysis of 63 cases. Am J Surg Pathol. 1987;11:835–45.

Hayes MC, Scully RE. Stromal luteoma of the ovary: a clinicopathological analysis of 25 cases. Int J Gynecol Pathol. 1987;6:313–21.

Irving JA, Alkushi A, Young RH, Clement PB. Cellular fibromas of the ovary: a study of 75 cases including 40 mitotically active tumours emphasizing their distinction from fibrosarcoma. Am J Surg Pathol. 2006;30:928–38.

Koukourakis GV, Kouloulias VE, Koukourakis MJ, Zacharias GA, Papadimitriou C, Mystakidou K, Pistevou-Gompaki K, Kouvaris J, Gouliamos A. Granulosa cell tumour of the ovary: tumour review. Integr Cancer Ther. 2008;7(3):204–15.

Kozan P, Chalasani S, Handelsman DJ, Pike AH, Crawford BA. A Leydig cell tumour of the ovary resulting in extreme hyperandrogenism, erythrocytosis, and recurrent pulmonary embolism. J Clin Endocrinol Metab. 2014;99(1):12–7.

Mancari R, Portuesi R, Colombo N. Adult granulosa cell tumours of the ovary. Curr Opin Oncol. 2014;26(5):536–41.

Numanoglu C, Guler S, Ozaydin I, Han A, Ulker V, Akbayir O. Stromal luteoma of the ovary: a rare ovarian pathology. J Obstet Gynaecol. 2015;35(4):420–1.

Prat J, Young RH, Scully RE. Ovarian Sertoli-Leydig cell tumours with heterologous elements. II. Cartilage and skeletal muscle: a clinicopathologic analysis of twelve cases. Cancer. 1982;50(11):2465–75.

Roth LM, Anderson MC, Govan ADT, et al. Sertoli-Leydig cell tumours: a clinicopathologic study of 34 cases. Cancer. 1981;48:187–97.

Scully RE. Juvenile granulosa cell tumour. Pediatr Pathol. 1988;8(4):423–7.

Shah SP, Kobel M, Senz J, et al. Mutation of FOXL2 in granulosa-cell tumours of the ovary. N Engl J Med. 2009;360:2719–29.

Shanthala PR, Saldhana P, Upadhyaya K. Gynandroblastoma: a rare ovarian tumour with an unusual clinical presentation. J Indian Med Assoc. 2014;112(2):128, 130.

Stellato G, Di Bonito M, Tramontana S. Primary fibrosarcoma of the ovary. Acta Obstet Gynecol Scand. 1995;74(8):649–52.

Stuart GC, Dawson LM. Update on granulosa cell tumours of the ovary. Curr Opin Obstet Gynecol. 2003;15(1):33–7.

Young RH. Ovarian sex cord-stromal tumours and their mimics. Pathology. 2018;50(1):5–15.

Young RH, Dickersin GR, Scully RE. Juvenile granulosa cell tumour of the ovary. A clinicopathological analysis of 125 cases. Am J Surg Pathol. 1984;8:575–96.

Zhang HY, Zhu JE, Huang W, Zhu J. Clinicopathologic features of ovarian Sertoli-Leydig cell tumours. Int J Clin Exp Pathol. 2014;7(10):6956–64.

Classification of germ cell tumour of ovary according to World Health Organization [1] has been highlighted in the Fig. 9.1.

Fig. 9.1 Classification of germ cell tumour of ovary

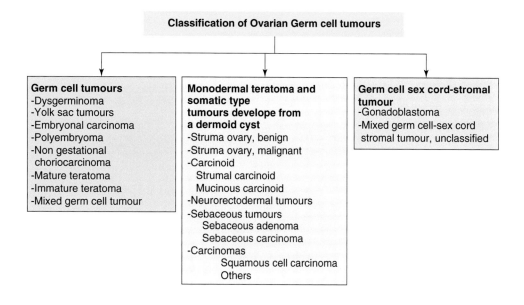

Classification of Ovarian Germ cell tumours

Germ cell tumours
-Dysgerminoma
-Yolk sac tumours
-Embryonal carcinoma
-Polyembryoma
-Non gestational
 choriocarcinoma
-Mature teratoma
-Immature teratoma
-Mixed germ cell tumour

Monodermal teratoma and somatic type tumours develope from a dermoid cyst
-Struma ovary, benign
-Struma ovary, malignant
-Carcinoid
  Strumal carcinoid
  Mucinous carcinoid
-Neurorectodermal tumours
-Sebaceous tumours
  Sebaceous adenoma
  Sebaceous carcinoma
-Carcinomas
    Squamous cell carcinoma
    Others

Germ cell sex cord-stromal tumour
-Gonadoblastoma
-Mixed germ cell-sex cord
 stromal tumour, unclassified

© Springer Nature Singapore Pte Ltd. 2019
P. Dey, *Color Atlas of Female Genital Tract Pathology*, https://doi.org/10.1007/978-981-13-1029-4_9

Dysgerminoma

Image gallery: Figs. 9.2, 9.3, 9.4, and 9.5.

Fig. 9.2 (**a**) Gross picture of dysgerminoma: Smooth outer surface. (**b**) Gross picture of dysgerminoma: Cut section showing grey white solid area with foci of necrosis

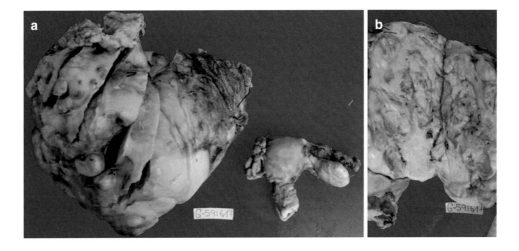

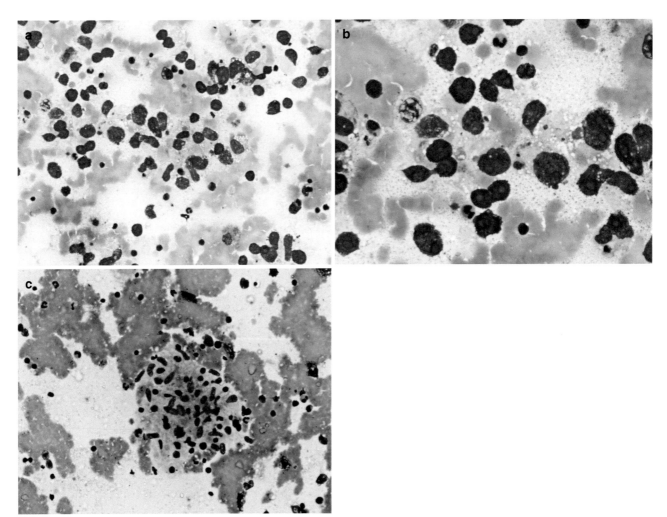

Fig. 9.3 (**a**) Cytology smear of dysgerminoma: Discrete tumour cells. (**b**) Cytology smear of dysgerminoma: The individual tumour cells with scanty deep blue cytoplasm and large nuclei with fine chromatin. (**c**) Cytology smear of dysgerminoma: Epithelioid cell granuloma

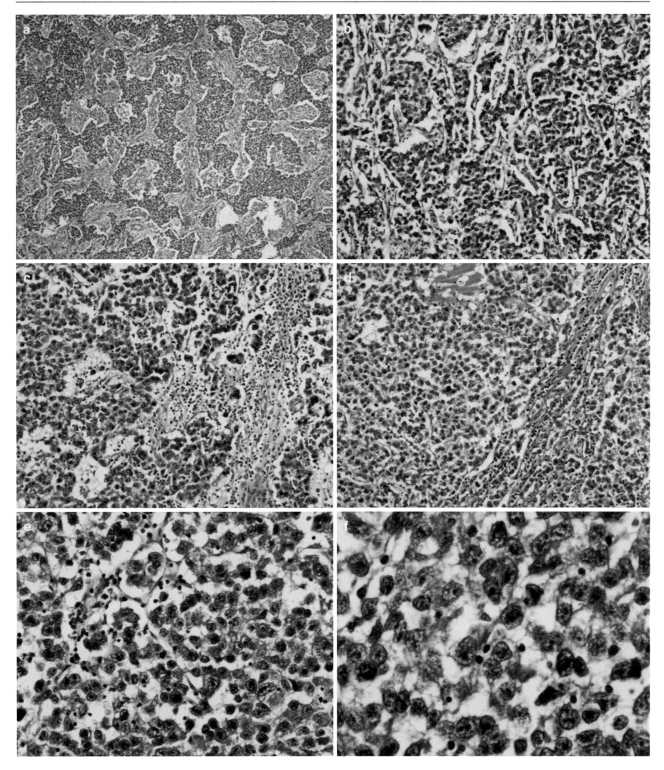

Fig. 9.4 (**a**) Dysgerminoma: Nests of cells with intervening thick fibrous septae. (**b**) Dysgerminoma: Small nests and cords of cells. (**c**) Dysgerminoma: Thick fibrous setae with lymphocytic infiltration. (**d**) Dysgerminoma: Diffuse sheets of cells. (**e**) Dysgerminoma: The tumour cells with sprinkling of lymphocytes. (**f**) Dysgerminoma: The cells with moderate amount of cytoplasm and centrally placed large nuclei having prominent nucleoli

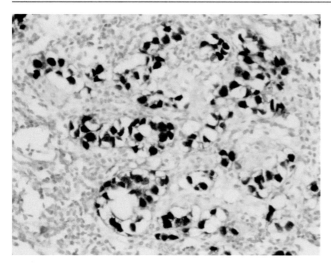

Fig. 9.5 Dysgerminoma: Tumour cells showing nuclear positivity of OCT 4

Epidemiology

- It constitutes 1% of all ovarian cancer
- The commonest malignant germ cell tumours of ovary
- Often admixed with other germ cell tumours (15%)

Clinical features

- Common in second and third decade of life
- Mean age 22 year
- About 25% patients present at the time of pregnancy
- Patient presents with a rapidly developing mass in pelvis
- Abdominal pain
- Serum lactate dehydrogenase level may be elevated
- Occasionally elevated level of human chorionic gonado-trophin level
- Rarely paraneoplastic syndrome may be seen

Gross features

- Predominantly unilateral and 20% tumours are bilateral
- Solid tumour
- Cut section: Firm, lobulated, greyish
- Foci of hemorrhage and necrosis may be seen

Cytology

- Discrete tumour cells admixed with lymphocyte
- Large round cells with deep blue cytoplasm having mod-erately pleomorphic nuclei with prominent nucleoli
- Occasional epithelioid cell granulomas

Histopathology

- Arrangement: Predominantly in diffuse sheet and nests, and in addition trabecular and insular patterns are also present
- Individual cells are large polygonal with abundant pale cytoplasm
- The cytoplasm contains glycogen that is PAS positive and diastase sensitive
- Centrally enlarged nuclei with vesicular chromatin and single prominent nucleoli
- High mitotic rate
- Intersecting fibrous septa with lymphocytes within it
- Epithelioid cell granulomas are present in 20% cases
- Syncytiotrophoblastic cells are also present in 2% cases

Immunohistochemistry

- *Positive*:
  - Placental alkaline phosphatase (PLAP) positive: Both cytoplasmic and also membranous
  - CD 117 (C- Kit)
  - D2-40
  - OCT-4, NANOG and CK

Molecular genetics

- Mutation of C-Kit
- 12p abnormality: isochromosome 12p

Key diagnostic features: See Box 9.1.

Box 9.1 Key Diagnostic Features of Dysgerminoma
- Predominantly diffuse sheet and nests of tumour cells
- large polygonal with abundant pale cytoplasm
- Large nuclei with vesicular chromatin and single prominent nucleoli
- Fibrous septa is infiltrated with lymphocytes
- Epithelioid cell granulomas often present
- High mitotic rate
- Frequently necrosis may be present
- Occasionally syncytiotrophoblastic cells present
- Immunohistochemistry: Positive for OCT 4, CD 117 (c-kit), and placental alkaline phosphatase

Differential diagnosis (Fig. 9.6).

- Yolk sac tumours
  - Presence of Schiller Duval bodies
  - Hyaline globules
  - Absent lymphocytic infiltration in the stroma
  - Nuclear pleomorphism is marked
  - High alpha feto protein
- Non Hodgkin lymphoma: Large cell type
  - Usually bilateral
  - Diffuse sheets of cells
  - CD 45 positive
- Clear cell carcinoma
  - Often associated with endometriosis
  - Glands and papillae may be present
  - Strong CK positivity (PLAP is not helpful)
- Sertoli cell tumour
  - Tubules present

- Lymphocytic infiltration is absent
- Inhibin and calretinin positive and negative for OCT4 and PLAP

Prognosis

- Good prognosis
- Five year survival of stage I tumour: 80–90%
- The tumour recurrence is seen usually in first few years after therapy

Treatment

- Fertility sparing surgery in early stage: Unilateral salpingo oophorectomy and contralateral ovarian biopsy
- If fertility of patient is not considered as an issue: hysterectomy and bilateral salpingo-oophorectomy

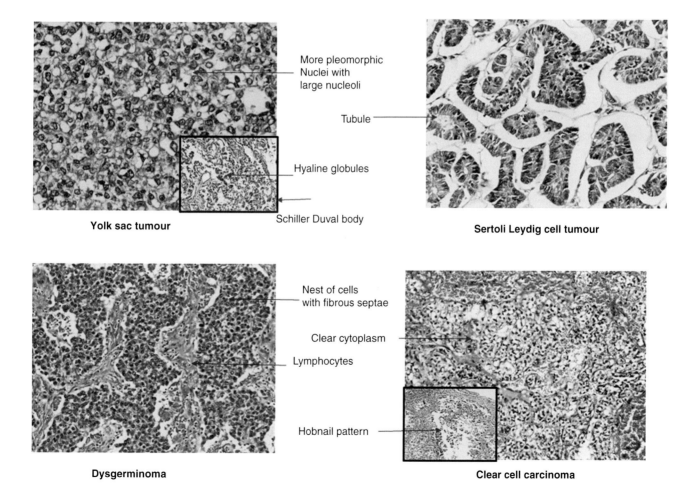

Yolk sac tumour   More pleomorphic Nuclei with large nucleoli   Tubule   Hyaline globules   Schiller Duval body   Sertoli Leydig cell tumour

Dysgerminoma   Nest of cells with fibrous septae   Clear cytoplasm   Lymphocytes   Hobnail pattern   Clear cell carcinoma

Fig. 9.6 Differential diagnosis of dysgerminoma

Yolk Sac Tumour

Image gallery: Figs. 9.7, 9.8, 9.9, 9.10, and 9.11.
  Synonyms: endodermal sinus tumour.
  Abbreviation: Yolk sac tumour (YST).
  Epidemiology

- Represents nearly 20% of all malignant germ cell tumours of ovary
- Represents about 1% of all ovarian malignancies

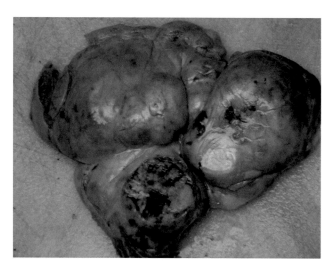

Fig. 9.7 Gross picture of Yolk sac tumour: Solid lobulated tumour. Cut section showing necrosis and haemorrhage

Clinical features

- Children and young females are commonly affected
- Mean age 19 years
- Chief complaints: Rapidly developing mass in abdomen and pain
- Uncommonly virilizing features due to gonadal dysgenesis
- Raised serum alpha fetoprotein level

Gross features

- Unilateral tumour
- Usually large mass and mean diameter 15 cm
- Cut section: solid, grayish yellow, foci of hemorrhage or necrosis may be present

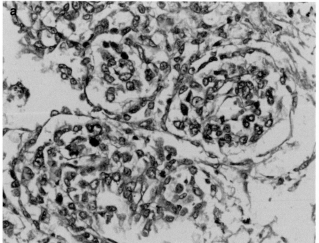
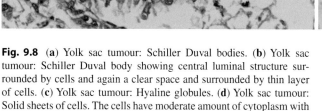
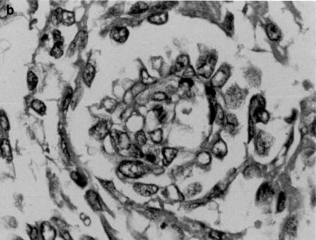

Fig. 9.8 (**a**) Yolk sac tumour: Schiller Duval bodies. (**b**) Yolk sac tumour: Schiller Duval body showing central luminal structure surrounded by cells and again a clear space and surrounded by thin layer of cells. (**c**) Yolk sac tumour: Hyaline globules. (**d**) Yolk sac tumour: Solid sheets of cells. The cells have moderate amount of cytoplasm with large pleomorphic nuclei. (**e**) Yolk sac tumour: Reticular pattern. (**f**) Yolk sac tumour: Reticular pattern showing interwoven spaces. (**g**) Yolk sac tumour: Microcystic pattern. (**h**) Yolk sac tumour: Higher magnification showing small cystic structures lined by tumour cells

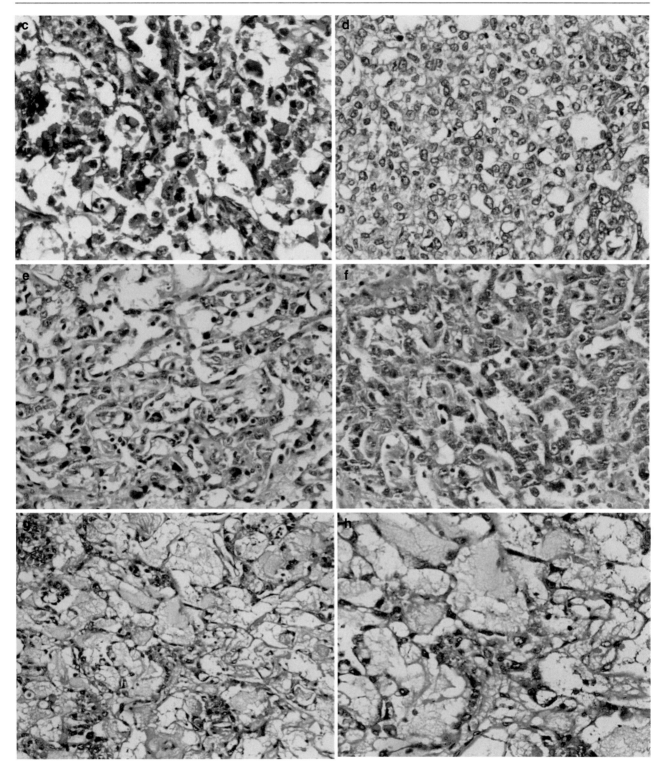

Fig. 9.8 (continued)

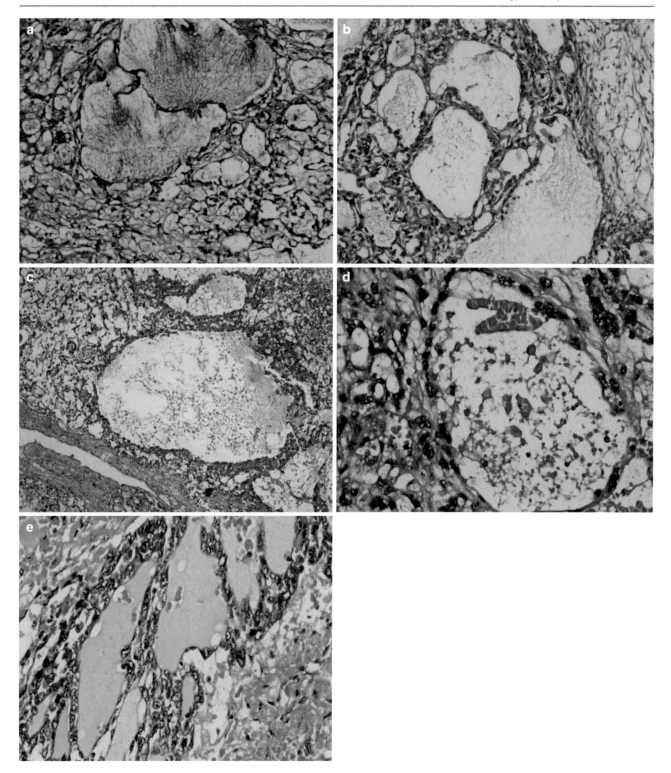

Fig. 9.9 (a) Yolk sac tumour: Macrocystic pattern showing large cystic spaces. (b) Yolk sac tumour: Macrocystic pattern. (c) Yolk sac tumour: Polyvesicular pattern. (d) Yolk sac tumour: Polyvesicular pattern show-ing numerous vesicular structures. (e) Yolk sac tumour: Polyvesicular pattern showing many vesicular structures containing thin fluid

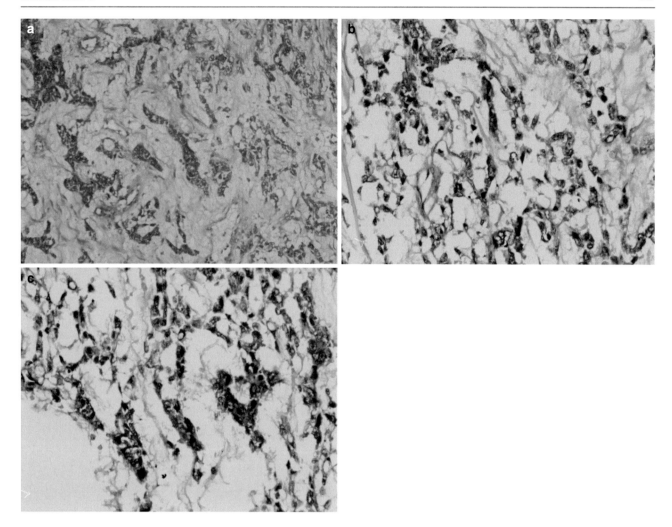

Fig. 9.10 (**a**) Yolk sac tumour: Multiple rows of cells. (**b**) Yolk sac tumour: The cells are arranged in thin rows. (**c**) Yolk sac tumour: Higher magnification of the same

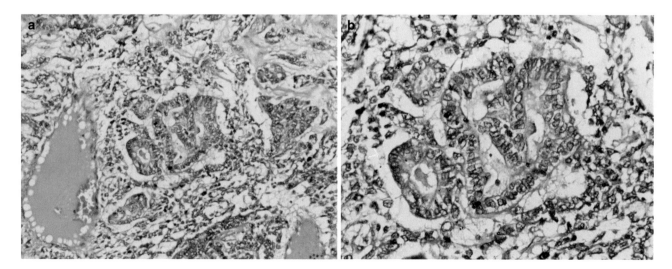

Fig. 9.11 (**a**) Yolk sac tumour: Endometrial gland like pattern. (**b**) Yolk sac tumour: Higher magnification of the gland pattern showing multiple glands lined by the tumour cells

Histopathology

Morphologic Pattern

YST shows various morphological patterns:

- Reticular:
  - Interanastomosing loose channel like spaces that look like honeycomb.
  - These spaces are lined by tumour cells that are flat to cuboidal containing atypical nuclei
  - Many reddish globules are present that are PAS positive and diastase resistant
- Endodermal sinus pattern
  - Many gland and papillae like structures
  - Characteristic Schiller Duval bodies present: Central capillaries surrounded by loose connective tissue and then peripheral rim of tumour cells
- Pseudopapillary
  - Multiple papillae with central fibrovascular core
  - Papillary lining cells show moderately pleomorphic nuclei having large prominent nucleoli
- Solid pattern
  - Solid sheets of tumour cells
  - Individual tumour cells are large with round moderately pleomorphic vesicular nuclei having prominent nucleoli
- Alveolar–glandular pattern
  - Alveolar, cystic spaces and glandular structures that are surrounded by myxomatous stroma
  - The lining cells of the alveoli are cuboidal with moderately pleomorphic nuclei
- Polyvesicular vitelline pattern
  - Many cysts or vesicles within the fibrocollagenous loose stroma
  - The cysts are lined by cuboidal cells having moderately pleomorphic nuclei
- Hepatoid pattern
  - It is composed of diffuse sheets of cells simulating hepatocytes
  - The tumour cells are polygonal with abundant eosinophilic cytoplasm having central nuclei
  - The tumour cells are positive for hepatocyte paraffin 1 antigen
- Hyaline globules
  - Eosinophilic round structures
  - Both intra and extracellular
  - These hyaline bodies are present in all the variants of YST
  - Also present in: Clear cell carcinoma
  - Positive for alpha feto protein (AFP) and occasionally alpha 1 antitrypsin

Immunohistochemistry

- *Positive for*
  - AFP: Dense cytoplasmic
  - CK
  - PLAP
  - CD 34
- *Negative for*
  - CD 117
  - EMA

Molecular Genetics

- Gain of chromosome 12i(12p)

Key diagnostic features: See Box 9.2.

Box 9.2 Key Diagnostic Features of Yolk Sac Tumour
- Predominantly reticular pattern, in addition various other patterns such as microcystic, pseudopapillary, solid, alveolar–glandular, polyvesicular vitelline and hepatoid present
- Tumour cells are large with clear cytoplasm
- Large pleomorphic nuclei with coarse chromatin
- Large nucleoli
- Characteristic Schiller Duval bodies
- Hyaline globules
- Immunohistochemistry: Positive for alpha fetoprotein, CK, PLAP, and CD 34

Differential diagnosis (Figs. 9.12 and 9.13).

- Sertoli leydig cell tumour (retiform variant)
  - No typical Schiller Duval bodies present
  - Individual tumour cell are less pleomorphic
  - Often androgenic manifestation
  - Inhibin positive and AFP negative
- Clear cell carcinoma
  - Most confusing because of overlapping histological features and this tumour often shows AFP positivity
  - No typical Schiller Duval bodies
  - Often shows associated endometriosis
  - Positive for EMA and CK 7
- Endometrioid carcinoma
  - Elderly patient
  - Squamous metaplasia
  - Endometriosis may also be seen

Fig. 9.12 Differential diagnosis of Yolk sac tumour with clear cell carcinoma

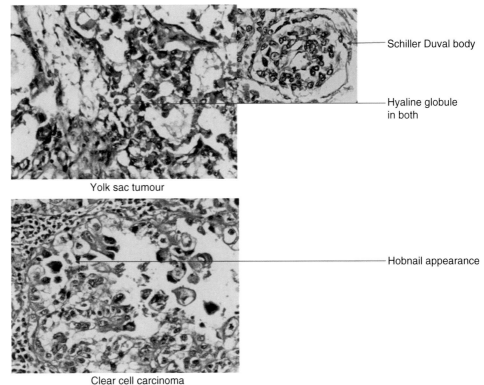

Schiller Duval body

Hyaline globule in both

Yolk sac tumour

Hobnail appearance

Clear cell carcinoma

- – Other characteristics of YST such as Schiller Duval bodies and hyaline globules are absent
- – AFP negative and positive for ER/PR, CK 7 and EMA
- Dysgerminoma
  - – Nuclear pleomorphism is comparatively less
  - – Presence of lymphocytes in the stroma
  - – Absence of the characteristic features of YST
  - – Immunostaining: OCT 4 positive and AFP negative
- Hepatocellular carcinoma (HCC)
  - – Metastatic HCC is usually bilateral
  - – The other pattern of YST missing

Prognosis

- Highly aggressive malignant tumour
- Metastasis in liver, peritoneal cavity and abdominal lymph nodes is common
- Different histological pattern has no impact on prognosis
- Unilateral salpingo oophorectomy followed by combination chemotherapy is the treatment protocol
- Serum AFP level is used for monitoring the patient

Fig. 9.13 (**a**) Differential diagnosis of yolk sac tumour with endometrioid carcinoma and sertoli leydig cell tumour. (**b**) Differential diagnosis of yolk sac tumour with dysgerminoma

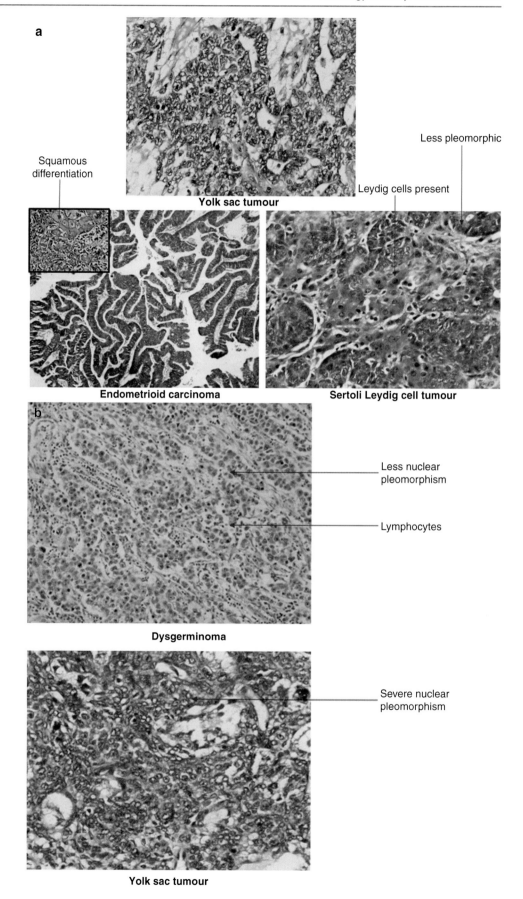

Embryonal Carcinoma

Image gallery: Fig. 9.14a–c.

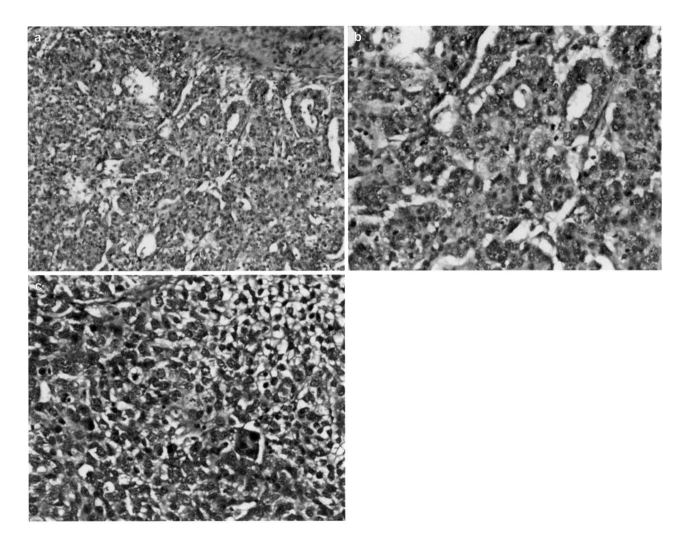

Fig. 9.14 (**a**) Embryonal carcinoma: Sheets of tumour cells with occasional ill formed glands. (**b**) Embryonal carcinoma: Higher magnification of the same. (**c**) Embryonal carcinoma: The sheets of tumour cells with polygonal appearance and central vesicular nuclei having prominent nucleoli

Epidemiology

- Rare malignant tumour
- Only 3% of all germ cell neoplasms of ovary

Clinical features

- Almost all patients are under 30 year
- Mean age 12 years
- Presents with abdominal pain and rapidly developing pelvic mass

Gross features

- Unilateral large tumour
- Mean size 15 cm
- Cut section: solid, greyish color with areas of hemorrhage and necrosis

Histopathology

- Diffuse sheets or nest of cells
- Large polygonal cells with abundant clear cytoplasm
- Centrally placed moderate to severely pleomorphic nuclei
- Large prominent nucleoli

Immunohistochemistry

- Positive for CK, OCT 4, SOX 2, CD 30 and PLAP

Differential diagnosis

- Dysgerminoma
  - Less nuclear pleomorphism
  - Mitotic rate is lower than embryonal carcinoma
  - Cytoplasmic border is distinct
- YST
  - Characteristic Schiller Duval bodies present
  - Negative for CD 30 and OCT 4
- Juvenile granulosa cell tumour
- Undifferentiated carcinoma
  - Elderly patient
  - EMA positive

Prognosis and treatment

- Highly aggressive tumour
- Unilateral salpingo oophorectomy followed by combination chemotherapy is the treatment of choice

Non Gestational Choriocarcinoma

Image gallery: Fig. 9.15a, b.
  Epidemiology

- Extremely rare tumour
- It represents less than 1% of malignant germ cell neoplasms of ovary
- Most of the time choriocarcinoma occurs as a part of other germ cell tumour

Clinical features

- Young patients
- Pain abdomen and pelvic mass
- Increased serum beta hCG level

Gross features

- Unilateral
- Large tumour
- Solid and foci of cystic changes
- Grey white with focal hemorrhage and necrosis

Histopathology

- Plexiform and diffuse sheets of cells
- Dual population of tumour cells: mononuclear cytotrophoblasts and multinucleated syncytiotrophoblast
- Cytotrophoblasts: Large oval to polygonal cells with distinct cytoplasmic border. Cells contain single large moderately pleomorphic nuclei and prominent nucleoli
- Syncytiotrophoblast: Large cells with moderate amount of cytoplasm having multiple hyperchromatic nuclei

Immunohistochemistry

- Positive: hCG, and PLAP

Differential diagnosis

- Undifferentiated carcinoma
- YST
- Embryonal carcinoma

Prognosis and treatment

- Aggressive malignancy
- Often spreads to the distant organs such as lung
- Unilateral salpingo-oophorectomy followed by combination chemotherapy is the treatment of choice

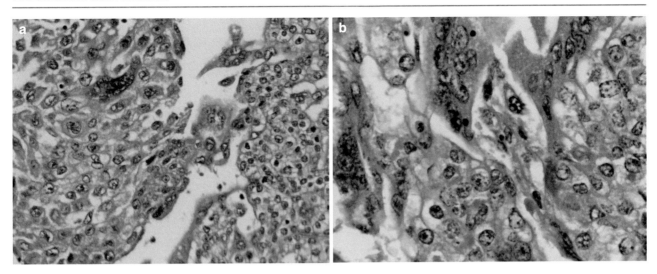

Fig. 9.15 (**a**) Choriocarcinoma: Both cyto and syncytiotrophoblasts present. (**b**) Choriocarcinoma: Large oval to polygonal cells with distinct cytoplasmic border

Teratoma

Mature Teratoma

Image gallery: Figs. 9.16, 9.17, and 9.18.
  Synonym: Dermoid cyst, mature cystic teratoma.
  Epidemiology

- Twenty five percent of all ovarian tumours
- About 90% of all germ cell neoplasms of ovary

Clinical features

- It occurs mainly in 20–50 years period
- Rare in postmenopausal patients
- Patients may be asymptomatic in 50% cases
- Pain abdomen and mass in pelvis

Gross features

- Unilateral in 85% cases
- Size varies from 2 to 40 cm
- Mean size 15 cm
- Cystic

- Uniloculated cyst
- It contains hair and sebaceous material
- Prominent solid area may be seen which is known as Rokitansky's protuberance

Histopathology

- All three germ layers present: ectodermal, endodermal and mesodermal
- Ectodermal elements: epidermis, sweat gland, sebaceous glands, hair follicles etc.
- Endodermal elements: Respiratory lining tissue, glands etc.
- Mesodermal elements: Cartilage, bone etc.
- Rarely carcinoma may develop from the germ cell components: Commonly squamous cell carcinoma, followed by adenocarcinomas and small cell carcinoma

Prognosis

- Benign tumour
- Young woman: Cystectomy
- Elderly woman: Unilateral salpingo oophorectomy

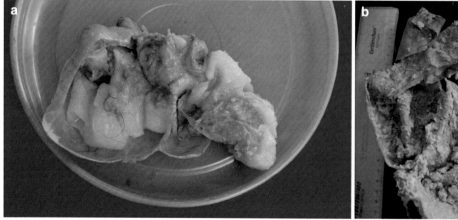
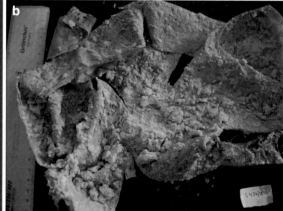

Fig. 9.16 (**a**) Gross picture of mature cystic teratoma showing heterogeneous texture. (**b**) Gross picture of mature cystic teratoma: The cut section showing cheesy material and also bunch of hair

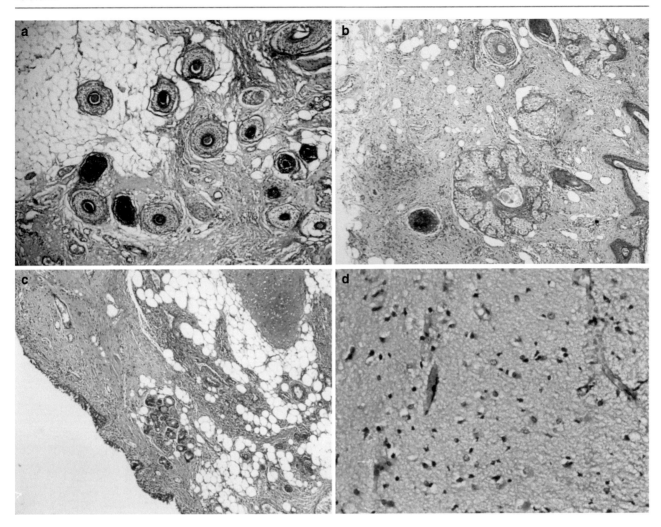

Fig. 9.17 (**a**) Mature teratoma: Multiple hair follicles and fat. (**b**) Mature teratoma: Hair follicles and sebaceous glands. (**c**) Mature teratoma: Fat, cartilage, and glands. (**d**) Mature teratoma: Mature glial tissue

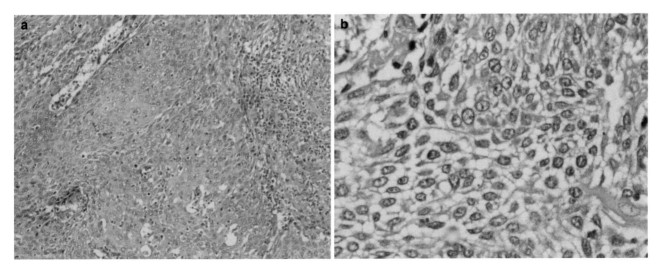

Fig. 9.18 (**a**) Squamous cell carcinoma in mature teratoma: Sheets of malignant squamous cells in a mature teratoma. (**b**) Squamous cell carcinoma in mature teratoma: Higher magnification showing polyhedral cells having large pleomorphic nuclei

Immature Teratoma

Image gallery: Figs. 9.19, 9.20, and 9.21.
  Epidemiology

- 1% of all malignant ovarian tumour
- 3% of ovarian teratoma

  Clinical features

- It is seen mainly under 30 years of age
- Mean age 19 years
- Pelvic mass and pain in abdomen

  Gross features

- Large unilateral mass
- Size varies from 8 to 30 cm, mean size 18 cm
- Solid tumour

- Cut section grey to tan color, lobulated, variegated fleshy
- Foci of hemorrhage and necrosis may be present

  Histopathology

- Haphazard arrangement of mature and immature elements
- Immature elements:
  - Immature neuroepithelial tissue with rosettes and tubules
  - The neuroepithelial rosette: Central lumen containing fibrillary material encircled by cuboidal cells
  - Immature glial tissue
  - Immature cartilage and bone
  - Primitive retinal tissue
- Mature components also coexist
- Immature teratoma are often mixed with other germ cell tumours: YST, embryonal carcinoma, dysgerminoma, choriocarcinoma etc. This

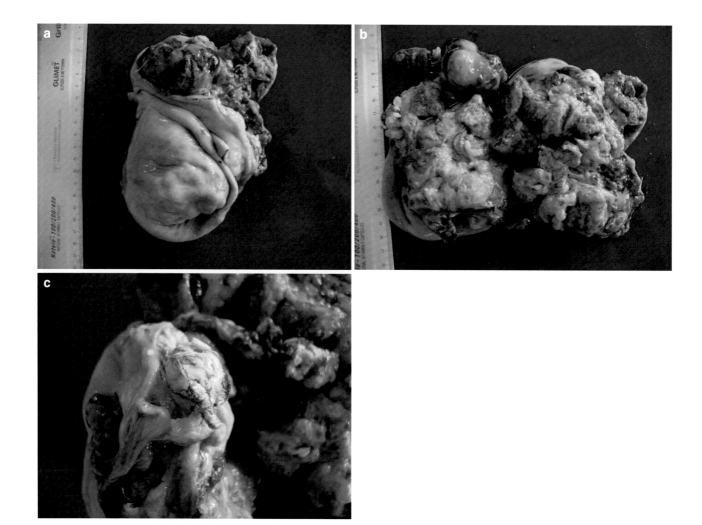

Fig. 9.19 (**a**) Immature teratoma: Outer surface is smooth and shiny. (**b**) Immature teratoma: Cut section of the gross specimen showing solid grey white area. (**c**) Immature teratoma: Bony hard area in the teratoma

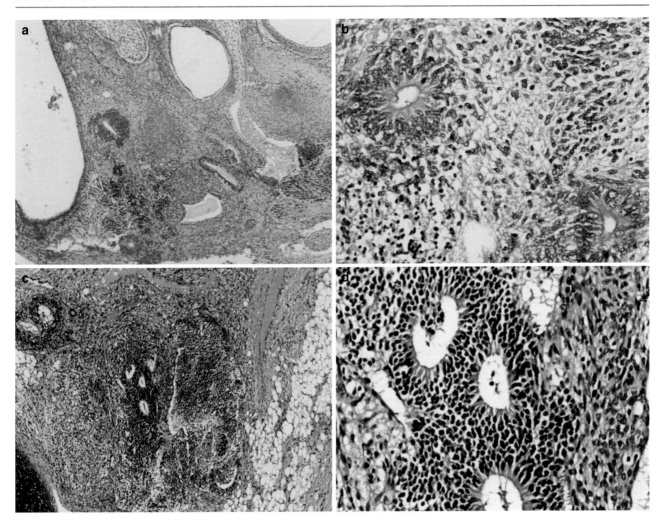

Fig. 9.20 (**a**) Immature teratoma: Immature neuroepithelial tissue. (**b**) Immature teratoma: Multiple rosettes. (**c**) Immature teratoma: Mature cartilage and glands along with immature neuroepithelial tissue in the form of rosettes. (**d**) Immature teratoma: Higher magnification of the same showing rosettes

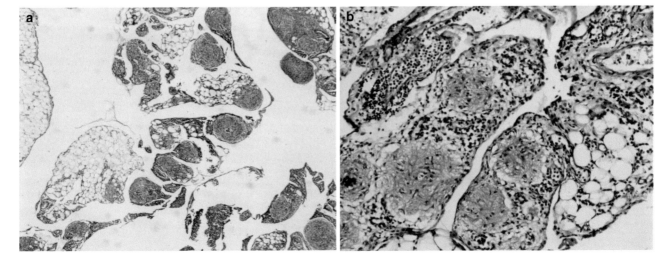

Fig. 9.21 (**a**) Immature teratoma: Peritoneal gliomatosis showing fat and glial tissue. (**b**) Immature teratoma: Peritoneal gliomatosis showing glial tissue

Grading of Immature Teratoma

Grading is based on the basis of frequency of immature neuroepithelial tissue. It is mentioned in the Table 9.1 below.

- Metastatic implant is considered as Grade 0: If no immature neural tissue seen
- Gliomatosis peritonei: Peritoneal implants that contain only mature glial element

Immunohistochemistry

- No good role
- Immature neural and neuroepithelial tissues: Positive for SALL 4, SOX 2, glypican 3
- Hepatic tissue: AFP

Differential diagnosis (Fig. 9.22).

- Mature cystic teratoma
  - Immature neuroepithelial component is mandatory for the diagnosis of immature teratoma
- Carcinosarcoma (malignant mixed Müllerian tumour) (see Table 9.2)
  - Elderly patient
  - Other germ cell components such as mature ectodermal, endodermal or mesenchymal components are absent
  - Carcinoma component: serous, high grade adenocarcinoma or adenosquamous carcinoma.
  - Not much variable histologic structures as seen in immature teratoma

Table 9.1 Immature teratoma grading

Grade	Frequency of immature neuroepithelial component
Grade 1	Occasional foci, less than 1 per LPF
Grade 2	1 to 3 per LPF
Grade 3	More than 3 per LPF

LPF Low power field, means 4 X Objective

Fig. 9.22 Differential diagnosis of immature teratoma

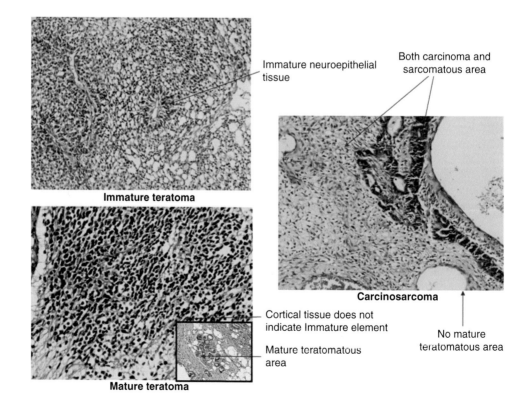

Immature neuroepithelial tissue

Both carcinoma and sarcomatous area

Immature teratoma

Carcinosarcoma

Cortical tissue does not indicate Immature element

Mature teratomatous area

No mature teratomatous area

Mature teratoma

Table 9.2 Distinguishing features between immature teratoma versus carcinosarcoma

Features	Immature teratoma	Carcinosarcoma
Age	Younger patient: 20–30 year	Elderly patient: 50–70 year
Mature teratomatous elements	Often present	Absent
Neuroectodermal element	Present	Usually absent
Malignant components	Malignant components are usually other germ cell tumours such as yolk sac tumour, dysgerminoma, choriocarcinoma etc	Carcinoma components are adenocarcinoma, squamous cell carcinoma Sarcoma components are chondrosarcoma, leiomyosarcoma, Fibrosarcoma etc

Prognosis

- Predominant prognostic factors are: Grade and stage of the tumour
- Grade 1 stage I tumour has very good prognosis compared to grade 2 and 3 tumour

Treatment

- Grade 1 tumour localized to one ovary only: unilateral salpingo-oophorectomy
- Grade 2/3 tumour localized to one ovary only: unilateral salpingo-oophorectomy followed by combination chemotherapy
- In the involvement of contralateral ovarian involvement: Total abdominal hysterectomy with bilateral salpingo-oophorectomy followed by adjuvant chemotherapy

Mixed Germ Cell Tumours

Image gallery: Fig. 9.23a–c.

Definition: The mixed germ cell tumour contains more than one germ cell tumour components.

Epidemiology

- Approximate 10% of germ cell tumour
- More number of such tumours are now reported due to the extensive examination

Clinical features

- Young patients
- Average age 15 year
- Serum tumour markers may be elevated: high AFP and beta HCG
- No other specific symptoms

Histopathology

- Dysgerminoma admixed with YST is the most frequent combination
- The individual tumour components are in variable amount and are admixed either homogenously or in separate areas
- Even the presence of minor foci of the other germ cell component should be mentioned

Prognosis

- Prognosis largely depends on the proportion of the high grade germ cell components such as YST and choriocarcinoma
- Tumours containing large areas of grade 3 immature teratoma or YST show worst prognosis

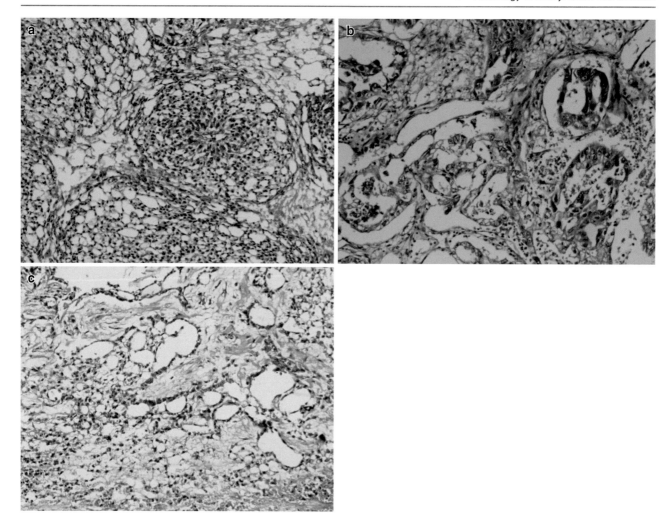

Fig. 9.23 (**a**) Mixed germ cell tumours: Immature teratoma showing neuroepithelial component along with yolk sac tumour component. (**b**) Mixed germ cell tumours: Yolk sac tumour component in the immature teratoma. (**c**) Mixed germ cell tumours: Microcystic spaces of Yolk sac tumour component in immature teratoma

Monodermal Teratoma

Struma Ovarii

Image gallery: Figs. 9.24 and 9.25.

Fig. 9.24 Gross picture of struma ovarii showing sloid waxy cut surface

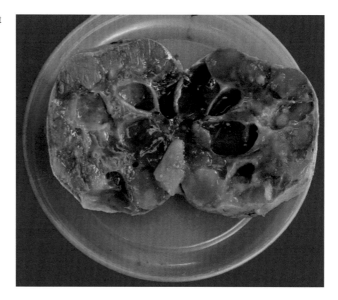

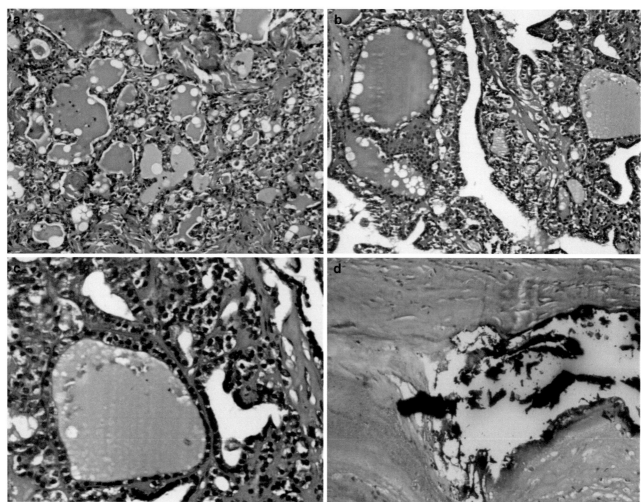

Fig. 9.25 (**a**) Struma ovarii: Micro and macrofollicles of thyroid. (**b**) Struma ovarii: Thyroid follicle filled with pinkish colloid material. (**c**) Struma ovarii: Micro and Macrofollicle of thyroid. (**d**) Struma ovarii: Calcification in struma

Definition: The type of mature teratoma that consists of predominantly thyroid tissue (more than 50%).

Epidemiology

- About 3% of all teratoma
- The commonest monodermal teratoma

Clinical features

- Women in reproductive age period
- Usually no specific symptoms
- Occasional patients may have hyperthyroidism
- Rarely: Meig's syndrome

Gross features

- Unilateral
- Size varies from 1 to 10 cm
- Solid
- Cut section: soft, gray to reddish

Histopathology

- Macrofillicular, microfollicular, trabecular and solid areas of thyroid tissue
- Intervening edematous stroma
- The thyroid follicles are lined by small cuboidal cells with monomorphic nuclei
- Calcification, and old hemorrhagic foci may be seen

Immunohistochemistry

- Tumour cells are positive: TTF 1, thyroglobulin

Differential diagnosis

- *Granulosa cell tumour*
    - Thyroid follicles are lined by cuboidal cells with bland nuclear morphology whereas Call Exner bodies are lined by granulosa cells.
- *Clear cell carcinoma*
    - Cells with abundant clear cytoplasm
    - EMA positive and thyroglobulin negative
- *Serous cystadenoma*
    - The glands are positive for CK 7 and negative for thyroglobulin

Prognosis

- Benign neoplasm
- Unilateral salpingo oophorectomy is the treatment of choice

Malignancy in Struma Ovarii

Image gallery: Fig. 9.26a–b.

Papillary thyroid carcinoma: Characteristic features of papillary carcinoma such as

- Papillae
- Nuclear features
    - Nuclear clearing
    - Nuclear longitudinal groove
    - Intranuclear inclusions

Follicular carcinoma

- Presence of vascular invasion
- Capsular infiltration
- Cells may show nuclear atypia and increased mitosis

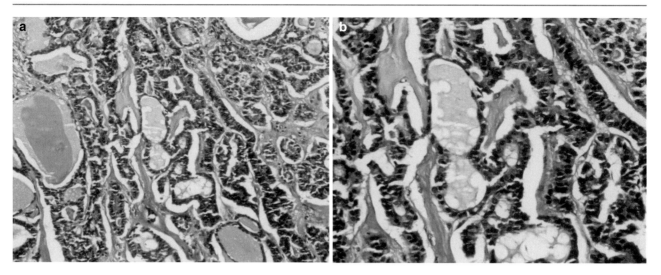

Fig. 9.26 (**a**) Follicular carcinoma in struma ovarii: Abundant microfollicles. (**b**) Follicular carcinoma in struma ovarii: Higher magnification of the microfollicles

Carcinoid

Image gallery: Fig. 9.27a, b.
  Synonym: Neuroendocrine tumour.
  Epidemiology

- Uncommon tumour in ovary
- Less than 1% of ovarian teratomas

Clinical features

- Mainly perimenopausal patients
- Mean age 53 years
- Most of the time incidental detection of the tumour
- One third patients present with carcinoid syndrome such as flushing, diarrhea, cardiac murmur, hypertension etc. The carcinoid syndrome predominantly occurs in insular carcinoid type.

Gross features

- Unilateral
- Solid tumour
- Often nodular mass on the wall of mature cystic teratoma
- Variable size
- Cut section: yellowish to brown color

Histopathology

- *Types*: Insular, trabecular, strumal, and mucinous carcinoid
- *Insular carcinoid*
  – Multiple nests and acini of cells separated by fibrocollagenous stroma
  – Acini are either in the periphery or central part of the nests and often gives a cribriform appearance
  – Individual cells are round to polygonal with abundant cytoplasm
  – Often reddish granulation in the cytoplasm
  – Central monomorphic round nuclei with "salt and pepper" chromatin
  – Low mitotic activity
- *Trabecular*
  – Tumour cells are arranged in trabeculae and cords
  – Long linear rows of cells that often anastomose within a fibrous stroma
  – Tumour cells have abundant eosinophilic cytoplasm
  – Long axis of nuclei is perpendicular to the axis of the cord
- *Strumal carcinoid*
  – Carcinoid tumour is mixed with thyroid tissue components
  – Carcinoid component is usually trabecular type
- *Mucinous carcinoid*
  – Many small glands within a loose edematous stroma
  – The glands often floats in acellular mucinous material
  – Around a central lumen the columnar to cuboidal cells are arranged. Goblet cells are also present.

Immunohistochemistry

- Overall the tumour cells are positive for CD 56, chromogranin and synaptophysin
- Insular and trabecular type: CK7 positive, CK 20 negative
- Mucinous type: CK 7 negative and CK 20 positive
- Strumal type: TTF 1 positive

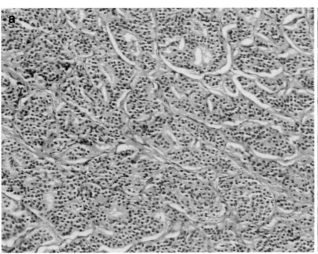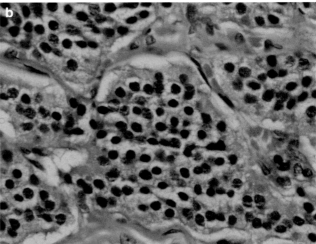

Fig. 9.27 (**a**) Insular carcinoid: Multiple nests of cells separated by fibrous septae. (**b**) Insular carcinoid: Round cells with moderate amount of cytoplasm

Differential diagnosis

- Metastatic carcinoid
  - History of primary
  - Usually carcinoid syndrome present
  - Both the ovaries involved
  - Lack of any dermoid cyst component
  - Predominantly insular or mucinous type
- Granulosa cell tumour
  - Call Exner bodies may simulate acinar type of carcinoid
  - Nuclear grooves present
  - Inhibin positivity
- Krukenberg's tumour
  - Always bilateral
  - Typical signet ring cells present
  - No components of teratoma

Prognosis

- Good prognosis as most of the carcinoids (95%) show benign course
- Overall 5 year survival: 95%
- Mucinous carcinoid often shows malignant behavior

Gonadoblastoma

Epidemiology

- Rare neoplasm of ovary

Clinical features

- The patients are phenotypically female having gonadal dysgenesis
- Mostly asymptomatic and incidentally detected
- Detected at the time of investigations for amenorrhea

Gross features

- More frequent in right gonads
- Variable size, usually small and less than 8 cm in diameter
- Solid, lobulated
- Cut section: gray white, firm to hard, often whitish calcified material

Histopathology

- Multiple nest of tumour cells
- The nest of cells contain germ cells and acinar like arrangement of primitive sex cord like cells.
- The sex cord cells form acini around a central eosinophilic material. These cells resemble sertoli and granulosa cells
- The germ cells resemble the tumour cells of dysgerminoma
- Foci of calcification and hyaline plaques are also noted

Immunohistochemistry

- Germ cell components are positive for PLAP, OCT-4, NANOG, C-Kit
- Sex cord elements are positive for inhibin, calretinin, FOXL2, and WT 1

Prognosis and treatment

- Benign tumour
- Surgical excision of the tumour is adequate treatment
- Gonadoblastoma with YST may need combination chemotherapy

Reference

1. Kurman RJ, Carcangiu ML, Herrington S, Young RH. WHO classification of tumours of female genital reproductive organs. 4th ed. Lyon: International Agency for Research on Cancer; 2014.

Suggested Reading

Alwazzan AB, Popowich S, Dean E, Robinson C, Lotocki R, Altman AD. Pure immature teratoma of the ovary in adults: thirty-year experience of a single tertiary care center. Int J Gynecol Cancer. 2015;25(9):1616–22.

Aslam MF, Choi C, Khulpateea N. Neuroendocrine tumour of the ovary. J Obstet Gynaecol. 2009;29(5):449–51.

Ayhan A, Aksu T, Selçuk Tuncer Z, Mercan R, Ozbay G. Immature teratoma of the ovary. Eur J Gynaecol Oncol. 1993;14(3):205–7.

Corakçi A, Ozeren S, Ozkan S, Gürbüz Y, Ustün H, Yücesoy I. Pure nongestational choriocarcinoma of ovary. Arch Gynecol Obstet. 2005;271(2):176–7.

Dällenbach P, Bonnefoi H, Pelte MF, Vlastos G. Yolk sac tumours of the ovary: an update. Eur J Surg Oncol. 2006;32(10):1063–75.

Fukunaga M, Endo Y, Miyazawa Y, Ushigome S. Small cell neuroendocrine carcinoma of the ovary. Virchows Arch. 1997;430(4):343–8.

Gallion H, van Nagell JR Jr, Donaldson ES, Hanson MB, Powell DF. Immature teratoma of the ovary. Am J Obstet Gynecol. 1983;146(4):361–5.

Gershenson DM. Update on malignant ovarian germ cell tumours. Cancer (Phila). 1993;71:1581–90.

Goffredo P, Sawka AM, Pura J, Adam MA, Roman SA, Sosa JA. Malignant struma ovarii: a population-level analysis of a large series of 68 patients. Thyroid. 2015;25(2):211–5.

Goyal LD, Kaur S, Kawatra K. Malignant mixed germ cell tumour of ovary--an unusual combination and review of literature. J Ovarian Res. 2014;7:91.

Guillem V, Poveda A. Germ cell tumours of the ovary. Clin Transl Oncol. 2007;9(4):237–43.

Monti E, Mortara L, Zupo S, Dono M, Minuto F, Truini M, Naseri M, Giusti M. Papillary thyroid cancer in a struma ovarii: a report of a rare case. Hormones (Athens). 2015;14(1):154–9.

Nogales FF, Dulcey I, Preda O. Germ cell tumours of the ovary: an update. Arch Pathol Lab Med. 2014;138(3):351–62.

Nogales FF, Preda O, Nicolae A. Yolk sac tumours revisited. A review of their many faces and names. Histopathology. 2012;60(7):1023–33.

Tsuji T, Togami S, Shintomo N, Fukamachi N, Douchi T, Taguchi S. Ovarian large cell neuroendocrine carcinoma. J Obstet Gynaecol Res. 2008;34(4 Pt 2):726–30.

Wang Y, Zhou F, Qian Z, Qing J, Zhao M, Huang L. Mixed ovarian germ cell tumour composed of immature teratoma, yolk sac tumour and embryonal carcinoma. J Coll Physicians Surg Pak. 2014;24(Suppl 3):S198–200.

Wei S, Baloch ZW, LiVolsi VA. Pathology of Struma Ovarii: a report of 96 cases. Endocr Pathol. 2015;26(4):342–8.

Classification of the various miscellaneous tumour of ovary according to World Health Organization [1] has been highlighted in Fig. 10.1.

Fig. 10.1 Classification of miscellaneous ovarian tumours

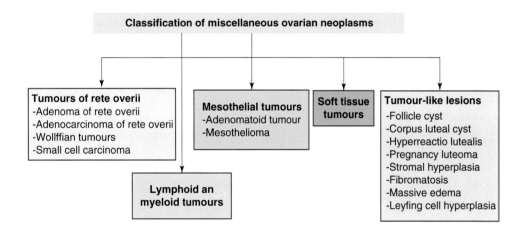

Metastatic Tumours in Ovary

Common sources of metastasis

- Intestine
- Stomach
- Appendix
- Pancreas
- Breast
- Uterus, cervix and fallopian tube

Features indicating metastasis

- Known primary site of malignancy
- Bilateral involvement of ovary
- Less than 10 cm diameter
- Superficial involvement with preserve normal ovarian parenchyma
- Lymphovascular invasion
- Infiltrative growth with marked desmoplastic reaction
- Abundant signet ring cells
- Extensive metastasis

Clinical features

- Age of the patients varies widely from young to old age
- Patients may present with abdominal pain and pelvic mass
- Incidentally the tumour may be detected at the time of other surgery
- In synchronous tumour: Both the primary tumour and ovarian tumour may be detected at the same time
- Rarely the primary tumour may not be detected for long period

Gross features

- Bilateral (70%)
- Smaller than 10 cm size
- Usually solid and nodular
- Uncommonly cystic and simulates primary cystic ovarian tumour
- Cut section: grey white, friable with areas of necrosis and haemorrhage

Individual Primary Sites

Intestinal Carcinoma

- *Common site*: Large intestine
- *Histopathology*
- Multiple small tubular to large glands
- Dirty necrosis surrounded by the glandular epithelial cell simulating garland pattern
- Focal necrosis of the lining epithelial cells
- Cribriform appearance of the crowded glands
- Stroma is desmoplastic or oedematous
- *Immunohistochemistry*
- Positive: CK 7, CDX-2, Dpc4
- Negative: CK 20, PAX 8

Stomach Carcinoma

(Krukenberg's tumour)
   Image gallery: Figs. 10.2, 10.3, 10.4, 10.5, and 10.6.
   Synonym: Krukenberg's tumour, signet ring cell carcinoma.
   Clinical features

- Mean age 43–45 years
- Non-specific complaints: Pain abdomen, pelvic mass
- Occasionally symptoms of gastrointestinal tumour

Gross

- Bilateral (85%)
- Variable size but it may be large (18 cm diameter)
- Solid
- Cut section: Soft to firm, white to reddish brown

Histopathology

- Pseudolobular pattern due to alternate hyper and hypocellular areas
- Glands, tubules, trabecular or nest like pattern may be present
- Stroma is often densely cellular
- Signet ring cells present: Cell with abundant cytoplasm and peripherally pushed nuclei

Immunohistochemistry

- Most of the cells positive for CK 7 than CK 20
- Dpc4 positive
- PAX8, ER/PR are negative

Fig. 10.2 (**a**) Gross of Krukenberg's tumour showing bilateral solid tumour. (**b**) Gross of Krukenberg's tumour showing maintained shape of the ovary. (**c**) Gross of Krukenberg's tumour showing: Solid greyish cut section

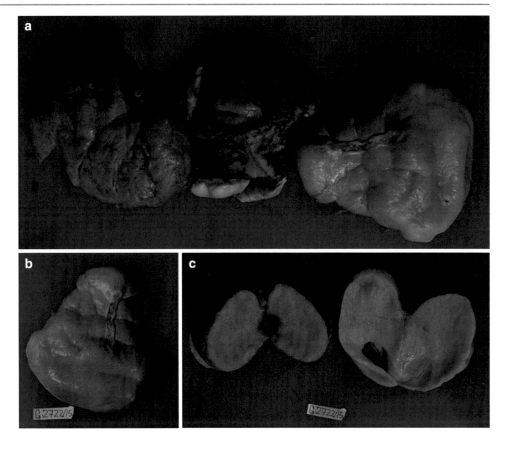

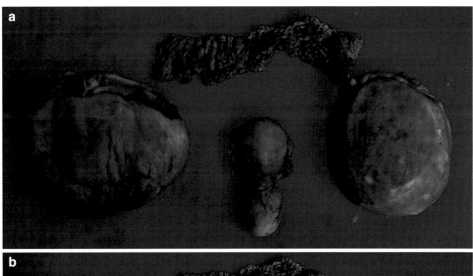

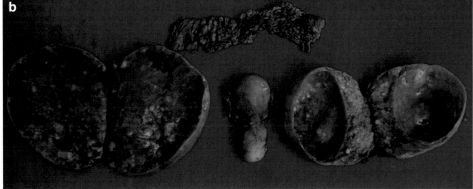

Fig. 10.3 (**a**) Metastatic carcinoma in ovary: Note the bilateral involvement of ovary. (**b**) Metastatic carcinoma in ovary: Solid growth in right ovary and partly solid partly cystic swelling of left ovary

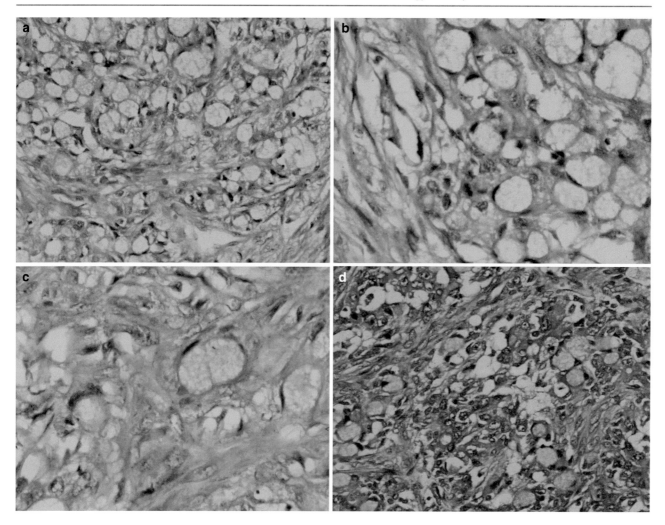

Fig. 10.4 (**a**) Krukenberg's tumour: Diffuse sheet of tumour cells. (**b**) Krukenberg's tumour: Signet ring cells with abundant cytoplasm and peripherally pushed nuclei. (**c**) Krukenberg's tumour: Higher magnification of the signet ring cells. (**d**) Krukenberg's tumour: Alternate hypo and hypercellular areas

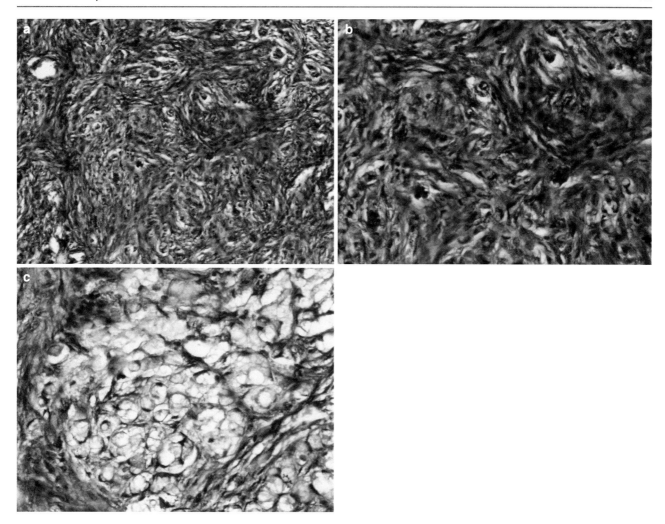

Fig. 10.5 (**a**) Krukenberg's tumour: Small fascicles of tumour cells giving a fibroma like appearance. (**b**) Krukenberg's tumour: Higher magnification of the same. (**c**) Krukenberg's tumour: Foci of signet ring cells in the fibromatous area

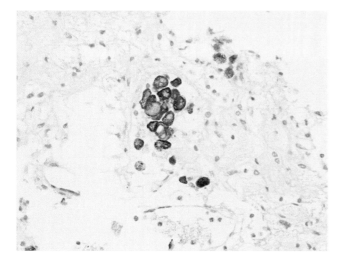

Fig. 10.6 Krukenberg's tumour: CK positivity in signet ring cells

Key diagnostic features: See Box 10.1.

Box 10.1 Key Diagnostic Features of Krukenberg's Tumour

- Alternate hyper and hypocellular areas give rise to pesudolobular pattern
- Small glands or tubules may be present
- Cellular areas contain large number of signet ring cells
- The signet ring cells have abundant vacuolated cytoplasm with eccentric nuclei
- At times stroma is cellular and shows spindle cells in small fascicles and gives rise to fibroma like appearance
- Immunohistochemistry: The tumour cells positive for CK 7 and Dpc4, and negative for PAX8 and ER/PR.

Differential diagnosis (Fig. 10.7).

- Sertoli leydig cell tumour
  - Lack of any signet ring cells
- Fibroma
  - Abundant spindle cells may simulate fibroma
  - Absence of signet ring cells
- Clear cell carcinoma
  - Occasional signet ring type of cells may be seen
  - Tubular gland and cystic space are present
  - Typical hobnail cells
- Mucinous type of carcinoid
  - Teratoma elements seen
  - Presence of goblet cells and Paneth cells

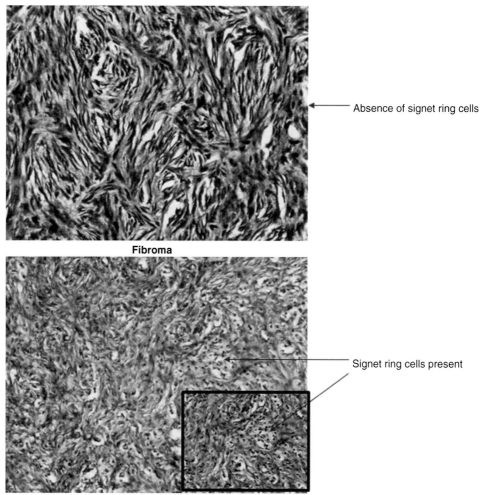

Absence of signet ring cells

Fibroma

Signet ring cells present

Krukenberg's tumor

Fig. 10.7 Differential diagnosis of Krukenberg's tumour and fibroma

Appendicular Carcinoma

Epidemiology

- Uncommon, only 1% of metastasis in ovary

Clinical features

- Patients are middle aged women
- Mean age: 52 years
- Mass in pelvis

Gross features

- Bilateral (80%)
- Large in size, mean diameter 15 cm
- Usually solid, however may have cystic component

Histopathology
Krukenberg's type

- Arrangement: Tubules, cords or trabecular
- Stroma is cellular and fibrous
- Signet ring cells are present and may give the appearance of Krukenberg's tumour

Intestinal type

- Intestinal type glands present
- Cribriform appearance of the glands
- Frequent mitosis

Immunohistochemistry

- Positive for CK 20 and Dpc4
- Negative for CK 7, p16, PAX 8

Pancreatic and Biliary Tract Tumour

Gall Bladder Carcinoma
Image gallery: Fig. 10.8.
   Epidemiology

- Rare primary sites for metastasis in ovary

Clinical features

- Wide age range: 30–85 year, mean age 63 year
- Non-specific symptoms: Abdominal pain, pelvic mas
- Often the patients may have history of primary pancreatic carcinoma

Gross features

- Bilateral tumour (80–100%)
- Mean size 8–12 cm
- Solid and partly cystic mass
- Multiloculated cyst

Histopathology

- Variable sized tubular and cystic glands
- Cribriform or Villoglandular pattern may be seen
- The glands are mucinous or endometrioid type
- Deep infiltration of the glands in the desmoplastic stroma
- The glandular epithelial cells show moderate to marked nuclear atypia

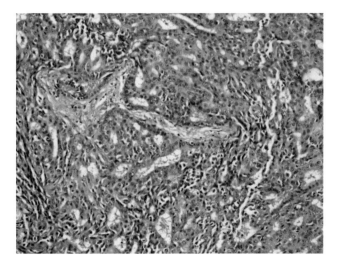

Fig. 10.8 Metastatic gall bladder carcinoma: Multiple glands like structures

Breast

Image gallery: Fig. 10.9.
   Epidemiology

- Represents 33% of primary source of metastasis
- Often incidentally detected

   Clinical features

- Age ranges widely from 30 to 80 year, Mean age: 49 years
- Most of the cases primary tumour is known at the time of ovarian metastasis

   Gross

- Bilateral
- Smaller in size and usually less than 5 cm in diameter
- Solid and occasionally cystic

   Clinical features

- Mostly incidental detection
- Rarely ovarian metastasis is detected before the detection of the primary tumour

   Histopathology
   Ductal carcinoma

- Diffuse sheets, nest and glandular arrangement
- Multinodular growth pattern

   Lobular carcinoma

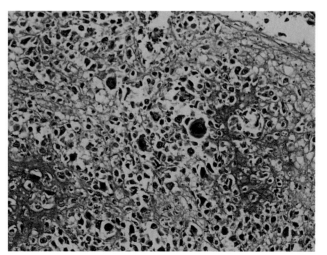

Fig. 10.9 Metastatic breast carcinoma in ovary: Discrete moderately pleomorphic tumour cells from the carcinoma of breast

- Single rows of cells arranged as Indian file
- Signet ring cells

   Immunohistochemistry

- Positive for ER, PR, GATA -3, GCDFP-15 (gross cystic disease fluid protein), and EMA

Uterine Tumours

Epidemiology

- About 15% of endometrial carcinoma metastasizes in ovary
- About 40% cases of endometrial carcinoma of uterus have been metastasized in autopsy studies

   Features suggestive of metastasis

- Deeper myometrial invasion
- Lymphovascular emboli
- Luminal involvement of the fallopian tube

Cervical Tumours

Epidemiology

- Only 1% of cervical carcinoma metastasizes in ovary
- Seventeen percent incidence of metastasis in autopsy cases

   Types of malignancy

- Predominantly cervical adenocarcinoma of usual types
- Squamous cell carcinoma metastasis is extremely rare

Tumours of Rete Ovarii

Adenoma of Rete Ovarii

Image gallery: Fig. 10.10a, b.
 Epidemiology

- One to six percent of all ovarian cystadenoma

Clinical features

- Age is widely variable 25–80 year, mean age 59 year
- Chief complaints: Pain abdomen, discomfort
- Occasionally virilization

Gross

- Bilateral (more than 90%)
- Usually cystic
- Mean size 9 cm

Histopathology

- Multiple closely spaced tubules
- Focal papillae formation
- Tubules are lined by low cuboidal cells with bland nuclei

Immunohistochemistry

- Positive for EMA, CAM 5.2, and CD 10

Differential diagnosis

- Adnexal tumour of probable Wolffian origin
  - Typical sieve like pattern

Prognosis

- Benign nature

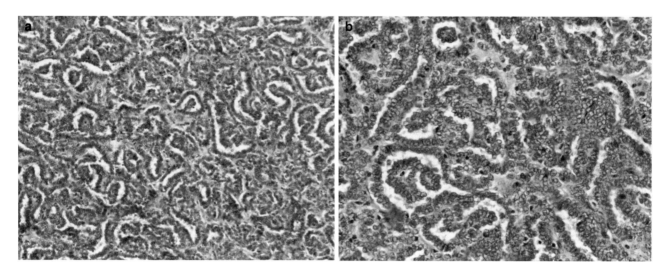

Fig. 10.10 (**a**) Rete adenoma ovary: Multiple closely packed slit like tubular structures. (**b**) Rete adenoma ovary: Higher magnification showing focal papillae formation. The tubules are lined by cuboidal cells

Wolffian Tumour

Image gallery: Fig. 10.11a, c.

Synonym: Female adnexal tumour of probable Wolffian origin (FATWO).

Epidemiology

- Uncommon tumour

Clinical features

- Wide age range 28–85 year, mean age is 46 year
- Abdominal pain, pelvic mass
- Postmenopausal bleeding

Gross features

- Unilateral
- Mean size 8 cm in diameter
- Solid or partly cystic
- Cut section: white to yellow

Histopathology

- Closely packed tubules and cysts resembling sieve like pattern
- Retiform, or trabecular arrangement may also be seen
- Tumour cells are cuboidal or occasionally spindle shaped
- The cytoplasm contain mucinous material
- The cells have bland nuclei with low mitotic activity

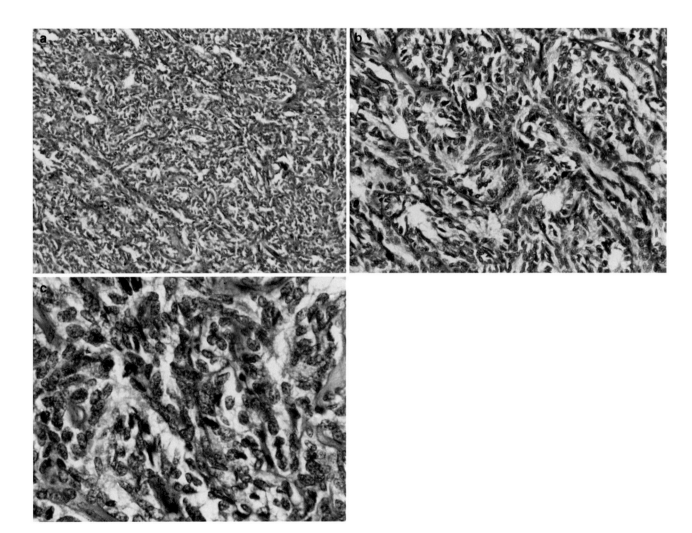

Fig. 10.11 (**a**) Wolffian tumour: Closely packed tubules resembling sieve like pattern. (**b**) Wolffian tumour: The tubules are lined by columnar shaped tumour cell. (**c**) Wolffian tumour: Higher magnification showing mildly pleomorphic columnar cells

Immunohistochemistry

- Positive: Pancytokeratin, vimentin, calretinin, and CD 10
- Occasionally positive: CK7 and inhibin
- Negative: CEA

Key diagnostic features: See Box 10.2.

Box 10.2 Key Diagnostic Features of Female Adnexal Tumour of Probable Wolffian Origin
- Tubules and cysts resembling sieve like pattern
- In addition, retiform, or trabecular arrangement
- Cuboidal or occasionally spindle shaped cells
- Nuclei are bland looking
- Low mitotic rate
- Immunohistochemistry: Positive for Pancytokeratin, vimentin, calretinin, and CD 10

Differential diagnosis

- Endometrioid carcinoma
  - True glands present
  - Squamous metaplasia
- Adenoma of rete ovarii

Prognosis

- Benign tumour
- Rarely malignant

Treatment

- Surgical resection is adequate treatment

Small Cell Carcinoma of Ovary

Image gallery: Fig. 10.12a–b.

Epidemiology

- Rare tumour

Clinical features

- Young patients; mean age 25 year
- Patients present with paraneoplastic syndrome (66%)
- Occasional patients may have hypercalcaemia
- Other complaints: pain abdomen and pelvic mass

Gross features

- Unilateral
- Predominantly large, mean size 15 cm
- Solid, cut section grey white with areas of necrosis and haemorrhage

Histopathology

- Mainly diffuse sheets, in addition nests, and trabecular arrangement
- Follicle like structures may also be present
- The tumour cells are small with scanty cytoplasm
- Nuclei are round and monomorphic with hyperchromatic clumped chromatin
- Occasionally rhabdoid like cells present: Large cells with moderate amount of cytoplasm and eccentric nuclei having prominent nucleoli

Immunohistochemistry

- Positive: CK 8/18
- Occasionally positive: Pancytokeratin, EMA, WT1,CD 10 and calretinin
- Negative: Inhibin, chromogranin, Mic 2

Prognosis

- Aggressive in behaviour
- Single important prognostic factor is stage of the tumour
- Unfavourable prognostic factors include
  - Age higher than 30 year
  - Tumour size less than 10 cm
  - Absence of hypercalcemia
  - Lack of large pleomorphic cells

Treatment

- Surgical removal of the tumour followed by chemotherapy

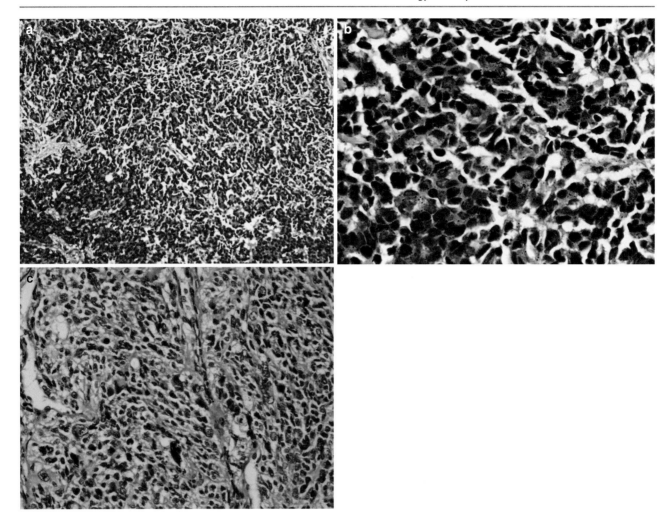

Fig. 10.12 (**a**) Small cell carcinoma of ovary: Small round cells with dark hyperchromatic nuclei. (**b**) Small cell carcinoma of ovary: Cell to cell compression causing nuclear molding. (**c**) Small cell carcinoma of ovary, hypercalcaemic type: Small mildly pleomorphic tumour cells

Paraganglioma

Image gallery: Figs. 10.13 and 10.14.

Epidemiology

- Extremely uncommon

Clinical features

- Wide variation: 15–68 year
- Incidental

Gross features

- Large size; more than 20 cm in diameter
- Solid, unilateral tumour

Histopathology

- Multiple nests of tumour cells separated by blood vessel (Zellballen pattern)
- Tumour cells are polygonal with abundant cytoplasm
- Nuclei are large round and central in location

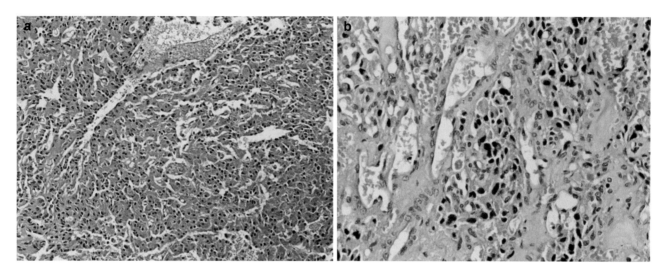

Fig. 10.13 (**a**) Paraganglioma: Multiple nests of tumour cells separated by blood vessel giving Zellballen pattern. (**b**) Paraganglioma: Higher magnification showing Groups of tumour cells surrounded by blood vessels

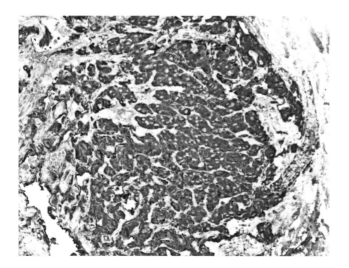

Fig. 10.14 Paraganglioma: Strongly positive chromogranin

Mesothelial Tumour

Adenomatoid Tumour

Image gallery: Fig. 10.15a, b.
  Epidemiology

- A rare tumour

  Clinical features

- Women from 20 to 30 year
- Incidental
- Asymptomatic patient

  Gross features

- Located in hilus of ovary
- Small size: 0.5–3 cm in diameter
- Solid tumour

Histopathology

- Multiple anastomosing cleft like spaces
- Tubular glands or solid aggregation of tumour cells
- The cleft and tubules are lined by cuboidal to flat cells
- Nuclei are round and monomorphic

Immunohistochemistry

- Positive for mesothelial cell markers: Calretinin, WT 1, thrombomodulin and CK 5/6
- Negative for: EMA, B 72.3

Prognosis

- Benign tumour

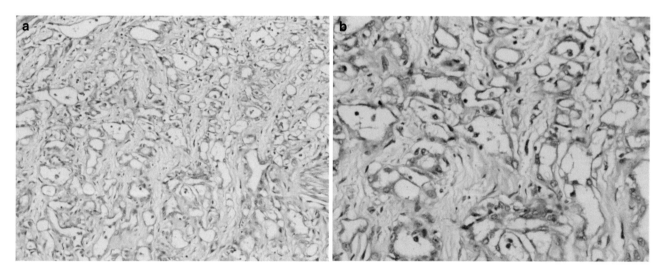

Fig. 10.15 (**a**) Adenomatoid tumour: Multiple anastomosing cleft like spaces. (**b**) Adenomatoid tumour: The cleft and tubules are lined by flat cells

Soft Tissue Tumours

Leiomyoma

Image gallery: Fig. 10.16.
  Epidemiology

- Rare tumour in ovary

  Clinical features

- Age range: 30–60 year
- Asymptomatic
- Occasionally non-specific symptoms: Pain abdomen, pelvic mass

  Gross features

- Variable size: 1–15 cm in diameter
- Solid
- Cut section: Gray white, whorled appearance

  Histopathology

- Oval to spindle cells arranged in short and long fascicles

  Prognosis
  Benign tumour
  Treatment

- Simple excision

Lipoleiomyoma Ovary

Image gallery: Fig. 10.17.
  Description

- Lipoleiomyoma is a variant of leiomyoma where the leiomyoma is admixed with significant amount of adipose tissue.
- The clinical features, gross appearance and prognosis are same as ovarian leiomyoma

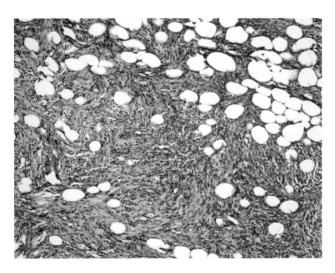

Fig. 10.17 Lipoleiomyoma ovary: Mature fat within the leiomyomatous area

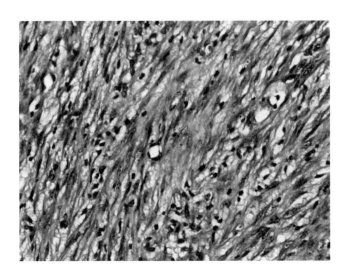

Fig. 10.16 Leiomyoma ovary: Fascicles of spindle cells

Leiomyosarcoma

Image gallery: Fig. 10.18a, b.
  Epidemiology

- Rare in ovary

  Clinical features

- Elderly woman; mean age 53 year
- Non-specific symptoms

  Gross features

- Unilateral
- Usually large

- Solid, grayish tumour with areas of haemorrhage and necrosis

Criteria of diagnosis: Any two features

- Moderate to marked nuclear atypia
- Coagulative necrosis
- More than 10 mitotic activity per 10 HPF

Differential diagnosis

- Immature teratoma with leiomyomatous component
  - Other components of teratoma present
- Metastatic leiomyosarcoma from uterus
  - History of primary tumour

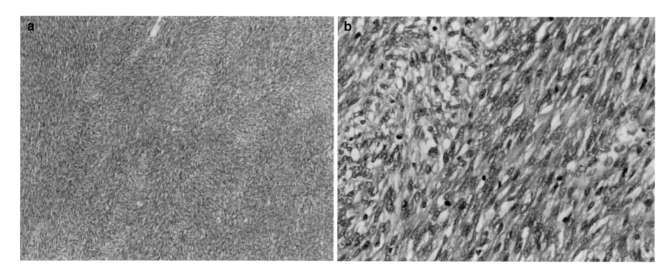

Fig. 10.18 (**a**) Leiomyosarcoma ovary: Fascicles of smooth muscle cells. (**b**) Leiomyosarcoma ovary: The cells showing frequent mitosis and nuclear pleomorphism

Fibrosarcoma Ovary

Image gallery: Fig. 10.19a, b.
  Incidence

- Uncommon tumour of ovary
- Represents less than 1% of ovarian neoplasms

Histopathology

- Oval to spindle cells arranged like herring bone pattern

- Nuclei of the cells are spindle shaped with moderate nuclear atypia
- Mitosis is usually more than 3 per 10 HPF

Differential diagnosis

- Cellular fibroma
  - It is very difficult to differentiate a mitotically active cellular fibroma from Fibrosarcoma. Often long term follow up is needed.

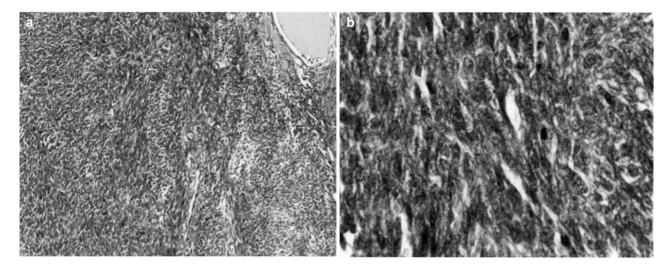

Fig. 10.19 (**a**) Fibrosarcoma ovary: Bundles of spindle cells. (**b**) Fibrosarcoma ovary: The tumour cells show frequent mitosis. The cells are negative for caldesmon and smooth muscle actin

Lymphoid and Myeloid Neoplasms in Ovary

Lymphoma

Image gallery: Figs. 10.20, 10.21, and 10.22.
Epidemiology

- Rare; Primary lymphoma represents less than 1.5%

Clinical features

- Wide age range 20–75 year
- Predominantly in 40–50 year
- Chief complaints: Non-specific symptoms such as abdominal pain and mass abdomen

Gross features

- Primary ovarian lymphoma
  - Unilateral
  - Variable size: small microscopic size to 20 cm diameter; mean diameter 10–15 cm
  - Solid
  - Cut section: soft, fleshy, white to gray

Histopathology

- Common types
  - Diffuse large B-cell lymphoma
  - Burkitt's lymphoma
  - Follicular lymphoma

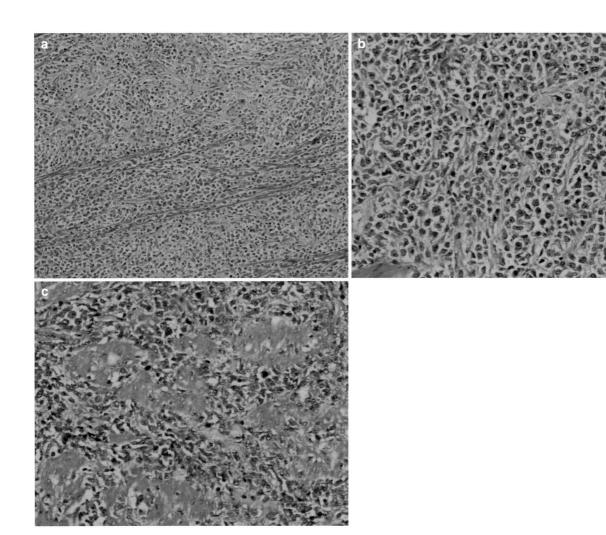

Fig. 10.20 (**a**) Non Hodgkin lymphoma, diffuse large B cell type: Diffuse sheet of round cells. (**b**) Non Hodgkin lymphoma, diffuse large B cell type: The cells are round and mildly pleomorphic. (**c**) Non Hodgkin lymphoma, diffuse large B cell type: Foci of hyalinization are present in between the tumour cells

- Morphology depends on the type of lymphoma
- The normal ovarian parenchyma may be focally preserved

Differential diagnosis

- Dysgerminoma
  - Nests of cells with mature lymphocytes in the stroma
  - CD 45 negative

- Metastatic carcinoma
  - CK and EMA positive
  - CD 45 negative
- Small cell carcinoma
  - Cohesive cells
  - Nuclear moulding
  - Positive for Cytokeratin

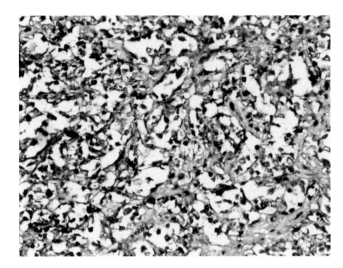

Fig. 10.21 Non Hodgkin lymphoma, diffuse large B cell type: The tumour cells are positive for CD 45

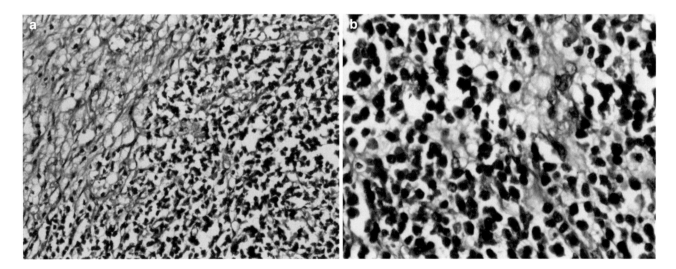

Fig. 10.22 (**a**) Plasma cell tumour: Diffuse infiltration of plasma cells within the ovary. (**b**) Plasma cell tumour: Higher magnification showing better morphology of the cells

Leukaemia of Ovary

Image gallery: Figs. 10.23 and 10.24.
   Incidence

- Ovarian involvement by leukaemia is rare
- Occasionally ovary is involved by acute myeloid leukaemia

Histopathology

- Discrete large round cells with focal preservation of the parenchymal structure
- Myeloblasts are large cells with large prominent nucleoli
- The cells often show granulocytes in the cytoplasm

Immunohistochemistry

- Positive for MPO and CD 117

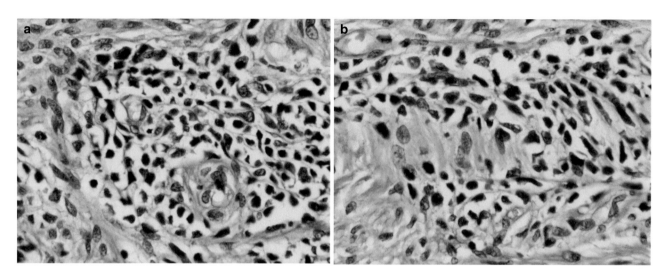

Fig. 10.23 (**a**) Leukaemia of ovary: Acute myeloid leukaemia in the ovary. (**b**) Leukaemia of ovary: Higher magnification showing better morphology of the blasts

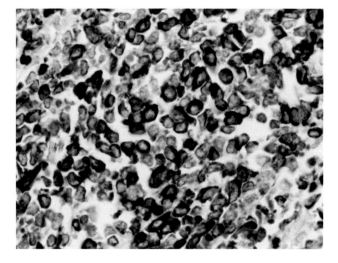

Fig. 10.24 Leukaemia of ovary: The malignant cells are strongly positive for myeloperoxidase

Reference

1. Kurman RJ, Carcangiu ML, Herrington S, Young RH. WHO classification of tumours of female genital reproductive organs. 4th ed. Lyon: International Agency for Research on Cancer; 2014.

Suggested Reading

Al-Agha OM, Nicastri AD. An in-depth look at Krukenberg tumour: an overview. Arch Pathol Lab Med. 2006;130(11):1725–30.

Elharroudi T, Ismaili N, Errihani H, Jalil A. Primary lymphoma of the ovary. J Cancer Res Ther. 2008;4(4):195–6.

Gupta AK, Srinivasan R, Nijhawan R. Female adnexal tumour of probable Wolffian origin. Indian J Pathol Microbiol. 2014;57(4):620–2.

Hirakawa T, Tsuneyoshi M, Enjoji M. Adenomatoid tumour of the ovary: an immunohistochemical and ultrastructural study. Jpn J Clin Oncol. 1988;18(2):159–66.

Kamiyama R, Funata N. A study of leukemic cell infiltration in the testis and ovary. Bull Tokyo Med Dent Univ. 1976;23(4):203–10.

Lash RH, Hart WR. Intestinal adenocarcinomas metastatic to the ovaries. A clinicopathological evaluation of 22 cases. Am J Surg Pathol. 1987;11:114–21.

Lerwill MF, Sung R, Oliva E, et al. Smooth muscle tumours of the ovary: a clinicopathologic study of 54 cases emphasizing prognostic criteria, histologic variants, and differential diagnosis. Am J Surg Pathol. 2004;28:1436–51.

Mira JL. Lipoleiomyoma of the ovary: report of a case and review of the English literature. Int J Gynecol Pathol. 1991;10(2):198–202.

Nogales FF, Carvia RE, Donné C, Campello TR, Vidal M, Martin A. Adenomas of the rete ovarii. Hum Pathol. 1997;28(12):1428–33.

Peccatori F, Bonazzi C, Lucchini V, Bratina G, Mangioni C. Primary ovarian small cell carcinoma: four more cases. Gynecol Oncol. 1993;49(1):95–9.

Schuldt M, Retamero JA, Tourné M, Nogales FF. Ovarian paraganglioma. Int J Surg Pathol. 2015;23(2):130–3.

Scully RE. Small cell carcinoma of hypercalcemic type. Int J Gynecol Pathol. 1993;12(2):148–52.

Singh SS, Chandra A, Majhi U. Primary fibrosarcoma of the ovary-report of two cases. Indian J Pathol Microbiol. 2004;47(4):525–8.

Stellato G, Di Bonito M, Tramontana S. Primary fibrosarcoma of the ovary. Acta Obstet Gynecol Scand. 1995;74(8):649–52.

Vierhout ME, Pijpers L, Tham MN, Chadha-Ajwani S. Leiomyoma of the ovary. Acta Obstet Gynecol Scand. 1990;69(5):445–7.

Yadav BS, George P, Sharma SC, Gorsi U, McClennan E, Martino MA, Chapman J, Chen LM, Prakash G, Malhotra P, Tantravahi SK, Glenn MJ, Werner TL, Baksh K, Sokol L, Morris GJ. Primary non-Hodgkin lymphoma of the ovary. Semin Oncol. 2014;41(3):e19–30.

Young RH, Gersell DJ, Roth LM, Scully RE. Ovarian metastases from cervical carcinomas other than pure adenocarcinomas. A report of 12 cases. Cancer. 1993;71(2):407–18.

Young RH. From Krukenberg to today: the ever present problems posed by metastatic tumours in the ovary. Part II. Adv Anat Pathol. 2007;14(3):149–77.

Zygouris D, Androutsopoulos G, Grigoriadis C, Arnogiannaki N, Terzakis E. Primary ovarian leiomyosarcoma. Eur J Gynaecol Oncol. 2012;33(3):331–3.

Pathology of Fallopian Tube

Classification of fallopian tube according to World Health Organization [1] is highlighted in Fig. 11.1.

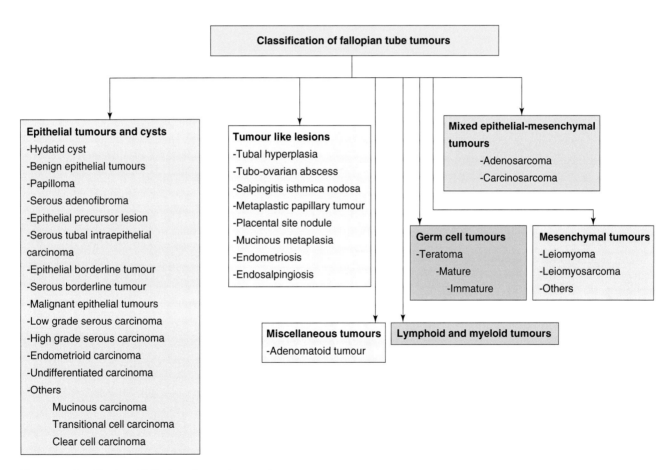

Fig. 11.1 Classification of fallopian tube neoplasms and cyst

© Springer Nature Singapore Pte Ltd. 2019
P. Dey, *Color Atlas of Female Genital Tract Pathology*, https://doi.org/10.1007/978-981-13-1029-4_11

Metaplasia of Fallopian Tube

Image gallery: Fig. 11.2a–c.
   Common types of metaplastic changes:

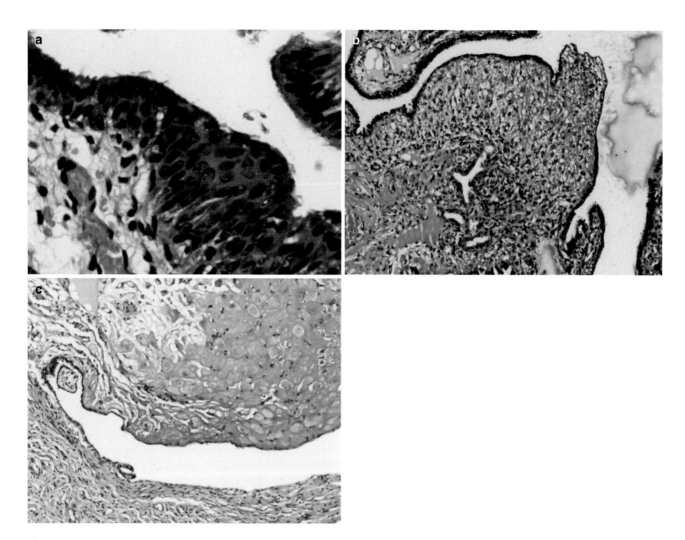

Fig. 11.2 (**a**) Transitional metaplasia: Tubal lining showing transitional epithelium. (**b**) Decidual metaplasia of fallopian tube: Extensive decidual change underneath the epithelium. (**c**) Decidual metaplasia of fallopian tube: Higher magnification of the same showing polygonal decidual cells

Transitional Metaplasia

- The tubal lining cells undergo transitional changes.
- No clinical importance

Decidual Metaplasia

- Incidentally detected at the time of postpartum tubal ligation
- Focal collection of the decidual cells underneath the epithelium

Mucinous Metaplasia

- The columnar mucus secreting cells replace the normal ciliated columnar cells
- Cribriform arrangement of the cells often resembles carcinoma

Salpingitis Isthmica Nodosa

Image gallery: Fig. 11.3a–d.
  Synonym: Adenomyosis of fallopian tube.
  Epidemiology

- Incidence varies from 0.6 to 11% in adult
- More frequent in ectopic pregnancy and infertile patients
- Isthmic part of the tube is commonly affected

Etiology

- Idiopathic
- Possibly related with inflammation

Clinical features

- Age range varies from 25 to 60 year; mean age is 30 years
- Incidentally detected

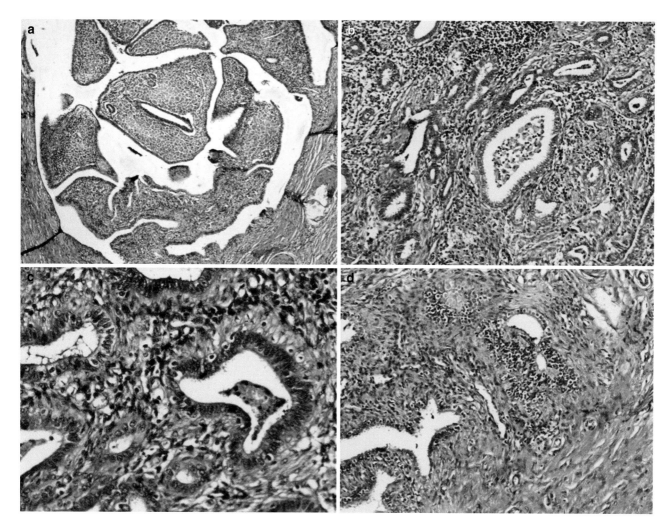

Fig. 11.3 (**a**) Salpingitis isthmica nodosa: Multiple infolding of the fallopian tube lining with many gland like structures surrounded by inflammatory cells. (**b**) Salpingitis isthmica nodosa: Multiple round to irregular infiltrating glands surrounded by disorganized and hyperplastic muscular tissue. (**c**) Salpingitis isthmica nodosa: Higher magnification showing the irregular gland like structure with peripheral muscle tissue. (**d**) Salpingitis isthmica nodosa: Irregular outpouching of the gland

Gross features

- Mostly bilateral
- Multiple small whitish nodules on the wall of the tube
- Size varies from 1 to 2 cm in diameter

Histopathology

- Multiple round to irregular infiltrating glands surrounded by disorganized and hyperplastic muscular tissue
- Serial section often reveals the communication of the glands with the lumen
- The lining epithelial cells of the glands are bland in appearance

Complications

- Ectopic pregnancy
- Infertility

Treatment

- Removal of the affected areas by microsurgery

Diagnostic key features: See Box 11.1.

Box 11.1 Diagnostic Key Features of Salpingitis Isthmica Nodosa
- Multiple irregular dilated glands infiltrate in the wall of the tube
- These glands are surrounded by disorganized and hyperplastic muscular tissue
- Lining epithelial cells are bland cuboidal and are arranged in a single layer
- Often associated with chronic inflammation
- There may be abundant endometrioid like stromal cells

Tubal Pregnancy

Image gallery: Fig. 11.4a–c.
   Definition: Implantation of the blastocyst resulting pregnancy in the tube.
   Epidemiology

- It represents 1% of all pregnancies
- Ninety five percent of extra uterine pregnancies are in the fallopian tube
- Eight five percent of the ectopic pregnancy is located in the ampulla of fallopian tube

Factors associated with tubal pregnancy

- Granulomatous inflammation such as tuberculosis
- Chronic salpingitis
- Salpingitis isthmica nodosa
- Application of intrauterine contraceptive device
- Congenital abnormalities of the fallopian tube

Clinical features

- Common complaints: Amenorrhea, abdominal pain and abnormal vaginal bleeding
- Rupture of the tube may present as acute abdomen
- Serum beta HCG level is high
- USG examination reveals the abnormal gestation in the tube

Gross features

- Dilated and enlarged tube resembles sausage
- Congested outer surface
- Cut section: Lumen filled with blood and friable fleshy grey white tissue

Histopathology

- Multiple chorionic villi in the lumen and wall of the fallopian tube
- Wall shows oedema, inflammation and haemorrhage
- Decidua and trophoblasts may also be noted

Prognosis

- Tubal rupture is a serious event as this may cause bleeding and death
- Unilateral salpingectomy is the treatment of choice

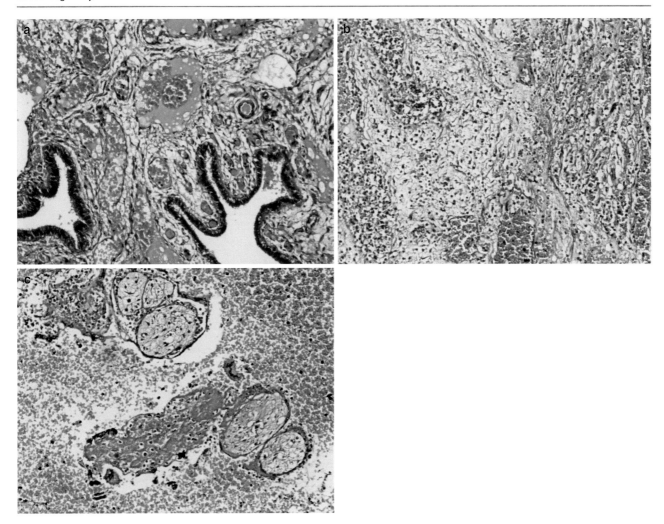

Fig. 11.4 (**a**) Tubal pregnancy: Congested vessels and oedema in the tubal wall. (**b**) Tubal pregnancy: Marked oedema in the wall. (**c**) Tubal pregnancy: Multiple first trimester chorionic villi in the tubal wall

Acute and Chronic Salpingitis

Image gallery: Fig. 11.5a, b.
  Salpingitis may be:

- Acute
- Chronic
- Granulomatous

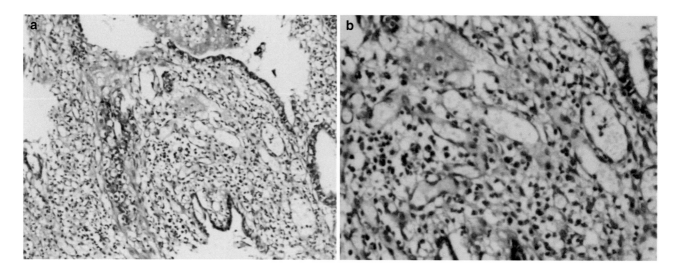

Fig. 11.5 (**a**) Chronic salpingitis: Diffuse infiltration of chronic inflammatory cells underneath the epithelium. (**b**) Chronic salpingitis: The inflammatory cells consist of lymphocytes and plasma cells

Acute Salpingitis

Causative organisms: Neisseria gonorrhoea, Chlamydia trachomatis and Mycoplasma genitalium.

Frequent association

- Multiple sex partner
- Use of intrauterine contraceptive device
- Intercourse started in early page
- Past history of sexually transmitted infection

Clinical features

- Patients are sexually active
- Reproductive age group patient
- Asymptomatic in one fourth cases
- Complaints: Pelvic tenderness, fever and leucorrhoea

Gross features

- Tube is swollen with oedematous wall
- Fibrinopurulent exudates over the surface
- Cut section: Pus in the tubal lumen

Histopathology

- Acute inflammation in the fallopian tube: Polymorphs and exudates
- Oedema
- Hyperplastic epithelium with crowding of the glands

Therapy

- Antibiotics

Chronic Salpingitis

Clinical features

- Pain in lower abdomen
- Infertility

Gross features

- Dilated tube
- Adhered with the neighbouring structures
- Tubal wall is hypertrophied
- Lumen contains thin pus

Histopathology

- Lymphocytes, histiocytes and plasma cells infiltration in the tubal wall
- Mucosal hyperplasia and plica formation due to adherence of the epithelium

Granulomatous Salpingitis

Causes:

- Tuberculosis
- Parasitic infection: *Enterobius vermicularis*, *Schistosoma*
- Fungal infection
- Rarely sarcoidosis

Tubercular Salpingitis

Image gallery: Fig. 11.6a–c.

   Causative organism: Mycobacterium tuberculosis.

   Epidemiology

- Widely variable incidence
- Overall incidence 5%
- In endemic countries: as high as 40% in infertile patients

   Clinical feature

- Predominantly latent infection
- Mostly infertile patient

   Gross features

- Usually bilateral
- Tube enlarged
- Small tubercles may be seen on the wall
- Cut section: Necrotic material in the lumen

Histopathology

- Multiple epithelioid cell granulomas in tubal wall
- Central caseation surrounded by epithelioid cells and multinucleated giant cells
- Hyperplasia of the mucosal lining epithelium

   Ancillary tests

- Ziehl Neelsen stain for acid fast bacilli
- Mycobacterial culture
- Polymerase chain reaction for mycobacteria

   Differential diagnosis

- Other causes of granulomatous inflammation
- Lipoid salpingitis due to chemical contrast substance

   Treatment

- Anti-tubercular therapy

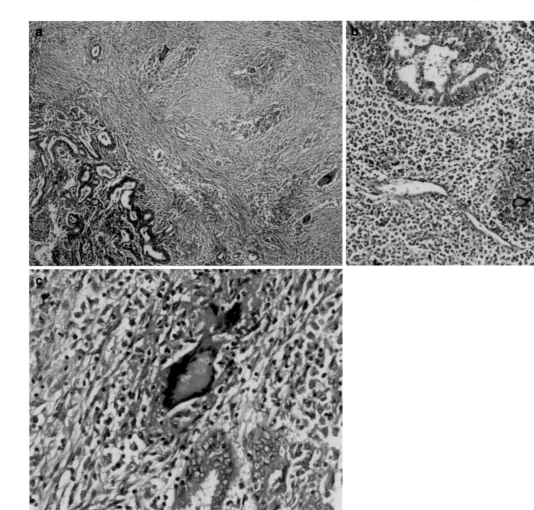

Fig. 11.6 (**a**) Tubercular salpingitis: Fallopian tube wall showing multiple epithelioid cell granulomas. (**b**) Tubercular salpingitis: The tubal epithelium along with well-formed granulomas. (**c**) Tubercular salpingitis: Higher magnification showing Langhan's giant cells along with lymphocytes and epithelioid cells

Xanthogranulomatous Salpingitis

Image gallery: Fig. 11.7a, b

- Many foamy histiocytes and inflammatory cell collection underneath the mucosa of the fallopian tube.
- No association with endometriosis

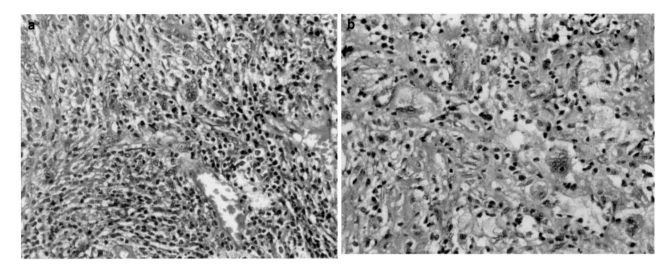

Fig. 11.7 (**a**) Xanthogranulomatous inflammation in fallopian tube: Abundant lymphocytes and foamy Histiocytes. (**b**) Xanthogranulomatous inflammation in fallopian tube: Higher magnification showing the foamy histiocytes

Endometriosis

Image gallery: Fig. 11.8a, b.
  Epidemiology

- About 10% of resected tube
- Fimbrial end is frequently affected

Clinical features

- Patients are always in reproductive age period
- Chief complaints: Abdominal pain, infertility and pain during menstruation

Gross features

- Small bluish nodules on the tubal wall
- Bilateral or unilateral

Histopathology

- Multiple endometrial glands embedded in the endometrial stroma
- Hemosiderin laden histiocytes

Differential diagnosis

- Endosalpingiosis
  - Only endometrial glands present, no stroma is seen
- Salpingitis isthmica nodosa
  - The glands are lined by ciliated columnar cells
  - No endometrial stroma

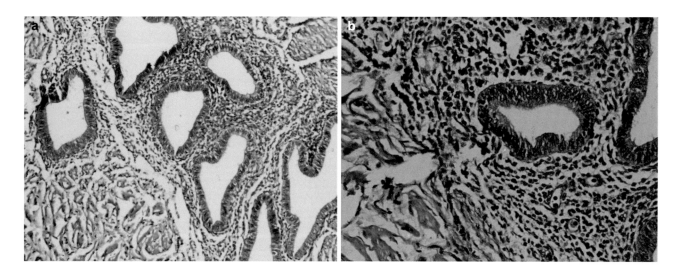

Fig. 11.8 (**a**) Endometriosis: Multiple endometrial glands and stroma in the tubal wall. (**b**) Endometriosis: Higher magnification showing endometrial glands in the endometrial stroma

Tumour

Adenomatoid Tumour

Image gallery: Fig. 11.9a, b.

Definition: Adenomatoid tumour is a neoplasm derived from mesothelial cells.

Epidemiology

- The most common benign neoplasm of the fallopian tube

Clinical features

- Middle aged female
- Incidentally detected

Gross

- Usually unilateral
- Small in size 1–2 cm
- Firm grayish well circumscribed nodule

Histopathology

- Multiple glands and branching cleft like spaces separated by connective tissue
- The lining epithelial cells are cuboidal to flat
- Nuclei of these cells are bland looing
- Scanty lymphocytes in the stroma

Immunohistochemistry
Positive: WT1, calretinin and thrombomodulin.

Negative: CEA, factor VIII,
Diagnostic key features: See Box 11.2.

Box 11.2 Diagnostic Key Features of Adenomatoid Tumour
- Multiple tubular and gland like spaces
- These cleft like spaces are surrounded by hyalinised connective tissue
- The lining epithelial cells are made by single layer of cuboidal to flat cells
- Multiple foci of lymphocytes in the stroma
- *Immunohistochemistry*: Positive for mesothelial markers such as WT1, calretinin, CK 5/6 and thrombomodulin; negative for CEA, Ber-EP4, B 72.3 and factor VIII

Differential diagnosis

- Lymphangioma
    - Negative for mesothelial cell markers (calretinin, WT 1)
    - Positive for CD 34
- Adenocarcinoma
    - Nuclear atypia
    - High mitotic activity

Prognosis

- Benign tumour

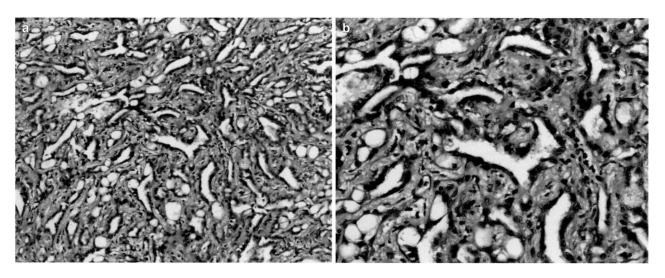

Fig. 11.9 (a) Adenomatoid tumour: Many slit like channels with intervening connective tissue. (b) Adenomatoid tumour: The slit like spaces lined by cuboidal to flat cells

Serous Tubal Intraepithelial Carcinoma (STIC)

Image gallery: Figs. 11.10 and 11.11.

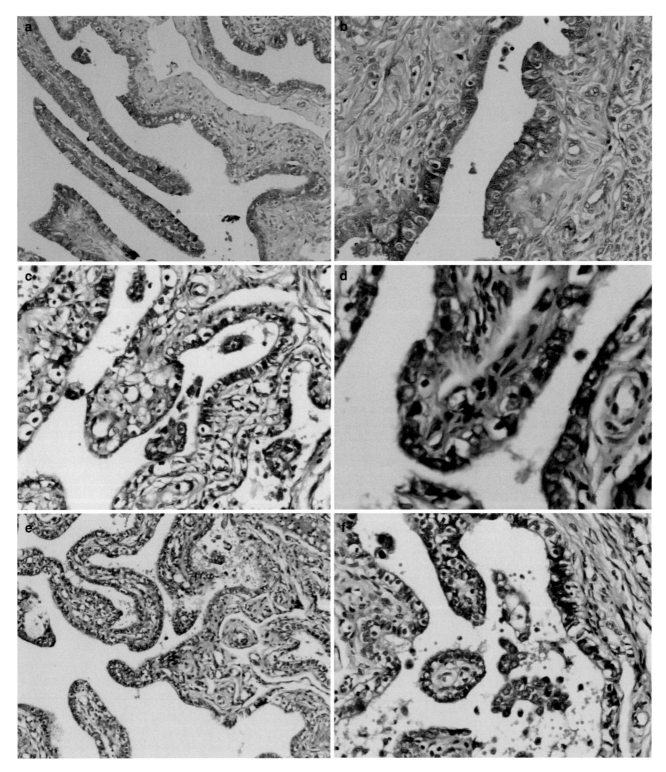

Fig. 11.10 (**a**) Serous tubal intraepithelial carcinoma: The lining epithelial cells are enlarged and mildly pleomorphic. (**b**) Serous tubal intraepithelial carcinoma: The cells have mild to moderate pleomorphism. Note the loss of cilia of these cells. (**c**) Serous tubal intraepithelial carcinoma: The epithelium showing focal tufting of the cells. (**d**) Serous tubal intraepithelial carcinoma: Higher magnification highlighting the nuclear enlargement and pleomorphism of the lining cells. (**e**) Serous tubal intraepithelial carcinoma: Multiple papillary folding. (**f**) Serous tubal intraepithelial carcinoma: The papillae are lined by single to multi-layered cells

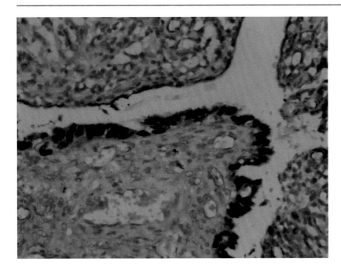

Fig. 11.11 Serous tubal intraepithelial carcinoma: The lining epithelial cells showing strong p 53 positivity

Definition: This is the early carcinoma of fallopian tube without any evidence of stromal invasion.
Epidemiology

- Incidence of STIC is 0.5–6% in BRCAI mutation cases
- Associated with 61% high grade serous carcinoma of ovary

Gross features: No visible macroscopic changes.
Histopathology:

- Cellular abnormality
  - The cells at first loose cilia
  - Nuclei enlarged with high nucleocytoplasmic ratio
  - Nuclei becomes hyperchromatic
  - Nuclear moulding noted
  - Irregularly clumped nuclear chromatin
  - Higher mitotic rate
- Multi layering of the epithelial cells and loss of polarity
  - The epithelial cells undergoes hyperplasia and shows focal stratification and loss of polarity
  - Clusters of exfoliated cells in the tubal lumen may be seen
- P 53 immunostaining
  - Strong and diffuse nuclear positivity
  - Deletion of p 53 gene may result complete negative p 53 staining
- Ki 67 index is high: Always more than 10% and usually more than 70%

Diagnostic key features: See Box 11.3.

Box 11.3 Diagnostic Key Features of Serous Tubal Intraepithelial Carcinoma

- Stratification of the epithelial cells and loss of polarity
- Exfoliated cells are seen in the lumen of the tube
- Cellular abnormalities
  - Loss of cilia
  - Enlarged hyperchromatic nuclei with high nucleocytoplasmic ratio
  - Nuclear moulding
  - Irregularly clumped nuclear chromatin
- Higher mitotic rate
  - Strong and diffuse nuclear positivity of P 53 immunostaining
- Ki 67 index is always more than 10%

Secretory Cell Outgrowth

- Outgrowth of secretory cell component in the fallopian tube
- No nuclear abnormality
- No true stratification
- PTEN and PAX 2 expression is deranged
- P 53 immunostaining is negative

P 53 Signature

- Normal appearing epithelium on microscopic examination
- Strong p53 positive cells: At least 12 consecutive cells show positivity
- Ki 67 index is less than 10%

Carcinoma of Fallopian Tube

Image gallery: Figs. 11.12, 11.13, 11.14, 11.15, and 11.16.
Epidemiology

- Uncommon tumour
- It constitutes less than 1% of all malignant tumour of the female reproductive organs

Clinical features

- Widely variable age from 25 to 85 year; mean age is 58 years
- Common complaints: Triad of
  - Mass in pelvis
  - Pain in abdomen and pelvis
  - Abnormal vaginal bleeding
- This triad is present in less than 5% patients

Gross features

- Unilateral tumour
- Located in the middle part to fimbrial side
- Size varies from 1 to 15 cm; mean size 7 cm
- Looks like hydrosalpinx
- Usually blocked fimbrial end
- Cut section: Gray white friable mass with areas of haemorrhage and necrosis

Histopathology
Types: Serous carcinoma, endometrioid carcinoma, transitional cell carcinoma and undifferentiated carcinoma

- Serous carcinoma
  - It represents 50–80% of carcinoma of fallopian tube
  - Multiple papillae with central fibrovascular core
  - The lining cells of the papillae are cuboidal to columnar cells
  - The tumour cells show moderate nuclear enlargement and pleomorphism
  - The tumours are graded from 1 to 3
  - The grade of the tumour depends on the predominant papillary or solid components, complex branching pattern of papillae and nuclear pleomorphism. The grade 1 tumours show predominantly simple papillae with mildly pleomorphic nuclei and grade 3 tumours show complex branching papillae with marked nuclear pleomorphism. Grade 2 tumour is in between the grade 1 and 3.
  - Majority of the tumours are grade 3 tumour.
  - Occasional tumour giant cells may be seen

- Endometrioid carcinoma
  - It represents near about 20% of carcinoma of fallopian tube
  - Simulates endometrioid carcinoma of ovary
  - Multiple endometrioid like glands
  - Tumour cells show moderate nuclear enlargement and pleomorphism
  - This tumour often resembles female adnexal tumour of probable Wolffian duct origin

- Transitional cell carcinoma
  - Origin is from metaplastic transitional cells
  - Solid growth or papillary like pattern
  - Round cells with scanty cytoplasm having moderately pleomorphic nuclei
  - Nuclear groove may be seen

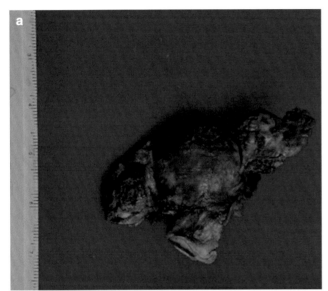

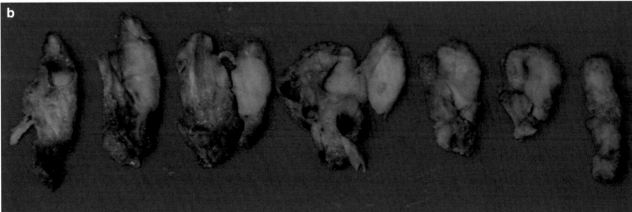

Fig. 11.12 (**a**) Gross photograph of the serous carcinoma of fallopian tube. The tube is enlarged. (**b**) Gross photograph of the serous carcinoma of fallopian tube. Solid grey white tumour occupying the whole of the lumen of the tube

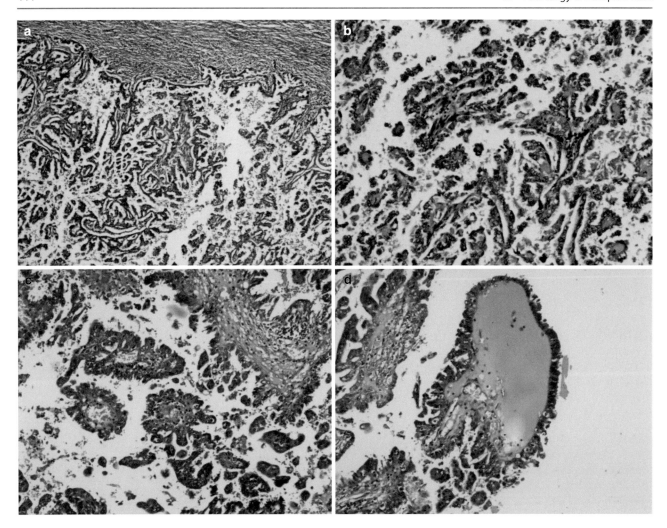

Fig. 11.13 (**a**) Serous carcinoma of fallopian tube, low grade: Predominantly simple papillary structures. (**b**) Serous carcinoma of fallopian tube, low grade: Multiple papillae with simple branching. (**c**) Serous carcinoma of fallopian tube, low grade: The papillae with fibrovascular core. (**d**) Serous carcinoma of fallopian tube, low grade: The papillae lined by mildly pleomorphic cells

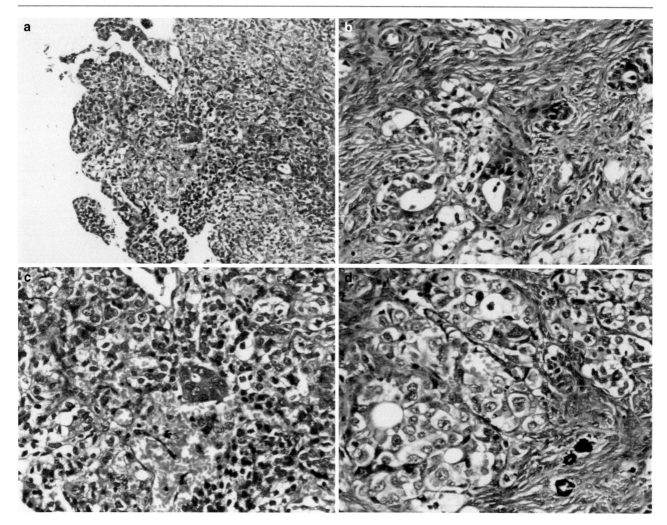

Fig. 11.14 (**a**) Serous carcinoma of fallopian tube, high grade: Occasional glands and predominantly solid component. (**b**) Serous carcinoma of fallopian tube, high grade: Occasional glands infiltrating in the wall. (**c**) Serous carcinoma of fallopian tube, high grade: Solid sheets of tumour cells and an isolated gland. (**d**) Serous carcinoma of fallopian tube, high grade: The cells are large with moderately pleomorphic nuclei having central prominent nucleoli. Foci of calcification are present

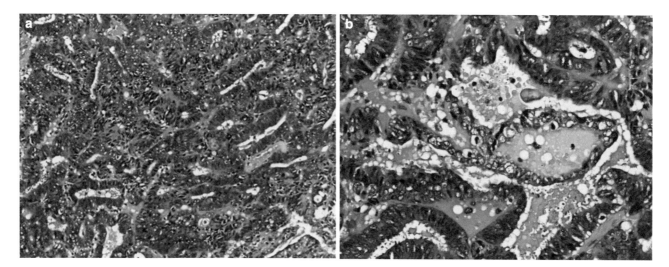

Fig. 11.15 (**a**) Endometrioid carcinoma: Multiple closely packed endometrioid like glands. (**b**) Endometrioid carcinoma: Tumour cells showing moderate nuclear enlargement and pleomorphism

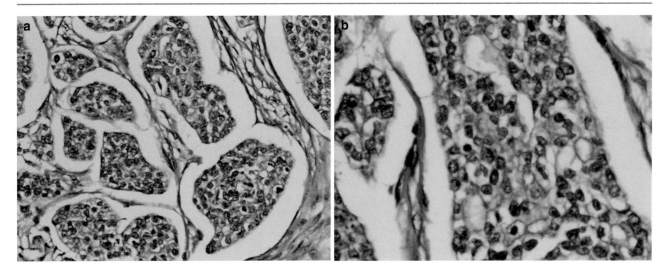

Fig. 11.16 (**a**) Transitional cell carcinoma: Multiple nests of tumour cells resembling transitional cells. (**b**) Transitional cell carcinoma: Round cells with scanty cytoplasm having moderately pleomorphic nuclei

Diagnostic key features: See Box 11.4.

Box 11.4 Diagnostic Key Features of Carcinoma of Fallopian Tube
Serous carcinoma

- Multiple broad papillae with central fibrovascular core
- Micropapillae with tufting
- Solid nests and irregular cleft like areas
- The lining cells of the papillae are cuboidal to columnar cells with moderate nuclear enlargement and pleomorphism
- The nuclei of the tumour cells are hyperchromatic with coarse chromatin and have prominent nucleoli
- Mitotic rate is high

Endometrioid carcinoma

- Multiple endometrioid like glands and villoglandular architecture
- Tumour cells have moderate nuclear enlargement and pleomorphism
- Squamous metaplasia
- Occasional bony metaplasia

Transitional cell carcinoma

- Solid tumour
- Exophytic papillary like pattern
- Round cells with scanty cytoplasm having moderately pleomorphic nuclei
- Nuclear grooves present
- Necrosis common

Differential diagnosis

- Female adnexal tumour of probable Wolffian duct origin (FATWO)
  - Endometrioid variety resembles this tumour
  - True lumen of the gland is lacking
  - FATWO is negative for EMA and positive for calretinin and inhibin

Prognosis

- Prognosis and management are almost same as ovarian serous carcinoma

Reference

1. Kurman RJ, Carcangiu ML, Herrington S, Young RH. WHO classification of tumours of female genital reproductive organs. 4th ed. Lyon: International Agency for Research on Cancer; 2014.

Suggested Reading

Ajithkumar TV, Minimole AL, John MM, et al. Primary fallopian tube carcinoma. Obstet Gynecol Surv. 2005;60:247–52.

Breen JL. A 21 year survey of 654 ectopic pregnancies. Am J Obstet Gynecol. 1970;106:1004–19.

Daya D, Young RH, Scully RE. Endometrioid carcinoma of the fallopian tube resembling an adnexal tumour of probable wolffian origin: a report of six cases. Int J Gynecol Pathol. 1992;11:122–30.

Egan AJ, Russell P. Transitional (urothelial) cell metaplasia of the fallopian tube mucosa: morphological assessment of three cases. Int J Gynecol Pathol. 1996;15:72–6.

Furuya M, Murakami T, Sato O, et al. Pseudoxanthomatous and xanthogranulomatous salpingitis of the fallopian tube: a report of four cases and a literature review. Int J Gynecol Pathol. 2002;21:56–9.

Kurman RJ, Shih I. Molecular pathogenesis and extraovarian origin of epithelial ovarian cancer–shifting the paradigm. Hum Pathol. 2011;42:918–31.

Majmudar B, Henderson PH III, Semple E. Salpingitis isthmica nodosa: a high-risk factor for tubal pregnancy. Obstet Gynecol. 1983;62:73–8.

Parikh FR, Nadkarni SG, Kamat SA, et al. Genital tuberculosis – a major pelvic factor causing infertility in Indian women. Fertil Steril. 1997;67:497–500.

Piek JM, van Diest PJ, Zweemer RP, et al. Dysplastic changes in prophylactically removed fallopian tubes of women predisposed to developing ovarian cancer. J Pathol. 2001;195:451–6.

Seidman JD. Mucinous lesions of the fallopian tube. A report of seven cases. Am J Surg Pathol. 1994;18:1205–12.

Young RH, Silva EG, et al. Ovarian and juxtaovarian adenomatoid tumours: a report of six cases. Int J Gynecol Pathol. 1991;10:364–72.

Placenta Reporting

Image gallery: Fig. 12.1a–c.
  Gross examination:
  Placenta should thoroughly examined for:

- Membrane: Colour, complete or torn
- Umbilical cord: Length, diameter, number of vessels, coiling, knots, insertion
- Placenta: Diameter, thickness, weight, presence of clot

© Springer Nature Singapore Pte Ltd. 2019
P. Dey, *Color Atlas of Female Genital Tract Pathology*, https://doi.org/10.1007/978-981-13-1029-4_12

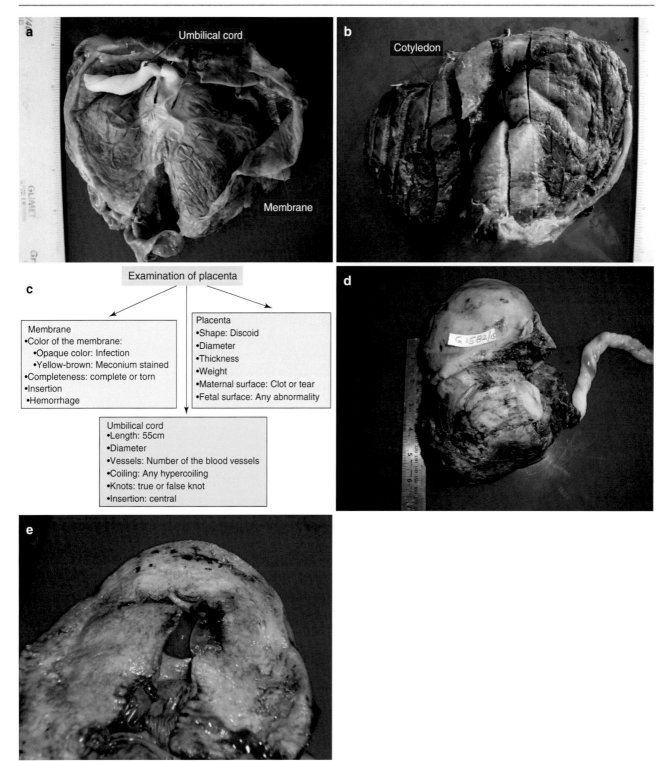

Fig. 12.1 (**a**) Fetal surface of the placenta. (**b**) Maternal surface of placenta. (**c**) Examination of placenta. (**d**) Placenta percreta: Gross picture showing adhesion of placenta with uterine wall. (**e**) Placenta percreta: Cut surface showing infiltration of placenta within the myometrium

Abnormal Adherence of Placenta

Image gallery: Figs. 12.1d–e and 12.2.
Classification

- Placenta accreta
  - Only superficial adherence of placenta
- Placenta increta
  - Deep myometrial infiltration of the chorionic villi
- Placenta percreta
  - The chorionic villi infiltrate the entire myometrial wall and reaches up to the serosa

Epidemiology

- Uncommon
- Incidence is nearly one in 7000 pregnancies
- The incidence has increased recently due to increased Caesarean section rate

Etiology

- Absence of decidua either partially or completely
- Normally the decidua works as barrier in the infiltration of villi in the myometrium. In absence of decidua the villi penetrates the myometrial tissue

Risk factors

- Past history of Caesarean section
- Placenta previa
- Cornual implantation
- Infection
- Instrumentation

Clinical features

- Antepartum bleeding
- Massive haemorrhage and uterine perforation may be presenting features in placenta percreta

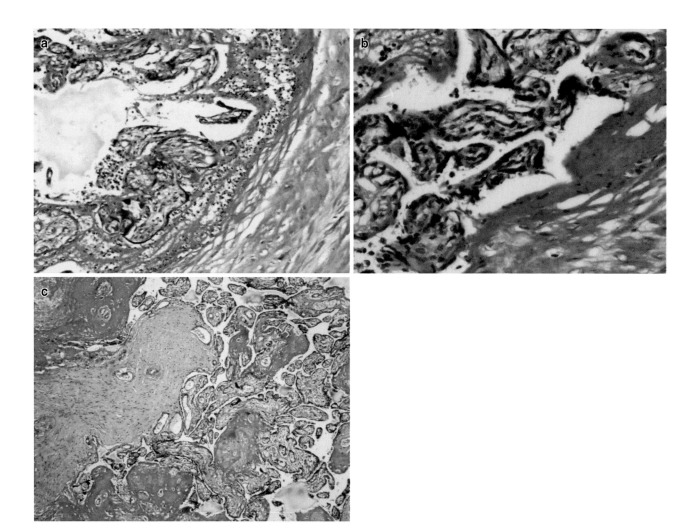

Fig. 12.2 (**a**) Placenta accreta: Villi are attached with the uterine wall. (**b**) Placenta accreta: No decidual barrier in between the chorionic villi and myometrium. (**c**) Placenta increta: The infiltration of the villi within the myometrium

Gross features

- Placenta accreta
  - The part of the placenta may be missing
- Placenta increta and percreta
  - Placenta is adhered with uterus
  - Thinned out myometrial wall
  - Grossly infiltrating placenta within the myometrium
  - Perforation of uterus is present in placenta percreta

Histopathology

- In placenta accreta
  - Chorionic villi is in direct contact with myometrium without any intervening decidual tissue
- In placenta increta and percreta
  - The chorionic villi infiltrate in the deeper myometrial tissue (increta) and may completely penetrate in the myometrium (percreta)

Complications

- Antepartum bleeding and death of fetus
- Severe postpartum bleeding and uterine rupture

Management

- Placenta accreta: Compatible with continuation of pregnancy
- Placenta increta and percreta: Placenta percreta needs hysterectomy

Inflammation

Infection in the Placenta

Image gallery: Figures.

Chorioamnionitis
Image gallery: Fig. 12.3a, b.

Definition: This is the inflammation of fetal membrane and umbilical cord.

Incidence

- Fifteen to twenty percent cases of term pregnancy
- Seventy percent cases of preterm delivery

Clinical features

- Patients may not any recognizable features
- Patients may have fever, tender uterus and high WBC count in blood
- Occasionally foul smelling vaginal discharge
- Fetal tachycardia

Pathways of infective organisms

- Ascending infection through vagina and cervix
- Direct inoculation of bacteria during instrumentation
- Haematogenous pathway
- Direct infiltration of organism through endometrium

Gross features

- Fetal membrane may not show any gross abnormality in mild inflammation
- Foul smelling, opaque brownish fragile membrane in severe long standing infection

Histopathology

- Neutrophilic infiltration in the membrane and chorion
- The inflammatory cells may be focal or diffuse with variable degree
- Necrosis may be present
- In long standing cases lymphocytes and histiocytes may appear

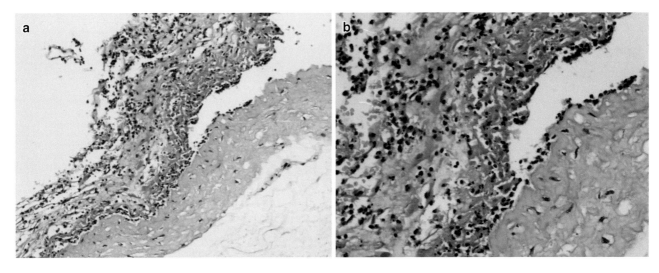

Fig. 12.3 (**a**) Chorioamnionitis: Acute inflammation in the membrane and chorion. (**b**) Chorioamnionitis: Higher magnification showing neutrophilic infiltration

Fetal Response of Chorioamnionitis (Fig. 12.4)

- Chorionic vasculitis: chorionic plate vessels are infiltrated by polymorphs of the fetus
- Umbilical phlebitis: Neutrophils of the fetus infiltrate within the umbilical veins
- Funisitis: The fetal polymorphs infiltrate in Wharton's jelly of the umbilicus and may cause necrosis

Clinical consequences

- Abortion
- Fetal death
- Fetal malformation
- Deafness of the baby

Villitis

Definition: This is defined as chronic inflammatory cells infiltrate within the stroma of the villi.

Etiology: Unknown.

Clinical feature: No specific clinical symptoms and signs.

Pathology

- Infiltration of lymphocytes, plasma cells and histiocytes within the villi
- Necrosis may be seen
- The degree of inflammation may varies from grade 1 to grade 4

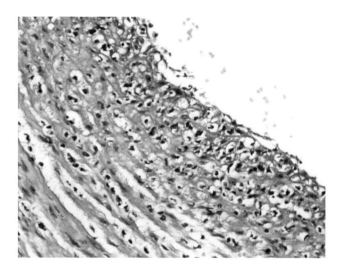

Fig. 12.4 Funisitis: Inflammation within the wall of the umbilical cord

Specific Infections of the Placenta

Viral Infections

Cytomegalovirus Infection
- Plasma cells and histiocyte infiltration in the villi
- Typical large eosinophilic Intranuclear inclusion in the trophoblastic cells
- Necrosis and foci of calcification
- PCR and immunocytochemistry may demonstrate CMV

Herpes Simplex Virus
- Inflammation and necrosis of the villi
- Herpes virus inclusion in the nuclei
- Ground glass nuclei
- In addition, decidual necrosis, vasculitis in chorion and funisitis may be seen

Rubella Infection
- Necrosis in the villi
- Vasculitis
- Inflammation in villi and sclerosis

Parasites

Toxoplasma Infection
- Lymphocytes and plasma cells infiltrate in villi
- Occasional granuloma formation with central necrosis surrounded by histiocytes
- Vascularity of the villi is raised
- Membrane and cord may also show inflammation

Malaria (Fig. 12.5a, b)
- Malarial pigment present
- Organism of *P. vivax* or falciparum within the RBCs

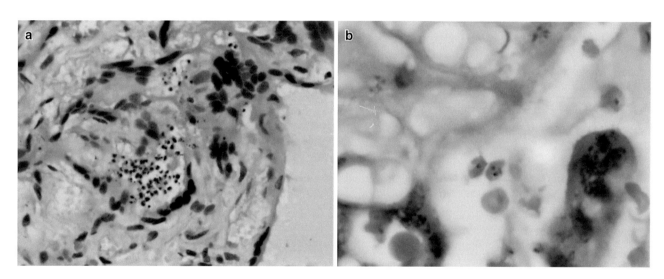

Fig. 12.5 (**a**) Plasmodium infection: Ring form of the *Plasmodium vivax*. (**b**) Plasmodium infection: Ring form of *Plasmodium vivax* within RBC

Bacteria

Syphilis
- Plasma cells infiltrate in the villi
- Vascular endothelial cells proliferation
- Villi enlarged
- Occasionally necrotizing funisitis

Tuberculosis (Fig. 12.6)
- Epithelioid cell granulomas and giant cells
- Necrosis present
- AFB may be demonstrated by Z-N stain

Circulatory Disorders

Image gallery: Fig. 12.7.

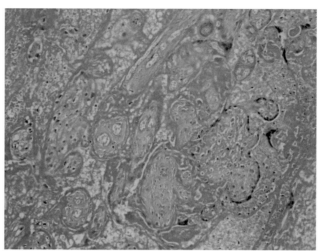

Fig. 12.7 Infraction: Ghost like villi

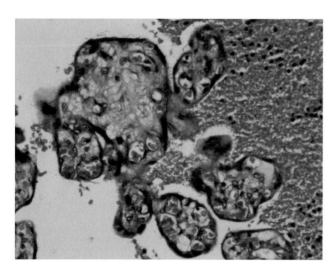

Fig. 12.6 Placental tuberculosis: Necrosis in the placenta

Infract

Incidence: About 10–20% of termed placenta.
   Significant infract

- If the size of infract more than 3 cm diameter
- If it is centrally located and multiple

   Etiology

- Spiral arterioles occluded by thrombi
- Atherosis of these vessels
- Large retroplacental haematoma

   Gross feature

- Wedge shaped
- Discoloured area, from red to tan brown followed by more yellowish colour
- Firm in consistency

   Histopathology

- Villi becomes crowded as the intervillous space is reduced
- Ghost like faint outline of the villi
- Slowly the dead villi are replaced by fibrosis

   Complications

- Fetal hypoxia
- Fetal growth retardation
- Large infract may cause fetal death

Maternal Floor Infract (MFI) and Massive Perivillous Fibrin (MPF)

Deposition
Image gallery: Figs. 12.8 and 12.9.
   Definition:

- Maternal floor infract (MFI): MFI is characterized by fibrin deposition only in the basal plate region of the placenta.
- Massive perivillous fibrin (MPF) deposition: In this condition the fibrin deposition occurs in the entire placenta.
- Both MFI and MPF are similar entities. The difference lies only in the distribution of fibrinoid material.

   Incidence of MFI: About 0.5% of deliveries.
   Etiology: Exactly not known, possibly

- Deranged blood circulation in the intervillous space such as in antiphospholipid antibody syndrome, thrombophilia, polymyositis etc.
- Various toxic substances

   Gross features

- Thickened maternal side of the placenta
- Hard and wax like material on the maternal surface that extends within the placenta

   Histopathology

- The villi are encircled by pinkish acellular fibrinoid material

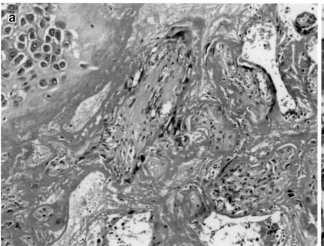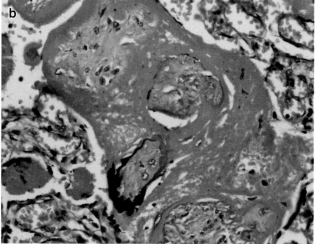

Fig. 12.8 (**a**) Maternal floor infract: The villi are encircled by pinkish acellular fibrinoid material. (**b**) Maternal floor infract: Higher magnification showing acellular pinkish material around the villi

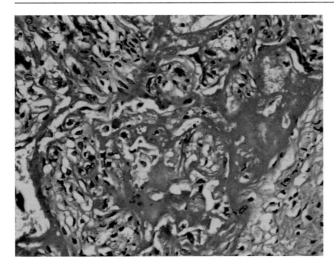

Fig. 12.9 Perivillous fibrin deposition: Extensive fibrin deposition around the villi

- The blood vessels of the villi is slowly lost however the peripheral outline of the villi along with the stroma is maintained

Significance

- Growth retardation of fetus
- Affection of the central nervous system

Retroplacental Hematoma

Image gallery: Fig. 12.10.

Definition: In this condition there is hematoma formation between the placental floor and myometrium.

Incidence: About 4% of placenta.

Etiology: Bleeding from the decidual artery may accumulate in the floor of placenta.

Association

- Preeclampsia
- Chorioamnionitis
- Smoking,
- Drug abuse
- Diabetes mellitus

Significance

- Large clot may cause accidental haemorrhage, growth retardation and even death of the fetus

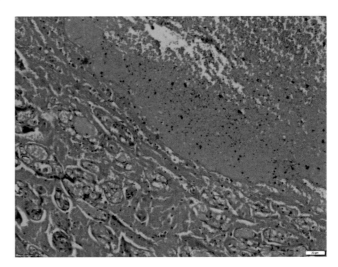

Fig. 12.10 Large retroplacental clot

Marginal Hematoma

Definition: This is characterized by the formation of hematoma in the peripheral margin of the placenta.
   Etiology: Tear of the uteroplacental veins.
   Gross features

- Crescent shaped clot in the lateral margin of the placenta
- Cut section: Triangular clot that makes an apex in the junction of the fetal membrane and chorion

Histopathology

- Location of the clot is outside the basal plate of the placenta
- Pigment laden histiocytes may be seen

Clinical significance

- Antepartum haemorrhage, however no adverse effect to fetus
- Chronic haematoma may develop circumvallation

Intervillous Hematoma

Definition: Here hematoma occurs in the intervillous space.
   Incidence: Common; 45% placenta.
   Gross features

- Small round to oval clots within the placenta
- Single to multiple in number
- Size varies from 1 to 3 cm in diameter

Histopathology

- Thrombi is seen as the collection of RBCs and fibrin
- The peripheral villi around the thrombi show features of infraction

Clinical significance

- No clinical significance if the haematoma is small
- Large clot may cause fetal anaemia and hydrops

Chorangiosis

Image gallery: Figs. 12.11 and 12.12.
   Definition: Chorangiosis is a diffuse process and is characterized by the increased number of blood vessels within the chorionic villi.

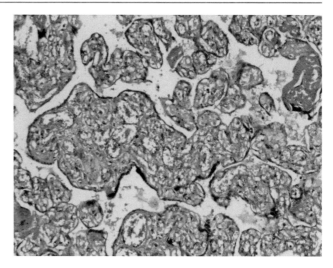

Fig. 12.11 Chorangiosis: Multiple villi with vascular proliferation

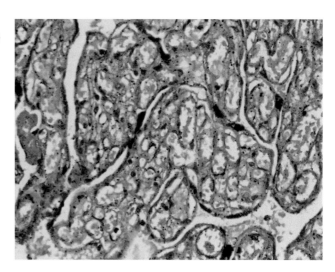

Fig. 12.12 Chorangiosis: The villous contains more than ten vessels

Incidence: Near about 5–7% of placenta.
Diagnostic criteria

- Ten or more capillaries should be present in more than ten terminal chorionic villi in more than ten low power field.

Etiopathogenesis

- Chronic hypoxemic conditions such as higher altitude, maternal anaemia and smoking

Clinical significance

- Increased perinatal mortality
- Abnormality of the cord
- Various abnormality of the placenta

Placenta in Maternal Disorders

Image gallery: Figs. 12.13, 12.14, 12.15, 12.16, 12.17, and 12.18.

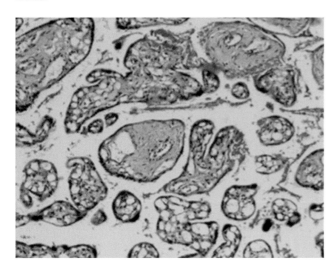

Fig. 12.13 Pre-eclampsia: Fibrosis within the villi

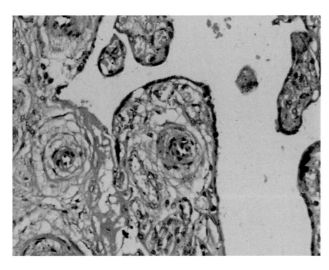

Fig. 12.14 Pre-eclampsia: Vascular wall thickening

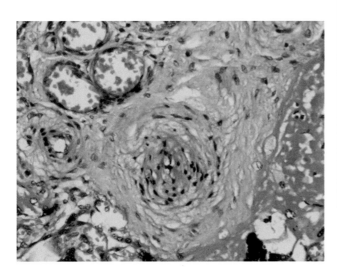

Fig. 12.15 Pre-eclampsia: Vasculitis

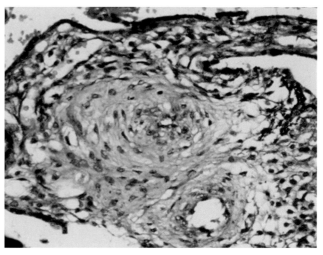

Fig. 12.16 Pre-eclampsia: Endothelial cell proliferation

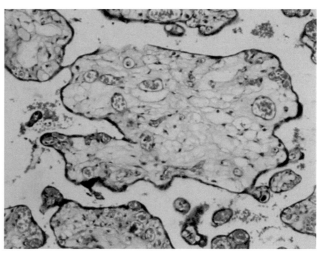

Fig. 12.17 Rh incompatibility: Large chorionic villi with less blood vessels and oedema within the villi

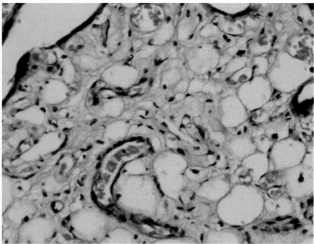

Fig. 12.18 Rh incompatibility: Oedematous villi

Preeclampsia

- The severity of preeclampsia is not correlated with changes in the placenta

Histopathology

- Decidual vasculopathy
  - Vasculitis: Lymphocytes and histiocytes infiltration in the vessel wall
  - Fibrinoid necrosis: Small vessels in the decidua shows hyalinization and fibrinoid necrosis
  - Atherosis: The vessel wall shows extensive fibrinoid changes and intima shows cholesterol containing histiocytes
  - Thrombosis: Small vessels show thrombi
  - Deficiency of physiological conversion of the decidual vessels: The muscular wall of the small vessels is retained in the midst of abundant trophoblasts
- Infraction: Multiple areas of infraction in the placenta
- Malformation of the chorionic villi and increased syncytial knots
  - The villi shows gross dis-correlation of gestational age and maturation. The villi are smaller is size due to hypoperfusion.
  - Abundant syncytial knots

Essential hypertension

- Thickened medial wall of the small vessels
- The intimal lining of the vessel wall shows hyperplasia
- Narrowed vascular lumen

Diabetes Mellitus

Gross features

- Large and heavy placenta
- Oedematous umbilical cord

Histopathology

- Chorangiosis
- Proliferation of cyto and syncytiotrophoblast
- Decidual vessel
  - Medial hypertrophy
  - Fibrinoid necrosis

Rh Incompatibility

Etiology and pathophysiology

- Rh negative mother develops antibody formation against RBCs of Rh positive fetus
- The anti Rh antibody destroys the fetal RBCs and produces anaemia
- The chronic destruction of fetal blood releases nucleated RBCs of the fetus into the fetal circulation
- In severe degree of destruction of fetal RBCs may cause congestive cardiac failure, ascites and generalized oedema of the fetus

Gross features

- Heavier placenta weighing more than 1 kg
- Bulky and oedematous placenta

Histopathology

- Large sized chorionic villi
- Intravillous blood vessels are reduced
- Abundant nucleated RBCs within the villi
- Oedema of the stroma of the villi and increased Hofbauer cells

Clinical implications

- Intranatal diagnosis of the hydrops fetalis requires intranatal blood transfusion

Pathology of the Membrane

Image gallery: Figs. 12.19 and 12.20.

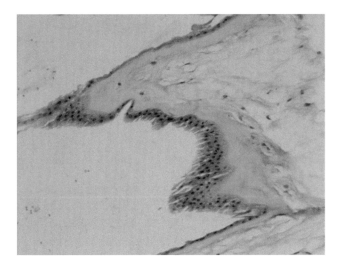

Fig. 12.19 Squamous metaplasia: The placental membrane is replaced by squamous epithelial cells

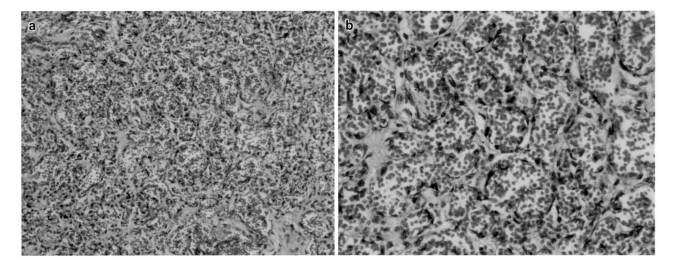

Fig. 12.20 (**a**) Chorangioma: Abundant blood capillaries with scanty connective tissue stroma. (**b**) Chorangioma: Higher magnification showing abundant blood capillaries

Squamous Metaplasia

Image gallery: Fig. 12.19

Gross features

- Multiple small white elevated lesion in the fetal membrane

Histopathology

- The placental membrane is replaced by squamous epithelial cells

Clinical implications

- No significance

Amniotic Nodosum

Gross features

- Multiple
- Small yellowish lesion

Etiology

- It occurs due to the lack of nutrition of the cells of the amniotic membrane resulting the death of the cells. This is often associated with oligohydramnios.
- This is followed by the deposition of the vernix over the dead cells

Histopathology

- Eosinophilic acellular material

Non Trophoblastic Tumour

Chorangioma

Image gallery: Fig. 12.20a and b.
Definition: This is a vascular neoplasm and is characterized by the proliferation of capillaries within the villi resulting a nodular lesion.
Incidence: About 0.1–1% of placenta.
Gross feature

- Single to multiple small, well defined nodule within the placenta.
- Brown to yellowish firm nodule
- The chorangiomas often resemble blood clot and it may be difficult to identify them

Histopathology

- Abundant blood capillaries with scanty connective tissue stroma
- Foci of necrosis and calcification

Clinical significance

- Small chorangioma has no clinical consequence
- Large chorangioma is frequently associated with hydramnios, preeclampsia and heart failure of the fetus

Acute Leukaemia

Image gallery: Figs. 12.21 and 12.22.
Rarely the placenta may be infiltrated by blasts of acute leukaemia from mother.

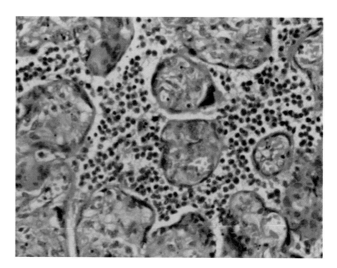

Fig. 12.21 Acute leukaemia: Immature myeloid cells in the perivillous space

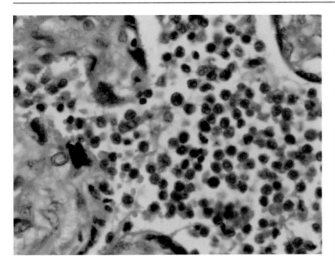

Fig. 12.22 Acute leukaemia: Higher magnification showing better morphology of the leukemic blasts

Umbilical Cord

Vestigial Remnants

Image gallery: Figs. 12.23 and 12.24.

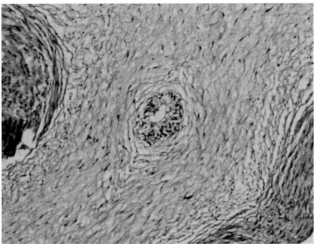

Fig. 12.23 Allantoic duct: The remnant of the duct in the umbilical cord

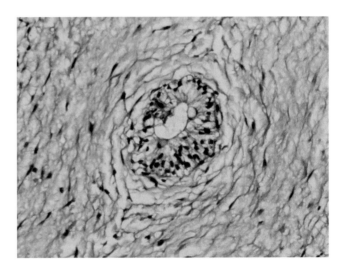

Fig. 12.24 Allantoic duct: The duct is lined by cuboidal to columnar epithelium

Allantoic Duct

Incidence: About 15% of placenta.

Location: Proximal part of the umbilical cord in between the two umbilical vessels.

Pathology: The duct is lined by cuboidal to columnar epithelium.

Omphalomesenteric Duct

Synonym: Vitelline duct.

Represent: It is the remnant of the connection between the fetal gut and yolk sac.

Incidence: Seven percent of the umbilical cord.

Location: Proximal part of the umbilical cord.

Pathology

- The duct is lined by columnar intestinal epithelial cells
- It has a muscular wall

Clinical significance: None.

Umbilical Knots

True Knots

Incidence: 0.4%.

Association

- Long umbilical cord
- Abundant amniotic fluid
- Multigravida

Complications

- Fetal asphyxia
- Thrombosis of the fetal blood vessels

False Knots

False knot occurs due to redundant umbilical vessels in focal area. This is easily identifiable grossly and it has no clinical significance.

Single Umbilical Artery

Image gallery: Fig. 12.25.

Definition: This is characterized by the presence of single umbilical artery in the umbilical cord.

Incidence: 2.5%.

Etiology: Atrophy or aplasia of the umbilical artery.

Clinical significance

- Increased perinatal mortality
- Fetal malformation
- Antepartum bleeding

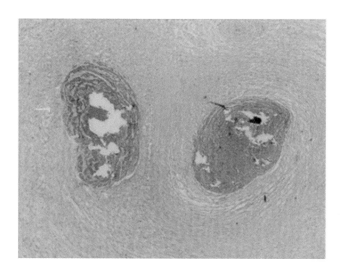

Fig. 12.25 Single umbilical artery: Only a single umbilical artery in the umbilical cord

Suggested Reading

Abramowsky CR, Gutman J, Hilinski JA. Mycobacterium tuberculosis infection of the placenta: a study of the early (innate) inflammatory response in two cases. Pediatr Dev Pathol. 2012;15(2):132–6.

Chen A, Roberts DJ. Placental pathologic lesions with a significant recurrence risk - what not to miss! APMIS. 2017; https://doi.org/10.1111/apm.12796.

Doritchamou JYA, Akuffo RA, Moussiliou A, Luty AJF, Massougbodji A, Deloron P, Tuikue Ndam NG. Submicroscopic placental infection by non-falciparum Plasmodium spp. PLoS Negl Trop Dis. 2018;12(2):e0006279.

Fan M, Skupski DW. Placental chorioangioma: literature review. J Perinat Med. 2014;42(3):273–9.

Naeye RL. Maternal floor infarction. Hum Pathol. 1985;16:823–8.

Redline RW, Faye-Petersen O, et al. Amniotic infection syndrome: nosology and reproducibility of placental reaction patterns. Pediatr Dev Pathol. 2003;6:435–48.

Salmani D, Purushothaman S, Somashekara SC, Gnanagurudasan E, Sumangaladevi K, Harikishan R, Venkateshwarareddy M. Study of structural changes in placenta in pregnancy-induced hypertension. J Nat Sci Biol Med. 2014;5(2):352–5.

Silver RM, Barbour KD. Placenta accreta spectrum: accreta, increta, and percreta. Obstet Gynecol Clin North Am. 2015;42(2):381–402.

Stanek J. Chorangiosis of chorionic villi: what does it really mean? Arch Pathol Lab Med. 2016;140(6):588–93.

Wortman AC, Alexander JM. Placenta accreta, increta, and percreta. Obstet Gynecol Clin N Am. 2013;40(1):137–54.

Classification of gestational trophoblastic disease according to World Health Organization [1] is highlighted in Fig. 13.1.

Prognostic classification of trophoblastic tumours is highlighted in Table 13.1.

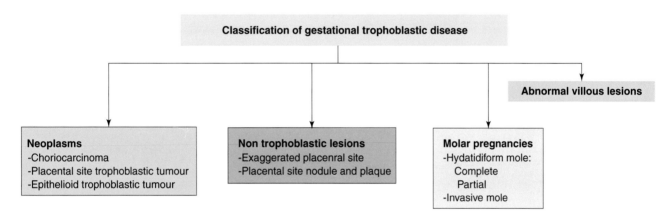

Classification of gestational trophoblastic disease

Neoplasms
-Choriocarcinoma
-Placental site trophoblastic tumour
-Epithelioid trophoblastic tumour

Non trophoblastic lesions
-Exaggerated placenral site
-Placental site nodule and plaque

Molar pregnancies
-Hydatidiform mole:
  Complete
  Partial
-Invasive mole

Abnormal villous lesions

Fig. 13.1 Classification of trophoblastic diseases

Table 13.1 Prognostic classification of trophoblastic tumours according to FIGO

Factors	Scoring points			
	1	2	3	4
Age in years	<40	More than 40	–	–
Previous pregnancy	Mole	Abortion	Term	
Interval of disease onset from pregnancy (in months)	<4	4–6	7–12	More than 12
Serum hCG level before the therapy (IU/ml)	$<10^3$	$10^3–10^4$	$10^4–10^5$	More than 10^5
The tumour size in uterus (largest one in cm)	<3	3–4	More than 5	–
Different locations of the metastasis	Lung	Spleen and kidney	GIT	Liver or brain
Total number of metastasis	–	1–4	5–8	More than 8
History of failed chemotherapy	–	–	One drug	Two or more than two drugs

Low risk: If the score is within 0–6
High risk: If the score is above 7
GIT: Gastrointestinal tract

© Springer Nature Singapore Pte Ltd. 2019
P. Dey, *Color Atlas of Female Genital Tract Pathology*, https://doi.org/10.1007/978-981-13-1029-4_13

Complete Hydatidiform Mole

Image gallery: Figs. 13.2, 13.3, 13.4, and 13.5.
    Abbreviation: Complete Hydatidiform Mole (CHM)
    Epidemiology

- In USA one in 1000 pregnancies

- Higher incidence in South East Asia: 4–13 in 1000 pregnancies
- It represents more than 50% of all molar pregnancies

Cytogenetics

- Normal karyotyping 46 XX

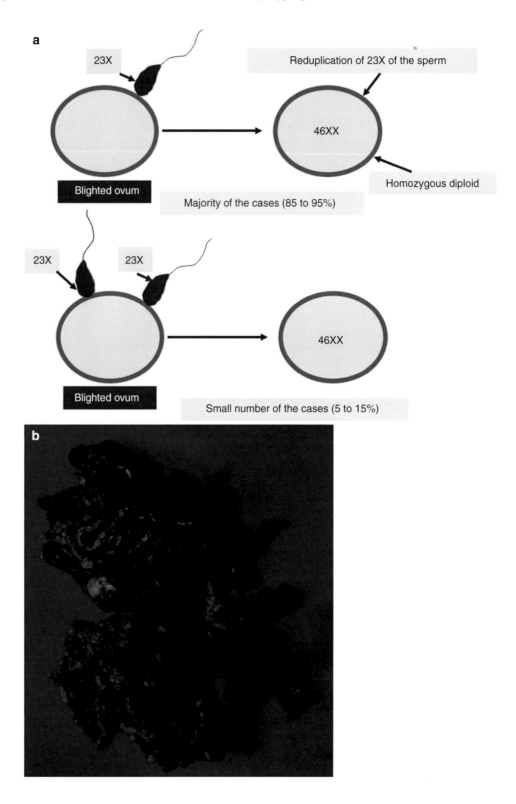

Fig. 13.2 (**a**) Chromosomal development of the hydatidiform mole. (**b**) Gross of Hydatidiform mole: Multiple small vesicles

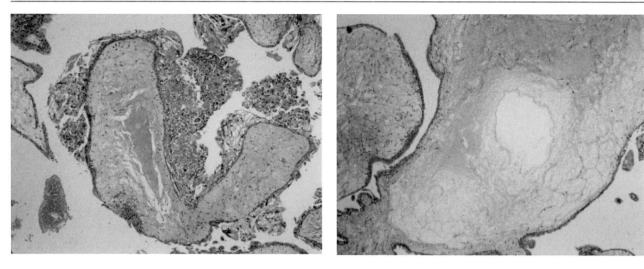

Fig. 13.3 Hydatidiform mole: Large villi with central hydropic changes

Fig. 13.4 Hydatidiform mole: Cystically dilated villi

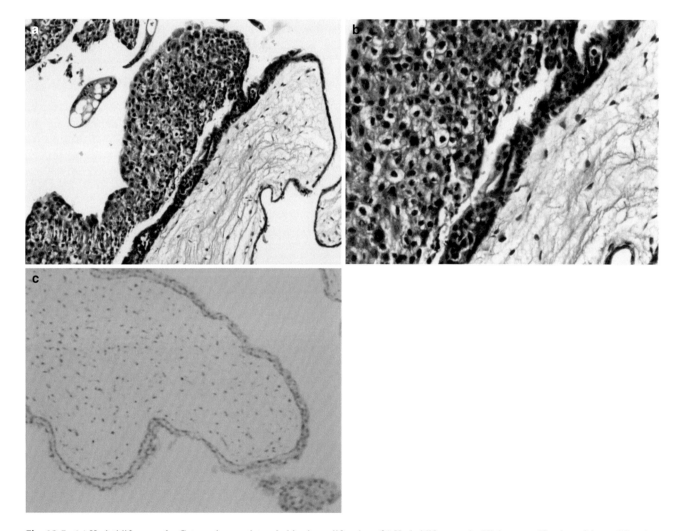

Fig. 13.5 (**a**) Hydatidiform mole: Cyto and syncytiotrophoblastic proliferation. (**b**) Hydatidiform mole: Higher magnification of the proliferating cells. (**c**) Hydatidiform mole: Negative p57 immunostaining

- Majority of the cases (85–95%): An empty ovum is fertilized by a single sperm (23 X) followed by the reduplication of the entire haploid chromosomes
- Remaining cases: an empty ovum is fertilized by two sperms (23 X).

Clinical features

- Patients are all in reproductive age period
- Peak incidence: 40 years
- Vaginal bleeding
- Disproportionate enlargement of uterus in comparison to gestational period
- High serum and urine Beta hCG level (more than 1,000,000 mIU/mL at the time of diagnosis)
- Early onset of toxaemia of pregnancy

Radiologic features

- Characteristic snow storm appearance

Gross features

- Multiple grape like transparent vesicles
- Size: 1–2 cm diameter vesicle
- Absence of fetus

Histopathology

- Multiple dilated villi with cistern like appearance
- Marked hydropic changes within villi
- Complete absence of blood vessels
- Circumferential proliferation of cyto and syncytio trophoblasts
- Cytological atypia of the trophoblastic cells
- No fetal tissue present

Immunohistochemistry

- Complete absence of p57 immunostaining
- Cytotrophoblast:
  - Positive for CD 10 and cytokeratin
  - Negative: HCG, HPL

- Syncytiotrophoblast:
  - HCG and PLAP

Key diagnostic features: See Box 13.1.

Box 13.1: Key Diagnostic Features of Complete Hydatidiform Mole
- Multiple dilated chorionic villi with cistern like appearance
- Central area of the villi is completely acellular
- Marked edematous villi with hydropic changes
- Complete absence of blood vessels
- Circumferential trophoblastic proliferation around the villi
- Cytological atypia of the trophoblastic cells
- No fetal tissue present

Differential diagnosis

- Hydropic changes in the aborted villi
  - No trophoblastic proliferation
- Choriocarcinoma
  - Complete absence of villi

Prognosis

- Persistent trophoblastic disease (PTD) is seen in about 20–30% patients
- Risk of choriocarcinoma is in 3–5% cases

Treatment

- Complete evacuation of hydatidiform mole and follow up investigation by serial Beta hCG estimation
- In case of persistent trophoblastic disease chemotherapy is administered. The cure rate of PTD is 100%.

Partial Hydatidiform Mole

Image gallery: Fig. 13.6a–d.
Epidemiology

- It occurs in 25–40% molar pregnancies

Cytogenetics

- Triploidy (69 XXY, 69 XXX or 69 XYY)
- A normal ovum is fertilized by two haploid sperms

Clinical features

- Almost same as that of CHM
- Uterus may be normal in size or small due to fetal death
- Serum and urinary Beta hCG may be either normal or low

Gross features

- The grape like vesicles are admixed with normal tissue
- The feus may show developmental anomalies

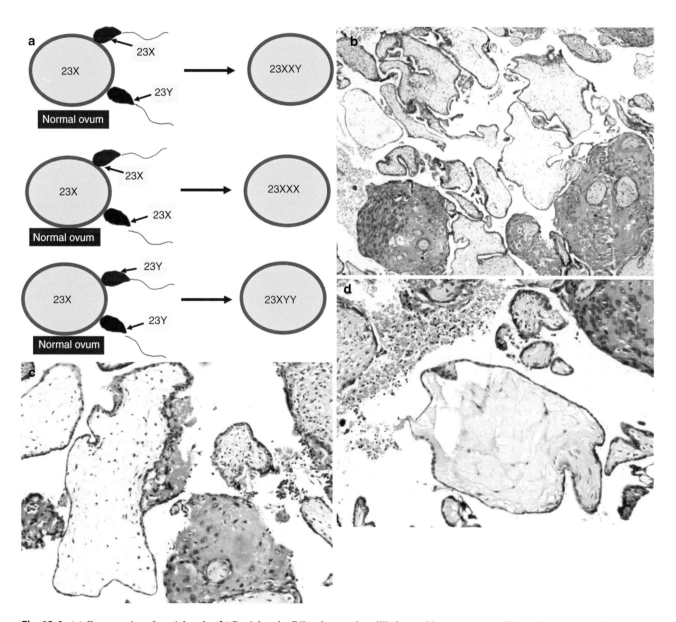

Fig. 13.6 (**a**) Cytogenetics of partial mole. (**b**) Partial mole: Dilated avascular villi along with many normal villi. (**c**) Partial mole: There is only focal trophoblastic proliferation present. d: Partial mole: Large villi with hydropic change

Histopathology

- Villi are dilated and mildly enlarged
- Hydropic degeneration is present but there may not be complete cistern formation
- The margin of the villi shows scalloping and focal invagination of the cytotrophoblast
- There is only focal proliferation of the cyto and syncytio trophoblasts and it gives a lacy appearance
- Cytological atypia is mild to absent

Immunohistochemistry

- Positive for p57 immunostaining

Key diagnostic features: See Box 13.2.

> **Box 13.2: Key Diagnostic Features of Partial Hydatidiform Mole**
> - Focal changes present
> - Relatively smaller villi
> - Villi are dilated and mildly enlarged
> - Stromal fibrosis
> - Occasional villi show hydropic degeneration
> - The margin of the villi shows scalloping and focal invagination of the cytotrophoblast
> - Focal proliferation of the cyto and syncytio trophoblasts
> - Cytological atypia is mild to absent
> - Immunohistochemistry: Diffusely positive for p57 immunostaining

Differential diagnosis: Complete Hydatidiform mole (see Table 13.2).

Prognosis and treatment

- Persistent trophoblastic disease may occur in 1–5% cases
- Choriocarcinoma may develop in <0.5% cases
- Complete evacuation of the mole

Table 13.2 Differential diagnosis of complete hydatidiform mole and partial hydatidiform mole

Features	Complete hydatidiform mole	Partial hydatidiform mole
Fetal part	Absent	Present
Outline of the villi	Round and regular	Scalloped due to trophoblastic invagination
Hydropic changes and cistern formation	Present	Occasional villi show cistern like dilatation. Normal appearing villi are also seen
Trophoblastic proliferation	Circumferential and more than the partial mole	Only focal part of the villi shows proliferation
Pleomorphism of the trophoblastic cells	Present	Mild
P57 immunostaining	Absent	Diffuse positivity

Invasive Hydatidiform Mole

Image gallery: Fig. 13.7a–c.

Definition: Invasive hydatidiform mole is characterized by the myometrial or uterine vascular invasion of complete or partial hydatidiform moles.

Clinical features

- Abnormal vaginal bleeding
- Persistently raised Beta hCG level in serum and urine even after evacuation of the mole

Gross features

- Hysterectomy is rarely done in invasive mole
- The uterus shows extensive haemorrhage in the endometrium

- There may be perforation of the myometrium

Histopathology

- Villi with hydatidiform changes are seen deep within the myometrium or in the extra uterine site
- The villi show molar changes

Prognosis and treatment

- The disease is cured in majority of the cases (80%) by chemotherapy

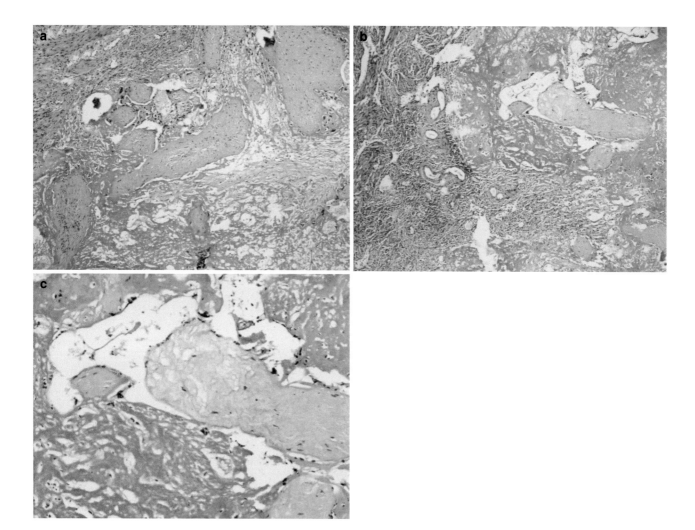

Fig. 13.7 (**a**) Invasive mole: Many large hydropic villi infiltrating deep in the myometrium. (**b**) Invasive mole: Large dilated villi within the myometrium with areas of haemorrhage. (**c**) Invasive mole: Higher magnification of the villi showing hydropic degeneration

Non Trophoblastic Lesion

Exaggerated Placental Site Reaction

Image gallery: Figs. 13.8 and 13.9.

Definition: It is characterized by marked proliferation of the intermediate trophoblasts in the placental site.

Clinical features

- It is seen in normal pregnancy and even in case of hydatidiform mole

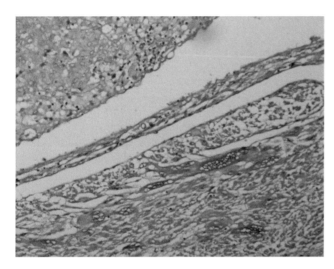

Fig. 13.8 Exaggerated placental site reaction: Abundant intermediate trophoblasts and many multinucleated giant cells in the endo-myometrium

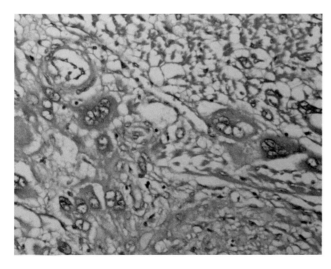

Fig. 13.9 Exaggerated placental site reaction: Higher magnification showing many multinucleated syncytiotrophoblast

Histopathology

- Abundant intermediate trophoblasts and many multinucleated giant cells in the endo-myometrium
- The normal anatomical arrangement of the tissue is maintained
- The trophoblastic cell infiltration is around the endometrial glands and small arterioles
- No mitotic activity

Placental Site Nodule

Definition: It is characterized by well circumscribed nodule in the placental site that contains intermediate trophoblasts.

Clinical features

- The patients are always in the reproductive age period
- Incidentally detected

Gross

- Small 1–3 cm nodule
- Cut section: Yellowish and may show haemorrhage

Histopathology

- Single to multiple well circumscribed nodule
- Central hyalinised stroma with embedded intermediate trophoblasts
- Nodules are encircled by lymphocytes and occasional multinucleated giant cells

Immunohistochemistry

- Positive: CK 18, PLAP, HCG and HPL
- Ki 67: Low labelling index (<10%)

Differential diagnosis

- PSTT
  - Cells are pleomorphic
  - Ki 67 labelling index is high

Prognosis and treatment

- Benign
- Surgical removal is possible as the lesion is well circumscribed.
- No recurrence occurs

Gestational Trophoblastic Tumours

Choriocarcinoma

Image gallery: Figs. 13.10, 13.11, 13.12, 13.13, 13.14, 13.15, 13.16, 13.17, 13.18, 13.19, and 13.20.

Epidemiology

- Incidence is two in 100,00 pregnancies
- Ten to 100 times higher in South-east Asian countries
- It is developed from:
  – CHM: 50%

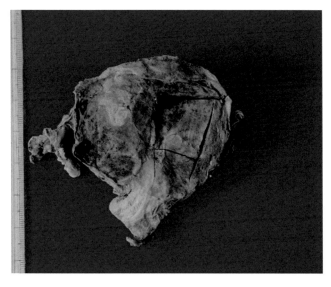

Fig. 13.10 Choriocarcinoma: Gross picture showing large tumour in the uterus with multiple foci of haemorrhage

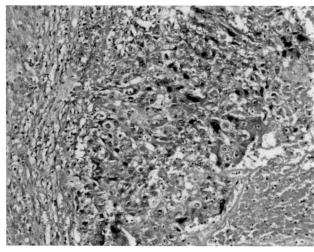

Fig. 13.11 Choriocarcinoma: Solid sheets of tumour cells

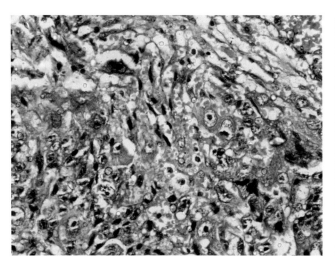

Fig. 13.12 Choriocarcinoma: Marked nuclear atypia of the tumour cells

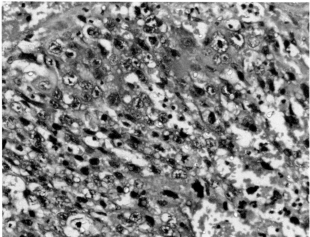

Fig. 13.13 Choriocarcinoma: Characteristic dimorphic pattern

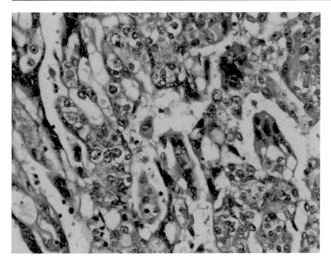

Fig. 13.14 Choriocarcinoma: The oval to polygonal tumour cells along with many multinucleated cells

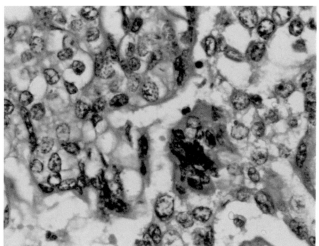

Fig. 13.15 Choriocarcinoma: Higher magnification showing large polygonal pleomorphic cells and multinucleated cells

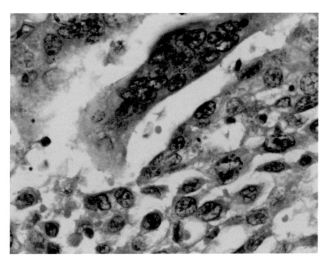

Fig. 13.16 Choriocarcinoma: Multinucleated large syncytial cells

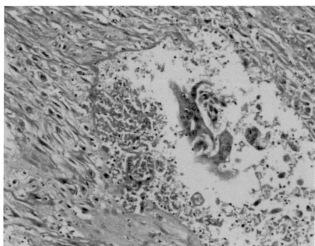

Fig. 13.17 Choriocarcinoma: Tumour cells infiltrating in the myometrium

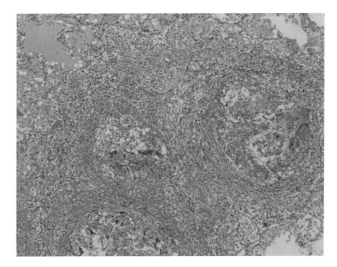

Fig. 13.18 Choriocarcinoma: Metastasis in lung as haemorrhagic tumour

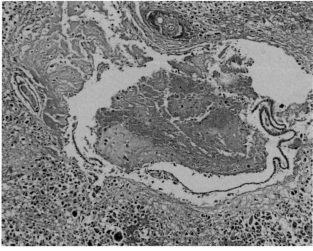

Fig. 13.19 Choriocarcinoma: Metastasis in pancreas

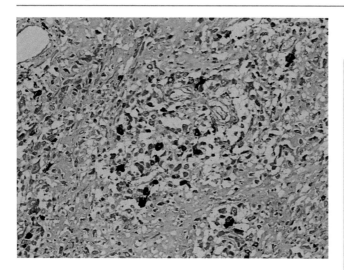

Fig. 13.20 Choriocarcinoma: Strongly positive for HCG

- Abortion: 25%
- Normal pregnancy: 22%
- Ectopic pregnancy: Uncommon

Clinical features

- Almost always occurs in reproductive age period
- Rarely seen in post-menopausal patients
- Chief complaints: Abnormal vaginal bleeding
- Very high serum and urinary HCG level
- Occasionally the patients may present with features of lung metastasis

Gross features

- The tumour makes the uterus bulky
- Red friable necrotic mass in the uterine cavity
- Areas of haemorrhage seen

Histopathology

- Solid sheets of tumour cells
- Characteristic bilaminar and dimorphic pattern
- Cytotrophoblasts and intermediate trophoblasts along with many syncytiotrophoblast are seen
- Marked nuclear atypia and very high mitotic activity are seen
- Large areas of haemorrhage present

Immunohistochemistry

- Beta hCG: Strong positive
- HPL: Weak positive
- cytokeratin 18, and inhibin: Positive
- Ki 67 labelling index: Very high (more than 9%)

Key diagnostic features: See Box 13.3.

> **Box 13.3: Key Diagnostic Features of Choriocarcinoma**
> - Diffuse solid sheets of tumour cells invading in the deeper myometrium
> - Complete absence of chorionic villi
> - Cytotrophoblasts, intermediate trophoblasts and many syncytiotrophoblast are present in sheet forming characteristic bilaminar and dimorphic pattern
> - Nuclei show marked pleomorphism, coarse chromatin and prominent nucleoli
> - Very high mitotic activity
> - Large areas of haemorrhage present and there may be blood lake formation surrounded by trophoblasts
> - Immunohistochemistry:
>   - Strongly positive Beta HCG and weak positive HPL
>   - Very high Ki 67 labelling index
> - Serum beta HCG level markedly raised

Differential diagnosis

- Early gestation
  - In case of early part of pregnancy there may be absence of villi and the presence of trophoblasts may be mistaken as choriocarcinoma
  - Nuclear atypia is absent
  - Beta hCG level is much low. Serial estimation of Beta hCG is more helpful
- Poorly differentiated carcinoma
  - In small biopsies occasionally only mononuclear trophoblastic cells may resemble carcinoma
  - Clinical history of molar pregnancy, abortion and pregnancy are helpful
  - Beta hCG level is a useful diagnostic marker
- Placental site trophoblastic tumour (see Table 13.3)
  - Only one type of cell population
  - Characteristic vascular invasion of the tumour cells and fibrinoid necrosis of the vessel wall
  - The tumour cells are strongly positive for HPL
  - Serum Beta hCG level is relatively low

Prognosis and treatment

- Highly aggressive malignancy
- Frequent metastasis in brain and lung
- About 100% survival rate after treatment
- Combination chemotherapy: Etoposide, methotrexate, actinomycin D, cyclophosphamide, and vincristine

Table 13.3   Distinguishing histopathological features between chorio-carcinoma and placental site trophoblastic tumour

Features	Choriocarcinoma	Placental site trophoblastic tumour
Tumour cells	Dimorphic cell population: Both cyto and syncytiotrophoblast	Monomorphic cells: Only intermediate cells
Cells	Cytoplasm is scanty to moderate amount	Cytoplasm is abundant eosinophilic
Necrosis	Marked	Absent
Infiltration of the tumour	Pushing margin	Infiltrating margin
Vascular invasion	Tumour emboli within the lumen of vessels	Tumour forming the wall of the vessels and infiltrate from the periphery
Mitotic rate	Very high (20 per 10 HPF)	Variable, but usually 6–10 10/HPF
Beta hCG	Strongly positive in tumour cells	Only 10% cells show weak positivity
hPL	Strongly positive in tumour cells	Weak positivity
Ki 67 index	High and usually more than 40	Usually low (<30)

Placental Site Trophoblastic Tumour (PSTT)

Image gallery: Figs. 13.21, 13.22, 13.23, 13.24, 13.25, 13.26, 13.27, and 13.28.

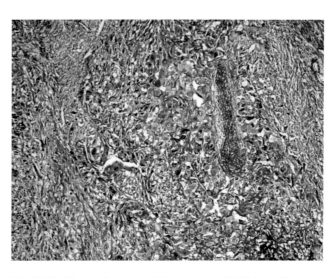

Fig. 13.21   Placental site trophoblastic tumour: Solid sheet of intermediate trophoblast cells

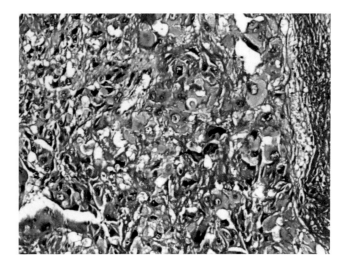

Fig. 13.22   Placental site trophoblastic tumour: Large polygonal cells with moderate cytoplasm and centrally placed nuclei

Definition: This is a trophoblastic tumour that is composed of intermediate type trophoblast.

Epidemiology

- Uncommon tumour
- Represents <3% of trophoblastic tumour
- It occurs mainly after normal pregnancy and may develop after abortion or molar pregnancy

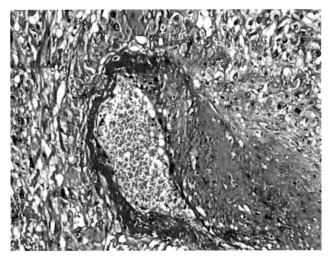

Fig. 13.23 Placental site trophoblastic tumour: The trophoblastic cells infiltrating and replacing wall of the blood vessels

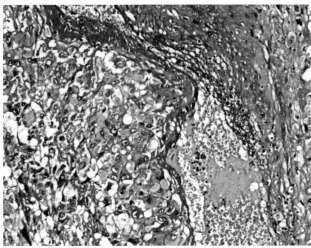

Fig. 13.24 Placental site trophoblastic tumour: Higher magnification showing the characteristic vascular invasion

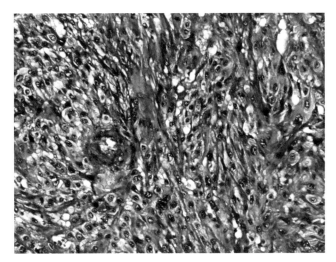

Fig. 13.25 Placental site trophoblastic tumour: Tumour showing infiltration in the myometrium

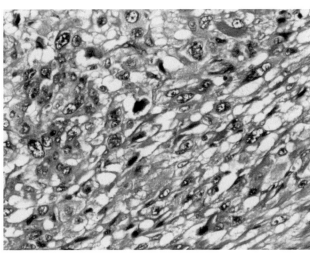

Fig. 13.26 Placental site trophoblastic tumour: Large pleomorphic tumour cells within the myometrium

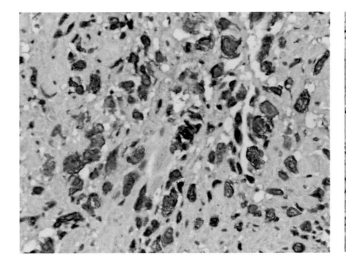

Fig. 13.27 Placental site trophoblastic tumour: The cells are strongly positive for HPL

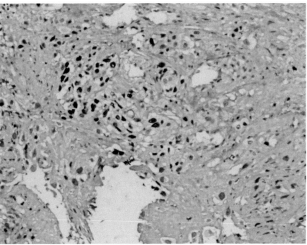

Fig. 13.28 Placental site trophoblastic tumour: High Ki 67 positivity of the tumour cells

Clinical features

- Placental site trophoblastic tumour (PSTT) occurs in the reproductive age period
- Mean age 30 years
- Chief complaints: Vaginal bleeding, amenorrhea and mildly enlarged uterus
- Serum and urinary Beta hCG is mild to moderately raised
- May occur after a prolonged gap of pregnancy

Gross features

- Well circumscribed nodular or polypoid mass in the endometrial cavity
- Size varies from 2 to 10 cm in diameter; mean 5 cm
- Tumour often infiltrate in the deeper myometrium
- Cut section: Soft, yellowish with focal necrosis and haemorrhage

Histopathology

- Solid sheet of intermediate trophoblast cells
- Large polygonal cells with moderate cytoplasm and centrally placed nuclei
- Nuclei may be monomorphic or mild to moderately pleomorphic
- Large multinucleated syncytiotrophoblastic cells may be seen
- Characteristic vascular invasion: The trophoblastic cells infiltrate and replace wall of the blood vessels
- Complete absence of chorionic villi

Immunohistochemistry

- Positive: HPL, Mel-CAM (CD 146), Mucin 4 and CD 10
- Weakly and focal positive: hCG

Key diagnostic features: See Box 13.4.

Box 13.4: Key Diagnostic Features of Placental Site Trophoblastic Tumour

- Monomorphic population of solid sheet of intermediate trophoblast cells
- Tumour cells are large polygonal shaped with moderate to abundant eosinophilic cytoplasm
- Nuclei: Monomorphic or mild to moderately pleomorphic
- Large multinucleated syncytiotrophoblastic cells may be seen
- Necrosis and haemorrhage less common
- The trophoblastic cells infiltrate and replace the wall of the blood vessels
- Complete absence of chorionic villi
- Immunohistochemistry: Strongly positive for hPL and Mel-CAM and weakly positive for beta hCG

Differential diagnosis

- Choriocarcinoma (see Table 12.2)
  - It develops predominantly from molar pregnancy
  - Beta hCG level is very high
  - Tumour has pushing margin in comparison to infiltrating growth in PSTT
  - Dimorphic population of cells
  - Vascular destruction occurs and tumour emboli rather than infiltrating tumour cells in the vessel wall
  - Extensive necrosis and haemorrhage
  - HPL weakly positive
  - Ki 67 labelling index very high
- Exaggerated placental site reaction
  - No mass like lesion
  - Absence of deep myometrial infiltration
  - Chorionic villi are present
  - Ki 67 labelling index low to absent

- Epithelioid trophoblastic tumour
  - Margin of the tumour is expansile
  - Nodular growth
  - Geographic type of necrosis
  - Extensive hyalinization is present
  - Tumour is p63 positive, whereas PSTT is p 63 negative
- Epithelioid leiomyosarcoma
  - More destructive infiltration pattern
  - SMA positive
  - HPL negative

Prognosis and treatment

- Mostly behaves like a benign tumour and 10–15% tumours are malignant
- Simple hysterectomy is the treatment of choice and it cures the patient
- Adverse prognostic factors are
  - Higher FIGO staging
  - Higher age group (>35 years age)
  - Long latent period between the pregnancy and tumour development
  - Metastasis at the time of presentation
  - Large size of tumour
  - Areas of necrosis
  - Deeper myometrial invasion
  - Tumour with clear cytoplasm
  - High mitotic rate: more than 5 per 10 HPF
  - High Beta hCG level
- Malignant PSTT is treated by multi agent chemotherapy

Epithelioid Trophoblastic Tumour

Epidemiology: A rare tumour.
  Clinical features

- It occurs only in reproductive age period
- Chief complaint: abnormal uterine bleeding
- Beta hCG level mildly raised
- Patient may have antecedent history of normal pregnancy (67%), molar pregnancy or abortion

Gross features

- Discrete solid nodule
- Size of the nodule is 1–5 cm
- Cut section: yellowish with foci of necrosis

Histopathology

- Well circumscribed growth
- The cells are arranged in nests, cords, or nodule
- Geographic necrosis is present in between the tumour cells
- Individual tumour cells are round with moderate amount of cytoplasm and central monomorphic nuclei
- Eosinophilic hyalinised material is often present
- Mitotic activity is low (0–9 per 10 HPF)

Immunohistochemistry

- Positive: p63 is characteristically positive, H3D3B1, E Cadherin, and cyclin E
- Occasionally positive: HPL, inhibin and CD 146 (Mel-CAM)

Key diagnostic features: See Box 13.5.

Box 13.5: Key Diagnostic Features of Epithelioid Trophoblastic Tumour
- Nodular growth
- Well circumscribed
- Nests, cords, or nodule of tumour cells
- The viable islands of tumour cells with extensive necrosis giving a "geographic pattern"
- Monomorphic population of tumour cells
- Round cells with moderate amount of cytoplasm and central monomorphic nuclei
- Nuclear chromatin is fine
- Eosinophilic hyalinised material is often present
- Calcification is often present
- Mitotic activity is low (2 per 10 HPF)
- Immunohistochemistry: Characteristically positive for p63 and focally positive for hPL and CD146

Differential diagnosis

- *PSTT*: Discussed before
- *Choriocarcinoma*
  - Bilaminar dimorphic cells
  - Marked nuclear pleomorphism
  - Very high Beta hCG
- *Squamous cell carcinoma of cervix*
  - In curetting or small biopsy they may simulate each other
  - Keratin pearl
  - Negative for CK 18 and inhibin

Prognosis and treatment

- Behaviour till not clear because only limited number of cases are reported
- Metastasis may occur (25% cases)
- In case of restricted tumour in uterus: 100% survival rate

Reference

1. Kurman RJ, Carcangiu ML, Herrington S, Young RH. Gestational trophoblastic disease. WHO classification of tumours of female genital reproductive organs, vol. 4. Lyon: International Agency for Research on Cancer; 2014.

Suggested Reading

Behtash N, Karimi Zarchi M. Placental site trophoblastic tumour. J Cancer Res Clin Oncol. 2008;134(1):1–6.

Berkowitz RS, Goldstein DP. Current management of gestational trophoblastic diseases. Gynecol Oncol. 2009;112(3):654–62.

FIGO Oncology Committee. FIGO staging for gestational trophoblastic neoplasia 2000. Int J Gynaecol Obstet. 2002;77(3):285–7.

Keser SH, Kokten SC, Cakir C, Sensu S, Buyukbayrak EE, Karadayi N. Epithelioid trophoblastic tumour. Taiwan J Obstet Gynecol. 2015;54(5):621–4.

Kim SJ. Placental site trophoblastic tumour. Best Pract Res Clin Obstet Gynaecol. 2003;17(6):969–84.

Mao TL, Kurman RJ, Huang CC, Lin MC, Shih I-M. Immunohistochemistry of choriocarcinoma: an aid in differential diagnosis and in elucidating pathogenesis. Am J Surg Pathol. 2007;31:1726–32.

McConnell TG, Murphy KM, Hafez M, Vang R, Ronnett B. Diagnosis and subclassification of hydatidiform moles using p57 immunohistochemistry and molecular genotyping: validation and prospective analysis in routine and consultation practice settings with development of an algorithmic approach. Am J Surg Pathol. 2009;33:805–17.

Moutte A, Doret M, Hajri T, Peyron N, Chateau F, Massardier J, Duvillard P, Raudrant D, Golfier F. Placental site and epithelioid trophoblastic tumours: diagnostic pitfalls. Gynecol Oncol. 2013;128(3):568–72.

Papadopoulos AJ, Foskett M, Seckl MJ, McNeish I, Paradinas FJ, Rees H, Newlands ES. Twenty-five years' clinical experience with placental site trophoblastic tumours. J Reprod Med. 2002;47:460–4.

Smith HO, Kohorn E, Cole LA. Choriocarcinoma and gestational trophoblastic disease. Obstet Gynecol Clin N Am. 2005;32(4):661–8.

Stevens FT, Katzorke N, Tempfer C, Kreimer U, Bizjak GI, Fleisch MC, Fehm TN. Gestational trophoblastic disorders: an update in 2015. Geburtshilfe Frauenheilkd. 2015;75(10):1043–50.